Neumann/Pfützner/Berbalk

Successful Endurance Training

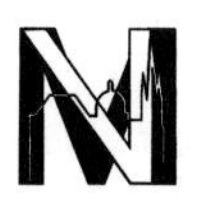

Meyer & Meyer Sport

Original title:
Optimiertes Ausdauertraining
- Aachen: Meyer und Meyer Verlag, 1999
Translated by Paul D. Chilvers-Grierson

British Library Cataloguing in Publication Data
A catalogue for this book is available from the British Library

Neumann, Georg:
Successful Endurance Training /
Georg Neumann ; Arnd Pfützner ; Anneliese Berbalk. [Transl.: Paul D. Chilvers-Grierson].
- Oxford : Meyer & Meyer Sport (UK) Ltd., 2000
ISBN 1-84126-004-5

Oxford, Aachen, Olten (CH), Vienna, Québec,
Lansing/Michigan, Adelaide, Auckland, Johannesburg, Budapest
Member of the world
Sportpublishers' Association
Cover photo: Polar Electro GmbH Deutschland, Büttelborn
Photos inside: See details under each photo
Cover design: Birgit Engelen, Stolberg
Cover, Litho and Type Exposure: frw, Reiner Wahlen, Aachen
Editorial: Dr. Irmgard Jaeger, Aachen; Harald Müller, Aachen
Printed and bound in Germany by
Druckpunkt Offset GmbH, Bergheim
ISBN 1-84126-004-5
e-mail: verlag@meyer-meyer-sports.com

Foreword

In industrial countries the affluence of the population is accompanied by an increasing lack of movement. The results are well-known civilisational illnesses such as cardiovascular and circulatory disorders, numerous metabolism disruptions and the consequences of false loading on the support apparatus and locomotor system of the body. Weight problems are often the first sign that one's lifestyle is going off the rails. Despite extensive health awareness propaganda, currently at least 30% of adults are overweight. Nevertheless, media campaigns against lack of exercise and excess weight are beginning to bear fruit. The results of major epidemiological studies show that regular physical exercise and leisure sport are a worthwhile preventive measure.

Sporting activity is no longer a privilege of the young. More and more people in the middle age-group are making an effort to fit suitable forms of physical and sporting activities into their lifestyle. Sport is capable of maintaining the quality of life for a long period of time.

In recent times there have been more and more warning voices that running in the field of fitness is too intense. Excessive lactate concentrations and/or heart rates during load are considered as evidence. This argument does not sufficiently take into account that the apparent temporary overload is an expression of insufficient basic performance capacity and can be sufficiently compensated by the following break of several days. With every beginning of training the biological effort in dealing with load is higher than the general recommendations for training control.

The time when the body is ready for a new load is regulated by the internal feeling of the muscles. In this way a brief overloading is compensated without problems. Brief anaerobic overloading is still better than no load at all.

Increasing numbers of young athletes strive to subject themselves to measures of training load that are hardly less than those required in performance sport. Only when they notice that the effort and the benefit of their training are fully out of proportion do they make an effort to find the level that suits them personally. Obviously everyone has to find their own insight with regard to the personal limits of load that can be dealt with.

In competitions divided according to age-groups, athletes of the same age often display major differences in performance. This phenomenon is explained by sporting talent and the effectiveness of training. Often athletes who subject themselves to lower training loads and maintain a balance between load and corresponding regeneration have better competition results than the "hard trainers". The latter often think they cannot allow themselves a break in training, they are addicted to load.

Increasing use is being made of the possibility to monitor one's own ability to handle load. Athletes no longer rely exclusively on their subjective feeling or their current physical condition to determine the amount of load they subject themselves to and use the heart rate (HR) to regulate load. Choosing subjective feeling as the basis for the choice of intensity of load (velocity) in long distance competitions has proved to be deceptive and in performance sport it often leads to overloading.

Every athlete, whether engaging in health, leisure (fitness), competitive or high-performance sport, has the opportunity to objectively measure the effect of training load. The most simple way of monitoring this is to write down the volume of training and the velocity achieved. These steps, however, assume measured distances.

The next step in self-monitoring is the use of biological indicators. The introduction of exact HR measurement via heart rate monitor ("Sporttester" range by POLAR) was a significant step forward for the self-monitoring of individual load and training control. By allowing athletes to directly and constantly monitor their HR during training and competitions it is possible to avoid overloading. Access to biochemical indicators only came with the introduction of dry chemical methods for self-measurement. For a long time there was no practical method of determining lactate levels. Lactate measurement was only possible with external assistance and the use of suitable laboratories. A significant breakthrough for athletes in the field was achieved with the development of Accusport® by BOEHRINGER. With the "paper strip method" any athlete can test their own blood lactate in the same way diabetics test their glucose levels.

On the basis of current knowledge, this book is designed to give athletes of all performance categories scientifically backed impulses which can be used practically. Many ideas on behaviour under load have changed drastically. One only needs to think of the unphysiological idea of runners that they should neither eat nor drink during physical exertion.

In order to plan and also to monitor one's own training better and more effectively, learning and thinking about the experiences of others can be advantageous. This requires one to look at the general principles of training methodology and to apply them to one's individual situation.

Faults and digressions of other athletes in training need not be repeated.

As the authors have been active for many years in the areas of competitive and leisure sport, they use their own comprehensive data and experiences in their presentation and argumentation and have summarised these into optimal training organisation for the endurance sports.

The views presented here on the structuring of training and load are based on the generally valid academic foundations of training methodology, sports medicine and performance physiology. They are intended to support the development of the reader's own positions and decisions when engaging in sporting activity. It is also intended to give athletes many practical tips in the individual performance categories. The planning and execution of training is seen particularly in close connection with the findings of sport methodology, performance physiology and sports medicine. In this book it is not intended to deal with detailed training schedules.

Training is carried out after planning, but it must always be remembered that the body functions according to the basic rules of biology and cannot be outwitted with abstract planning. This elementary starting point is often underestimated. Anyone who trains must always be prepared to make corrections when signals from the body or objectively measured indicators suggest this is necessary. Training objectives are very diverse, they can range from training for health or fitness up to high-performance training. As loads at the limits can rarely be sustained by a person over longer periods of time, preference should be given to moderate loads over longer phases of one's life. Even the objectives of sporting talents in high-performance training can only be realised over limited periods of time.

This book is designed to provide athletes, trainers, instructors, students and sports doctors with a diversity of impulses and ideas on individually optimal training. The authors are glad to receive critical comments, on the assumption that not all views and interests have been captured in this book.

Finally a note on gender use:
To make reading easier, the male form has been used throughout the book. It goes without saying that in all cases the female form is meant as well.

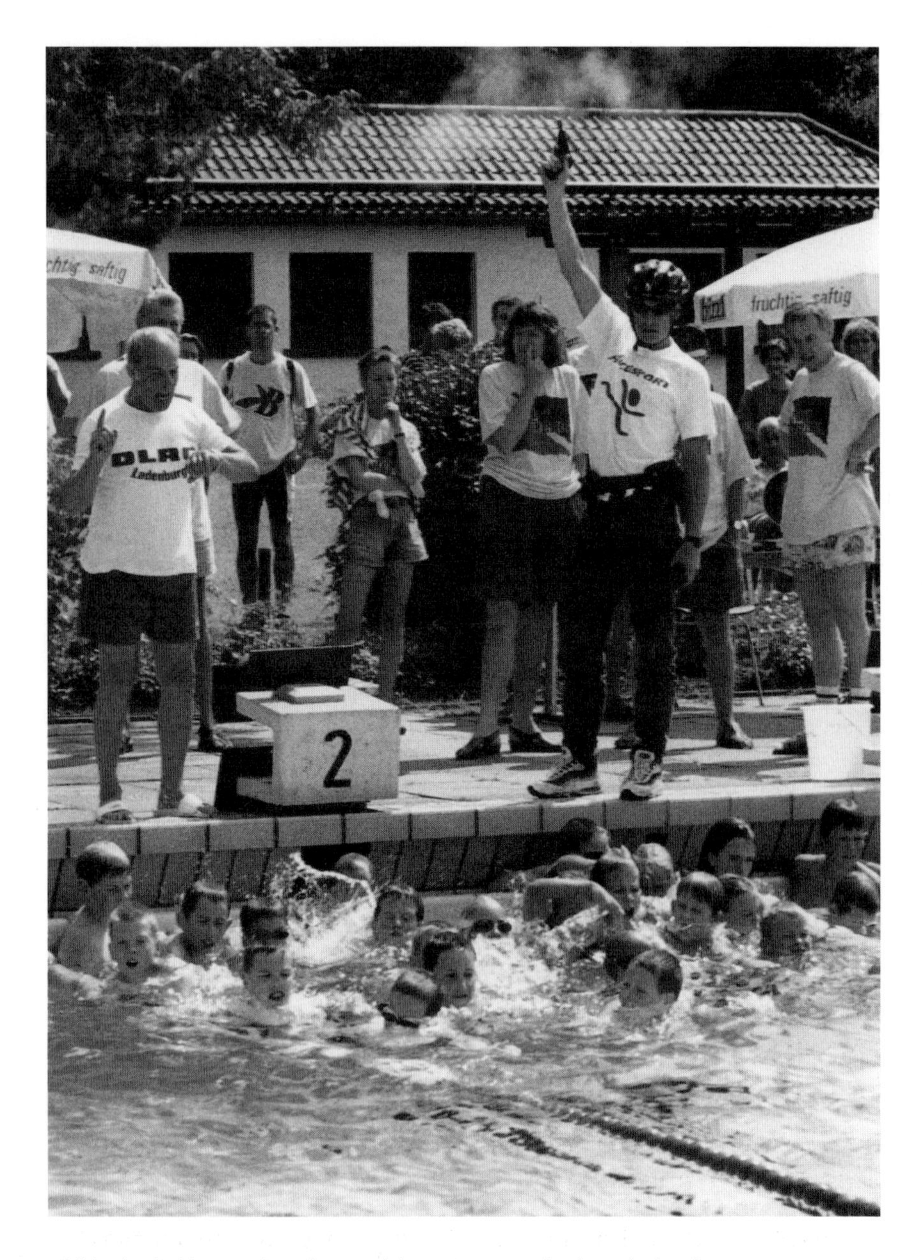

Children's triathlon. Jostle at the start (Photo: Georg Rombach, Cadenburg)

1 Development Trends in Endurance Performance

Endurance achievements are characterised by constant new developments in the fields of world records, conspicuous change in competition systems, the introduction of new techniques and innovative renewal of competition equipment.

Development of Top Performances

The international tendency in endurance sports is towards the constant development of world-class achievements.

In many sports and disciplines there are sometimes sensational improvements in top performances (Fig. 1/1, see p. 12).

The competition results of the Olympic Games and World Championships document the further development of world-class performances in almost all endurance sports. In a number of sports and events new dimensions of performance have been reached which are sometimes beyond the prognosis of development rates. The dynamics and the diversity of performance development in the individual sports and events as well as between the sexes also increased.

In the athletic endurance events in particular, such as the men's and women's 1500 m, 5000 m and 10,000 m run and the 3000 m hurdles, new performance dimensions were achieved that only a few years ago would hardly have been considered possible. The endurance sports are an example of the dynamics and complexity of the development in performance at world-class level. In the individual sports/events there has been an alternation between constant development, rapid development, performance stagnation and decrease in performance (FRANZ/PFÜTZNER, 1997).

The spectacular improvement in the world hour record in track cycling (Fig. 2/1, see p. 12) is a very good example of the complexity of the physical prerequisites, the sporting technical transfer and the optimal adjustment of competition equipment to the athlete. In cycling touring there has also been a constant increase in the average velocity (Fig. 3/1, see p. 13).

In sports which are greatly influenced by climatical and geographical conditions, figures measured over many years show a constant increase in performance (Fig. 4/1, see p. 14).

In triathlon as well, in which there have only been World and European Championships since 1989, a progressive performance trend can be identified (Fig. 5/1, see p. 15).

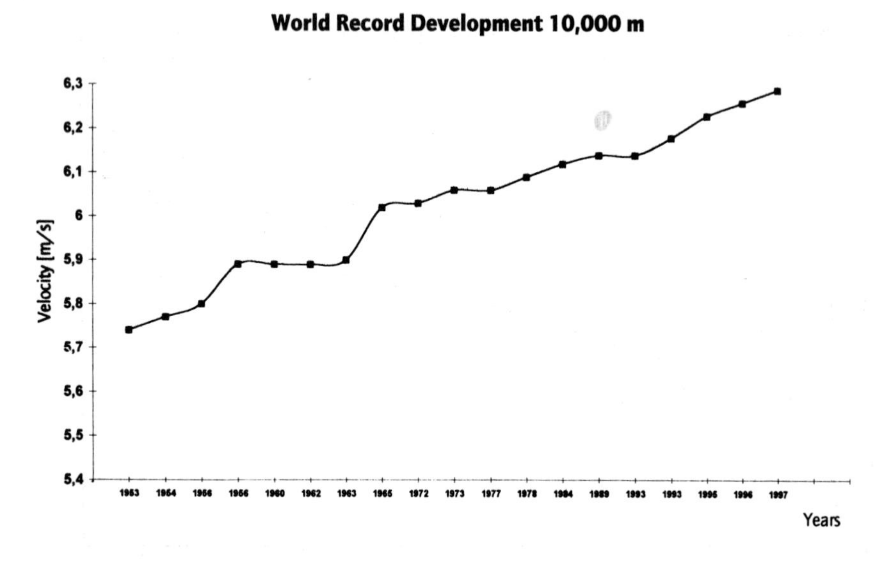

Fig. 1/1: Development of the 10,000 m world record

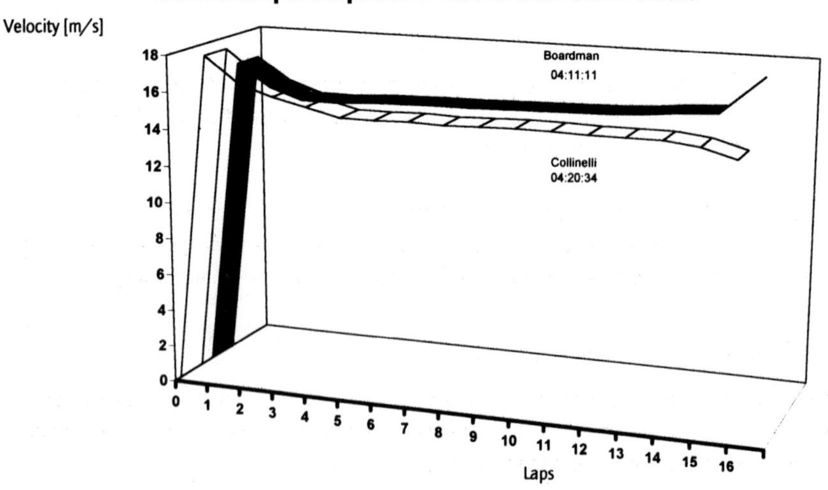

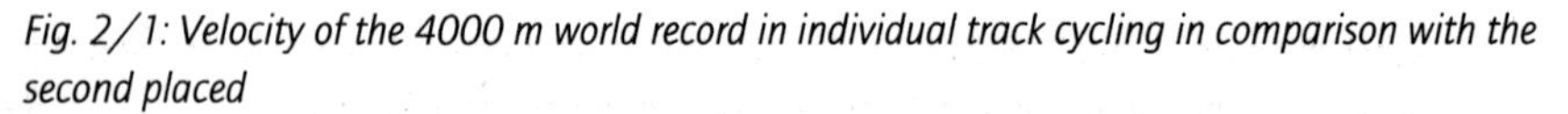
Fig. 2/1: Velocity of the 4000 m world record in individual track cycling in comparison with the second placed

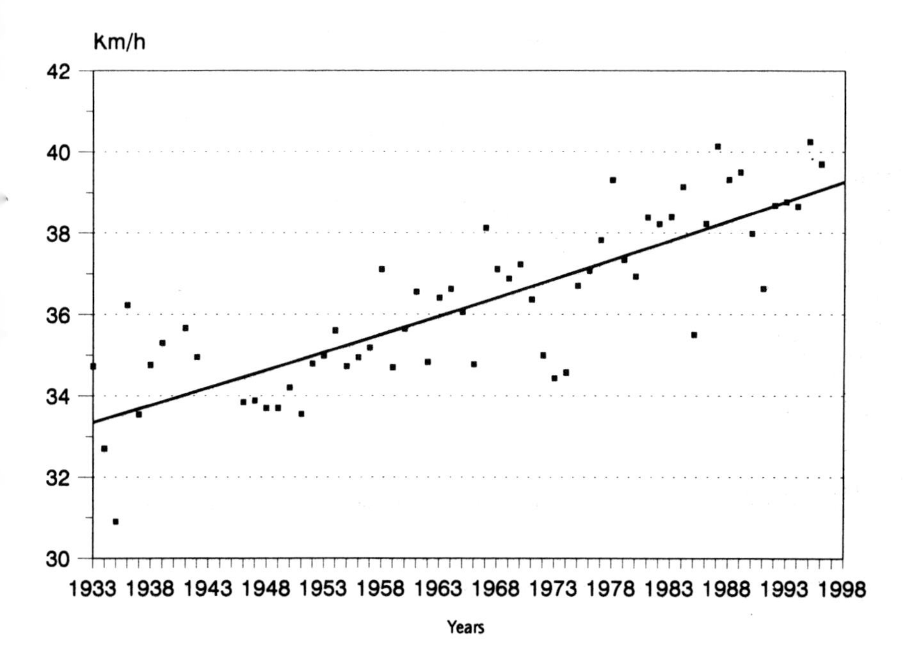

Fig. 3/1: Increase in average velocity in the Tour de Suisse. Each year the velocity increased by 0.3%.

With regard to this data the theory is again substantiated that there are currently no performance limits. In the future too, further improvements in world best performances and extreme performances are to be expected.

Of particular note is the relationship between the high pace in the development of performances and the degree of marketing of the individual sport through sponsors and the media. This applies especially to athletics, cycling, triathlon and cross-country skiing.

Development of Competitive Systems

In all sports the development of training systems is increasingly affected by the development of the competitive systems, including their strong differentiation between the sports and events. Trends in the development of the competitive systems include:

- A further increase in the number and frequency of international competitions, e.g. in athletics, swimming, cycling and triathlon as well as in the nordic skiing events.

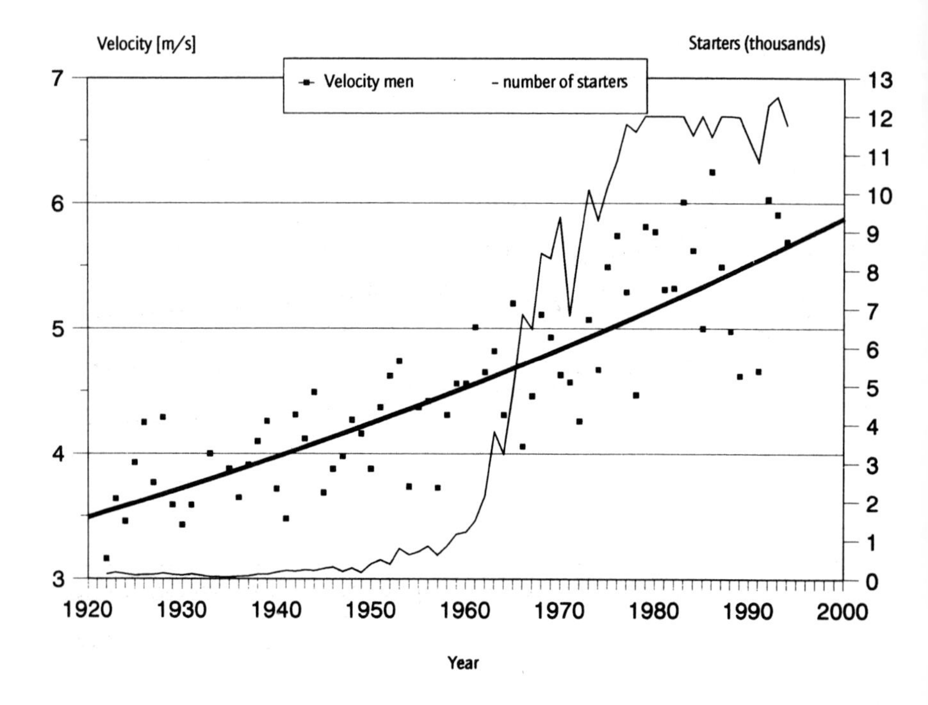

Fig. 4/1: Performance development of the Vasa Ski Cross-Country in Sweden (85.8 km). From the 1970s onwards there is a drastic rise in the number of participants.

- The development of new competitive events, such as team competitions in biathlon as well as reductions or extensions of the competition distances in swimming to 50 m or 5 km and 25 km amongst others.
- Changes in competition rules and conditions, e.g. removal of the slipsteam regulation in triathlon and covering the racing areas in speed skating.
- The introduction of additional international championships during the year (indoor competitions in triathlon, similar to indoor athletics competitions).
- Continuing commercialisation with increased striving for wins and records as well as spectacular performances. In sports that lend themselves to media presentation there is an increase in the athletes' willingness to do their best and to take risks.
- A clear differentiation of competition programmes into the top and youth areas in the individual sports.
- Spectacular extreme situations in running, cycling and mountaineering, among others.

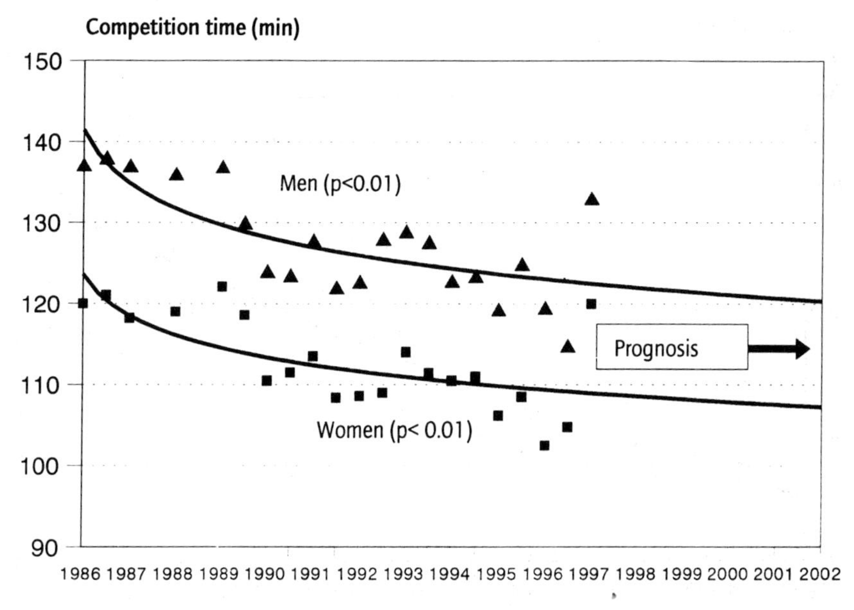

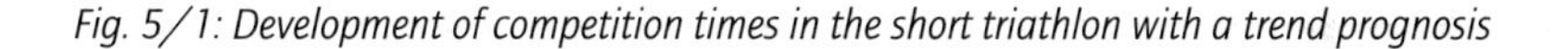

Fig. 5/1: Development of competition times in the short triathlon with a trend prognosis

From these developments, consequences are to be extrapolated for the structuring of annual performance and training, for the development of the prerequisites for performance and the markedness of performances. The sports methodological ideals for performance in competition are being changed considerably, not always to the advantage of the athletes.

New demands have arisen regarding the preparation and structuring of competitions, especially in competing with sporting opponents and the increase in performance density. As a result a greater stability of the performance prerequisites coupled with an increased variation of competition organisation has become necessary.

Performance development in recent years has also been characterised considerably by the development of new techniques. The emphasis is on optimal and energy-saving techniques. Athletes are constantly offered new competition equipment, materials and clothing that help them to improve propulsion.

Summary

In the near future no limits are to be expected in the development of top performances both in the elite categories of the endurance sports and the age-groups. In some endurance sports the pace of development is linked very closely to the degree to which they are marketed. Top performances require professional preparation. In addition to records, there is also an increase in extreme performances of individual athletes which encourage imitation.

1.1 Human Performance Capacity in the Aging Process

Age and growth have a clear influence on sporting performance. Depending on the sport, the age of top performance generally begins at 20 years. Retracing the number of training years required to reach top performance usually shows that athletes had to train for an average of ten years (eight to twelve years). In some endurance sports the top-level is so high and so close together that it takes until the age of 25 to 30 to reach it. Currently the phenomenon can be observed that athletes who have achieved top performances at national or world-class level try to stay at the top for as long as possible. Evidence of this are notable performances by athletes aged over 40 years in endurance but also in sprinting events. The moment of leaving the sport is a social event and not necessarily based on biological demands. Top-level sport also offers a way of earning a living over longer periods of an athlete's life.

The high-performance capacity of athletes in middle age is emphasised here because it also has an exemplary effect for leisure and fitness athletes. For the moment, performance limits are not to be expected in many sports; internationally, top performances are spread over an increasing number of athletes. Instead of a previously expected flattening out of performance development with regard to world records, in numerous sports there is an almost linear progression upwards (see Fig. 1/1).

In this connection it can be observed that the accepted limits and norms in training load are being reached by more and more athletes and there is still no end in sight to the imitation of high levels of load.

The typical example of a volume-orientated training is the marathon. If, for example, an athlete develops the goal of covering the distance of 42.2 km in three hours, then running training of over 80 km per week for several months is necessary. If the best performances in the marathon are compared with age, these differ little in the age-group of 20 to 40 years (Fig. 1/1.1: see p. 22).

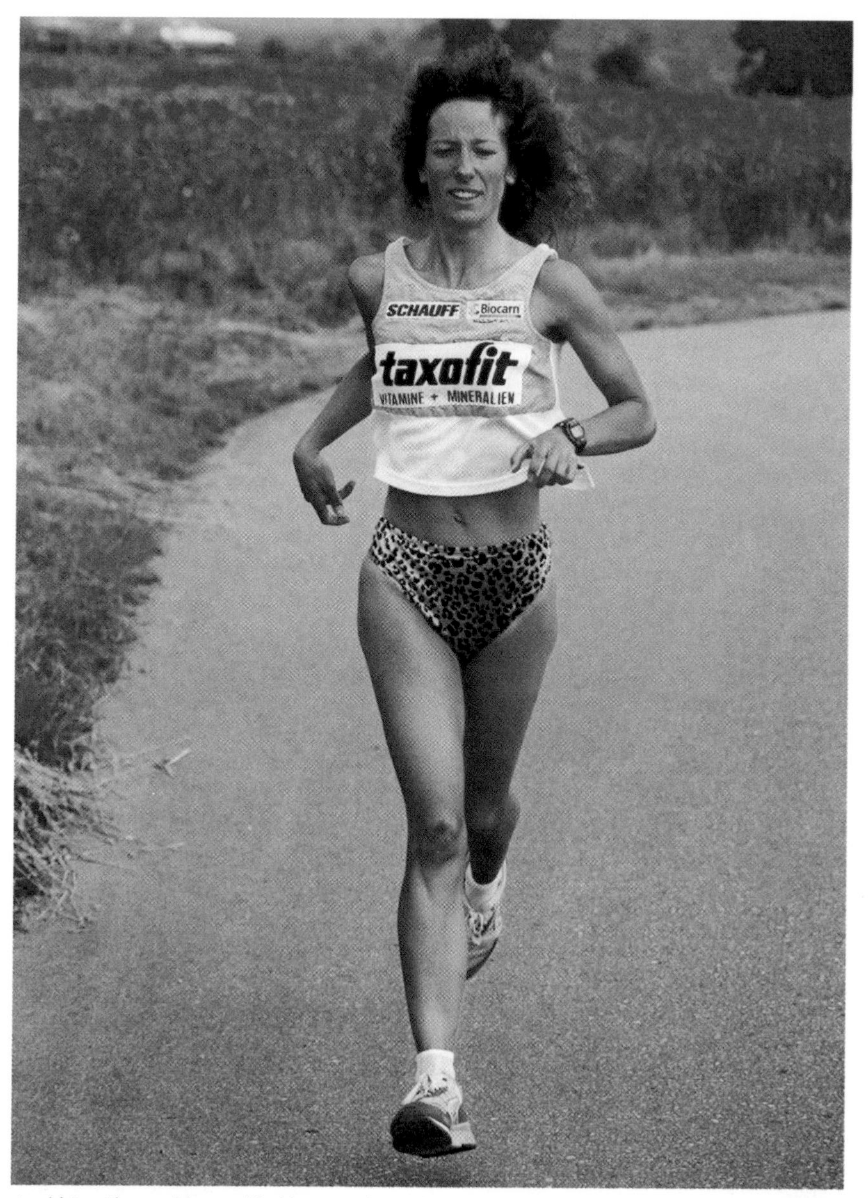

Astrid Benöhr, world record holder over three-, four- and five-times ultra triathlon, while running (Photo: Karsten Karbaum)

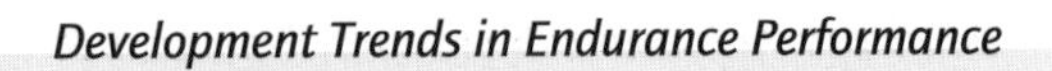

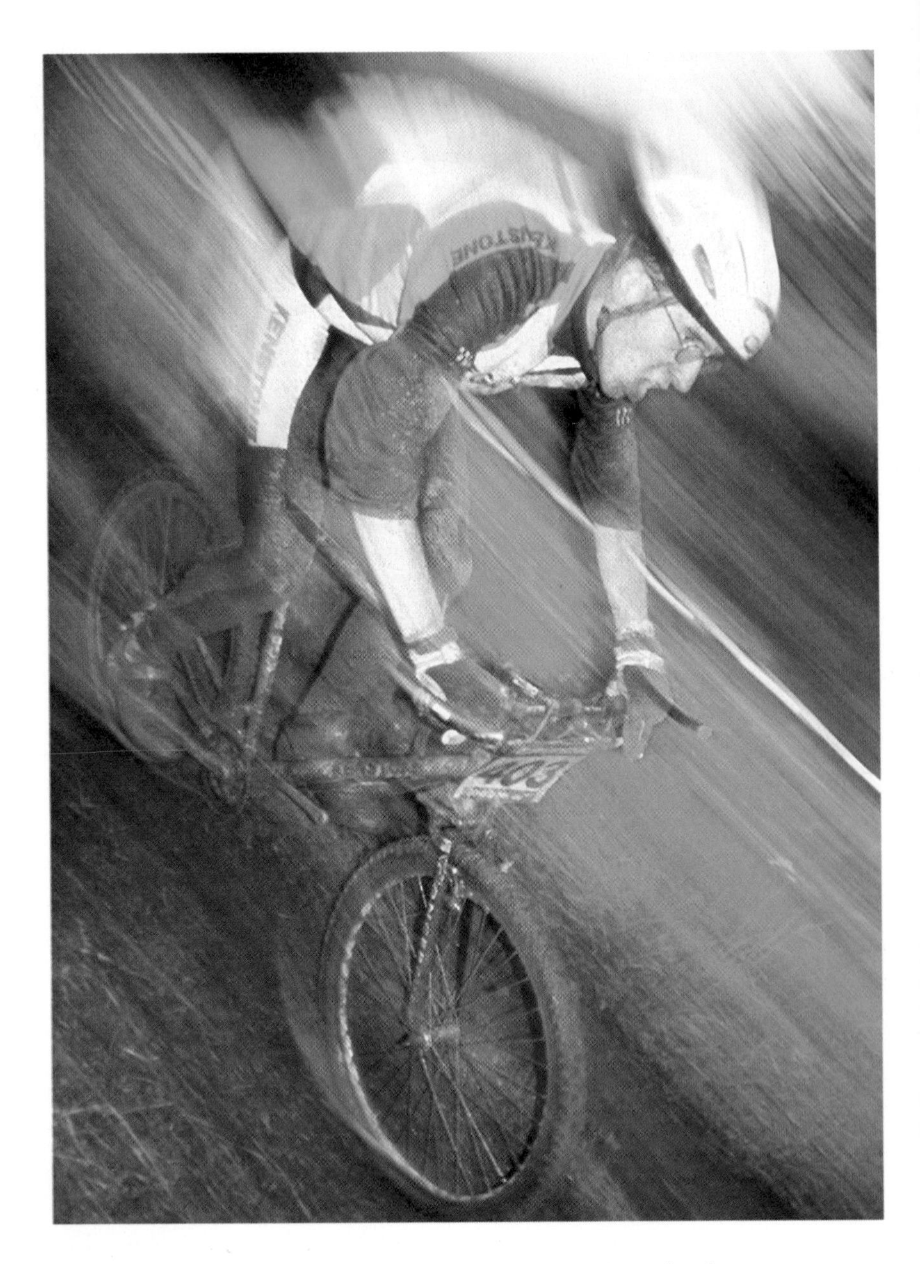

WAG's Picture and Text Agency, Freiburg (Photo: Armin Schirmaier, Freiburg)

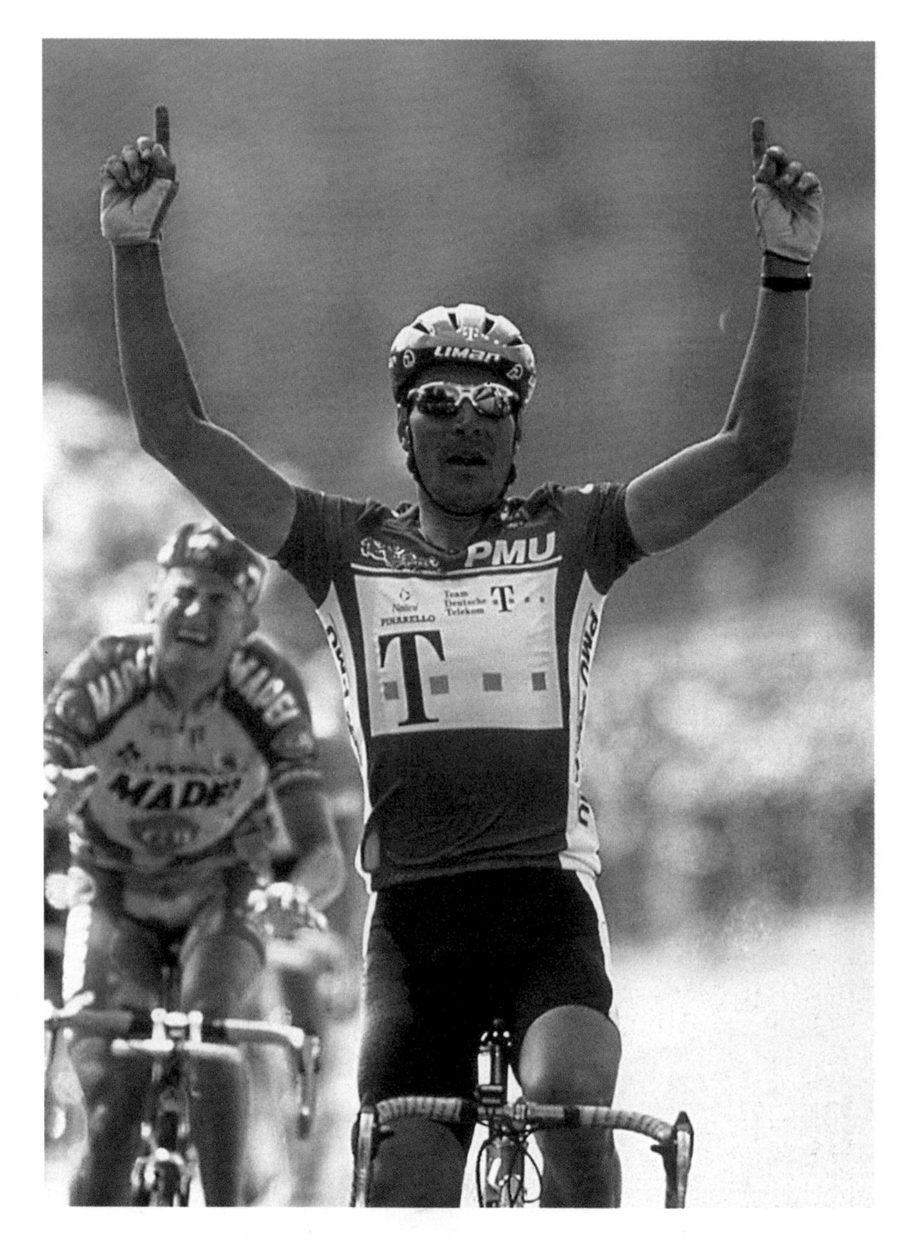

Finishing of Erich Zabel (Photo: Polar)

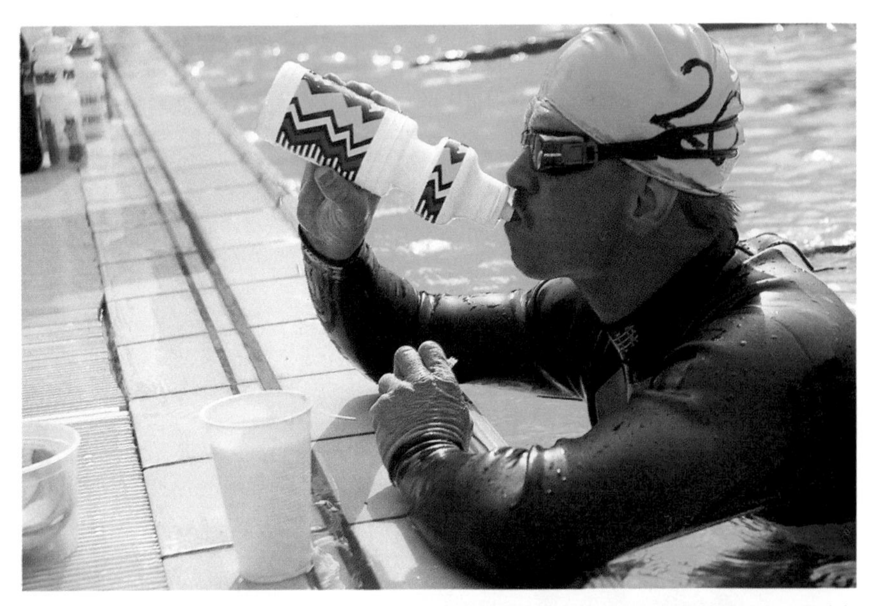

Intake of nutrition during long distance swimming over 11.4 km (Photo: Georg Neumann, Leipzig)

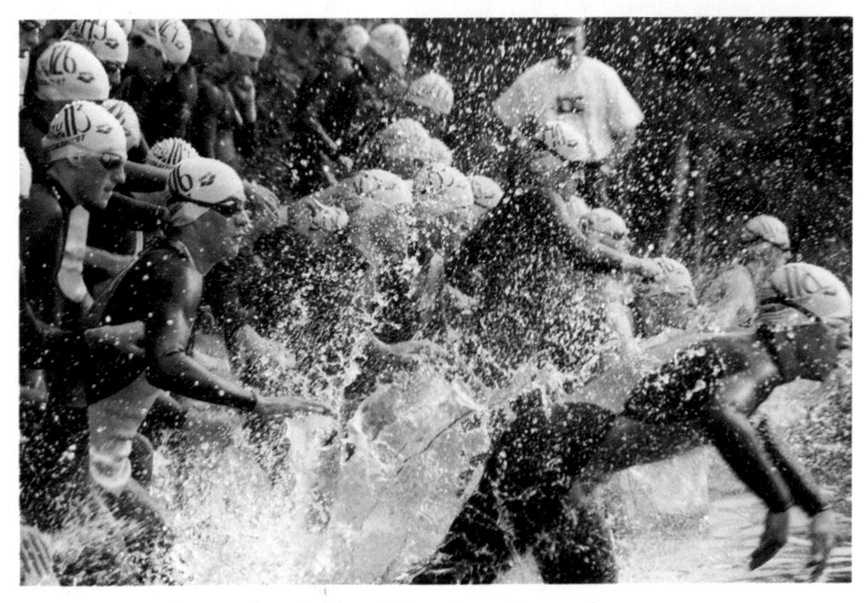

Triathlon: Swimming start from the shore (Photo: Georg Neumann)

The degeneration of motor abilities with increasing age varies as well as the possibility of training abilities when training is taken up again (Fig. 2/1.1, see p. 22). Obviously performance in running competitions often varies in the individual age-classes, which can be coincidence and dependent on the individual training opportunities; at any rate, 80-year-old runners still manage 50% of the performance of 20-year-olds (Fig. 3/1.1, see p. 23). The large numbers of participants in the popular mass sports (running, cross-country skiing, triathlon, swimming etc.) show the capabilities with increasing age and also the amount of training time put in.

Only after the age of 45 does a gradual reduction in performance set in. In the 1970s the trend towards mass races (running, cross-country skiing) evaluated in age-classes began (Fig. 4/1.1, see p. 23). The diagram shows that a 70-year-old triathlete achieves about 55% of the winning performance.

The big question is how does society or the athlete himself organise access to the mastery of a popular sport. If it is assumed that endurance sport is the most effective alternative as a preventive health measure, then these sports should technically be learned during childhood.

From a social point of view the early development of skills for technical mastery of a sport, such as swimming, cycling, cross-country skiing or running, is imperative. If the prerequisites for motor learning of a sport are not available then these can hardly or only unsatisfactorily be made use of later in a preventive way. The biomotor abilities of endurance, strength, speed and co-ordination cannot be stored, but when the sport is taken up again in middle age they must be retrievable. Warnings from experts about overloading the support apparatus and locomotor system when learning new sporting techniques have often proved to be a false conclusion. One only needs to think of the advent of the freestyle technique in cross-country skiing. This skating technique is increasingly used by older people and has proved to be easier on the joints than the classical skiing technique (Fig. 5/1.1, see p. 24). There is also a trend for women's performances to come closer to men's, but without being able to objectively achieve these. In long-distance swimming competitions a clear fluctuation can be observed in the gap between the women over 800 m and the men over 1500 m (Fig. 6/1.1, see p. 25).

After the introduction of tests for forbidden substances in competitions and training, the real physiological performance gap of 6-8% between women's and men's performances in swimming reappeared. In an average of all endurance performances the difference between women and men at comparable top performance levels is 8-12% (10%). The physiological causes of these performance differences are to be found in differences in body structure, hormones, muscular aerobic performance prerequisites and strength potential.

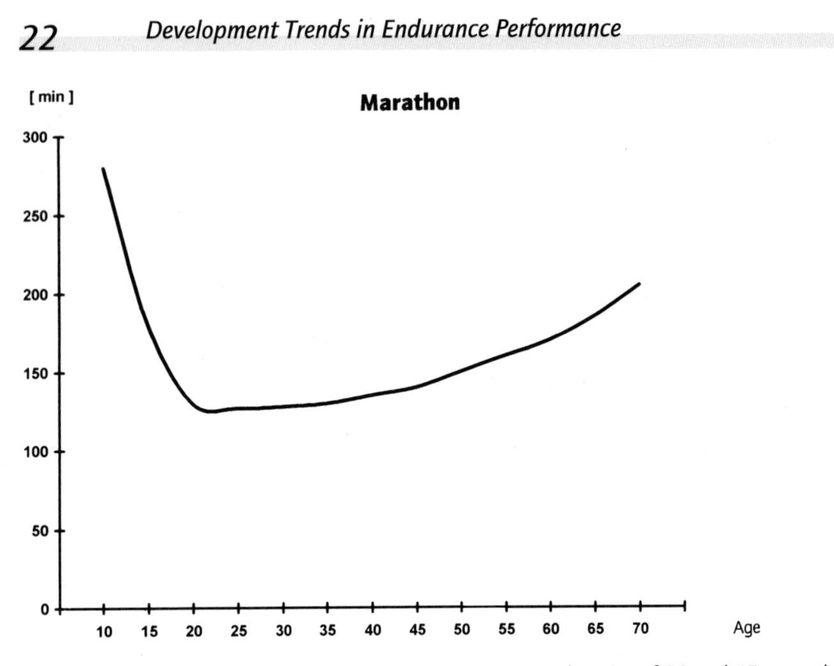

Fig. 1/1.1: Marathon best times in relation to age. Between the ages of 20 and 45 years there are only minor differences in performance.

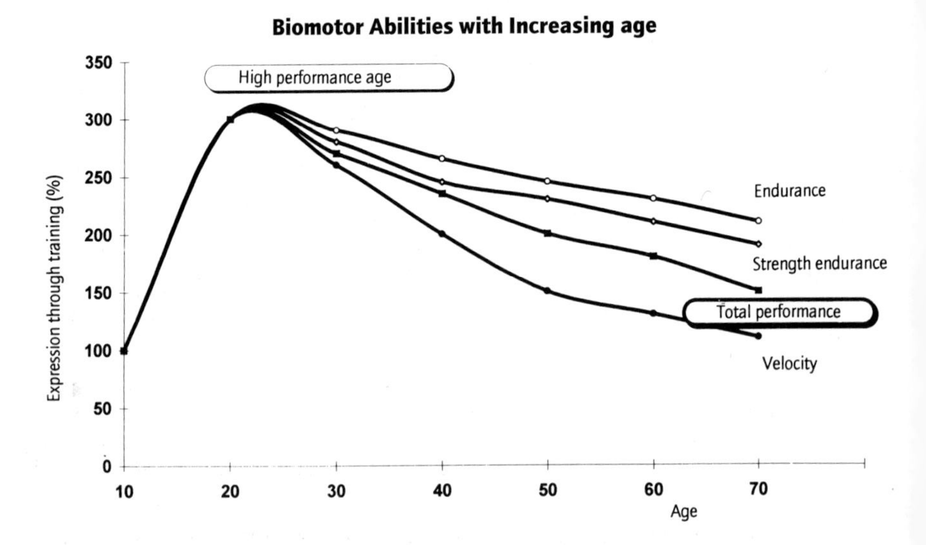

Fig. 2/1.1: Training of biomotor abilities with increasing age. With increasing age, endurance abilities can be trained best.

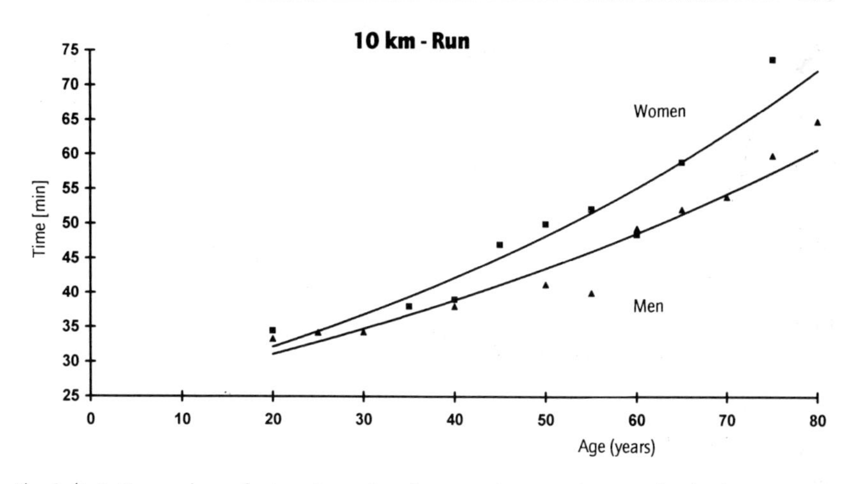

Fig. 3/1.1: Comparison of winner's results of men and women in a randomly chosen popular run over 10 km at increasing ages.

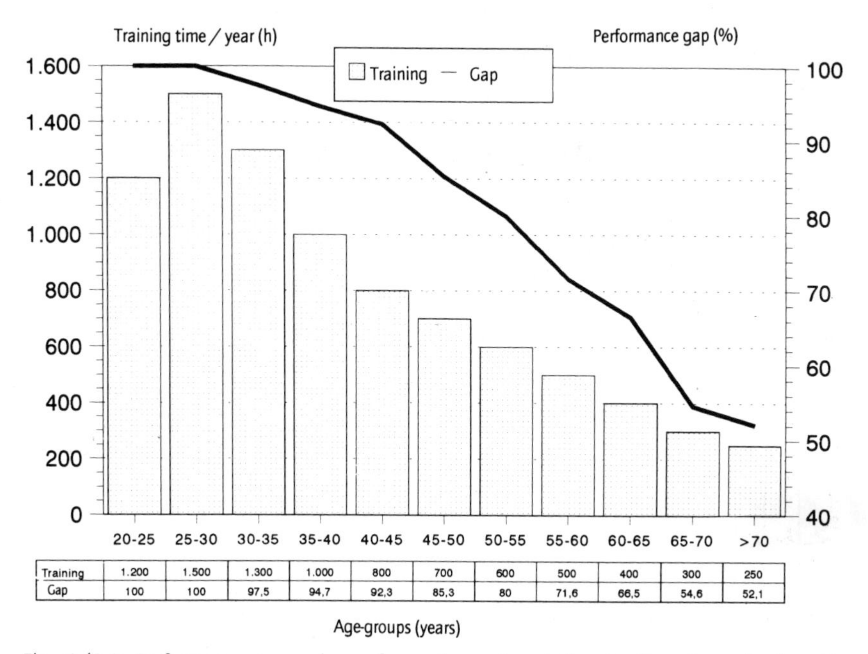

	20-25	25-30	30-35	35-40	40-45	45-50	50-55	55-60	60-65	65-70	>70
Training	1.200	1.500	1.300	1.000	800	700	600	500	400	300	250
Gap	100	100	97,5	94,7	92,3	85,3	80	71,6	66,5	54,6	52,1

Fig. 4/1.1: Performance comparison of age-classes in relation to the winner in the ultra triathlon (3.8 km swimming, 180 km cycling and 42.2 km running) in Hawaii. The graph shows the five best triathletes in each class according to the amount of training.

Through training maximum oxygen uptake (VO_2 max) increases, but with women it is always 10% lower than with men in the same sport. It is a representative unit for the rates of aerobic energy flow which are available during a load. In performance training one can double the VO_2 max (Fig. 7/1.1, see p. 26). With increasing age, maximum oxygen uptake gradually reduces and with it endurance performance (Fig. 8/1.1, see p. 26).

Summary

The high-performance age stretches over a wide range, on average from 18 to 38. The number of exceptions is increasing, and it seems that the human biological performance potential has been underestimated. Nevertheless there is a natural regression in performance capacity after the age of 40. Of the various abilities, endurance can best be trained at a higher age, followed by strength and speed. Endurance training has the greatest preventive effect in health terms.

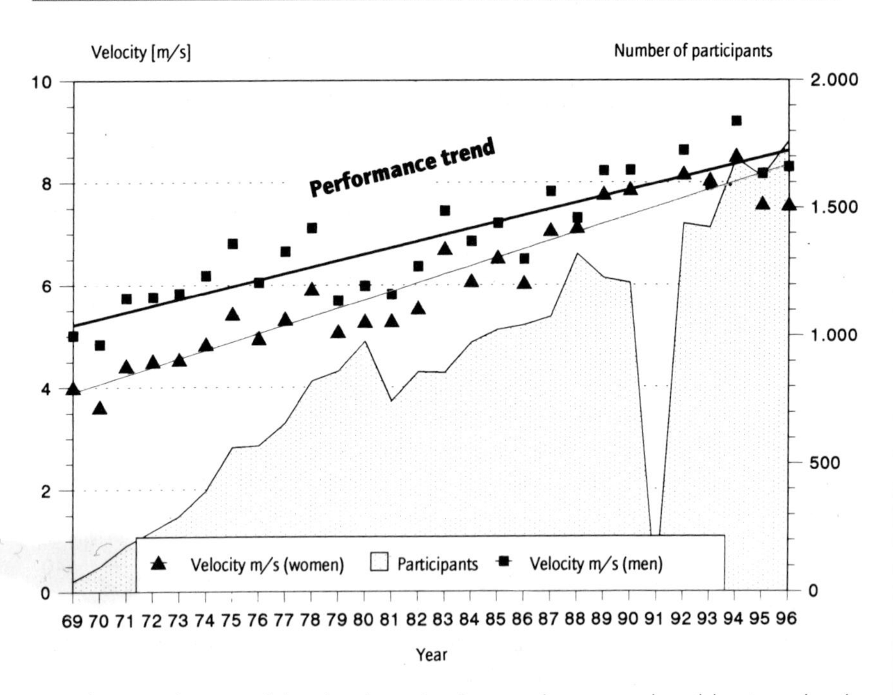

Fig. 5/1.1: Development of the winner's results of men and women and participant numbers in the Engadine Ski Marathon (42 km). From 1986 classical cross-country skiing was replaced by the freestyle technique.

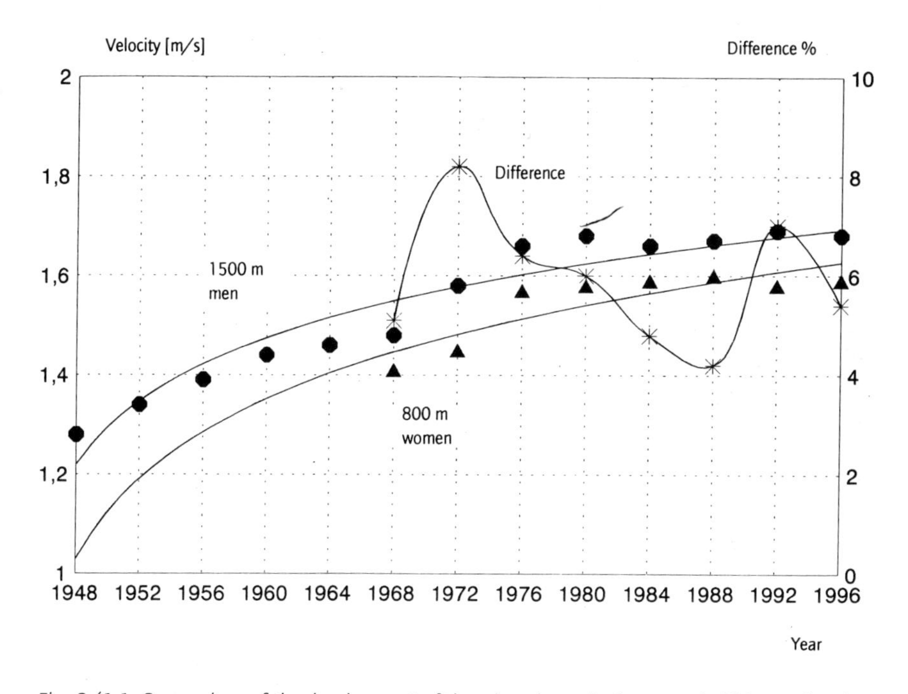

Fig. 6/1.1: Comparison of the development of the winner's results in women's 800 m swimming and men's 1500 m swimming at the Olympic Games. The gender specific performance differences between 1968 and 1996 have been emphasised.

1.2 Endurance Training and Health

In view of increasing life expectancy and the associated rising health costs, measures for maintaining health and preventing illness are of central social significance. Promoting health has always been an important objective of sport and is reflected in the term "health sport". Everyone active in sport can confirm that regular physical activity improves general well-being and gives one a feeling of increased performance capacity and stable health. In ancient times and the Middle Ages important doctors pointed out the positive influence of physical exertion on health. PLATO already recommended a mediumly effective level of exertion – "not too much and not too little" – as a sure path to health. The positive effects of regular sporting activity apply not only to healthy people, but to the same extent to people with illnesses e.g. of the cardiovascular system, metabolism, respiratory tracts, kidneys, nervous system among others. Sport is especially effective regarding impairments to the support apparatus and locomotor system. These days

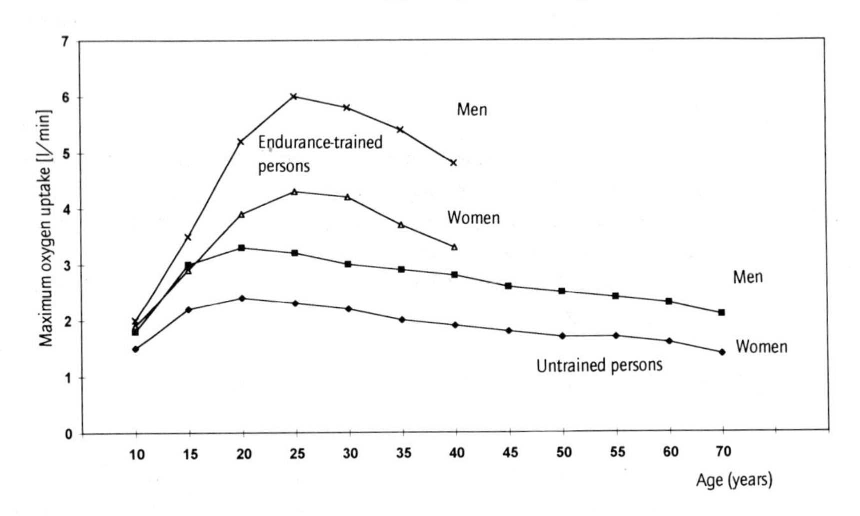

Fig. 7/1.1: Comparison of oxygen uptake (l/min) with increasing age of untrained and trained persons of both sexes

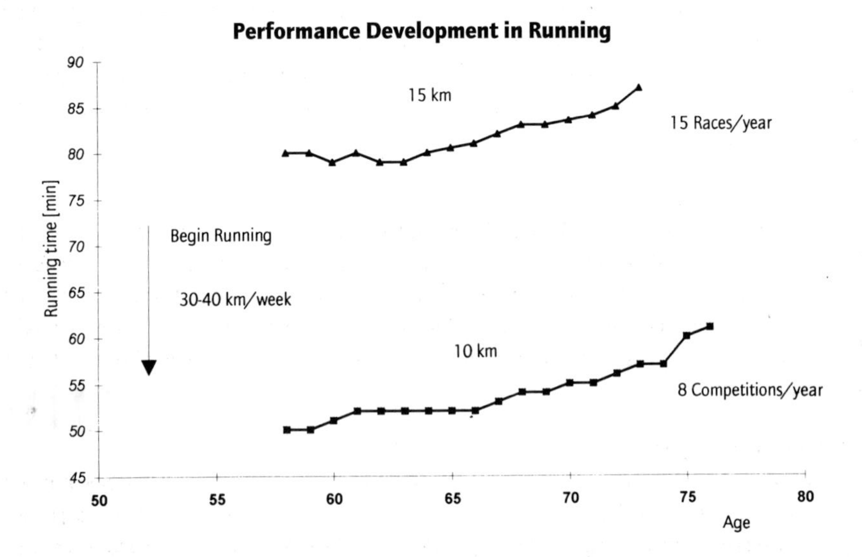

Fig. 8/1.1: Performance deterioration and average number of competitions per year of a hobby runner who first began training at the age of 57.

physical activity in the form of dosed sporting exertion has established itself in preventive, curing and rehabilitative medicine. Sport alone, however, is not a guarantee of health but must be integrated sensibly into one's lifestyle. This applies to both healthy and ill people.

Health Sport

Health sport can be summarised as regular, individual physical exertion with the aim of improving one's health or maintaining or regaining it. Thus health sport encompasses preventive sport, movement and sports therapy as well as rehabilitation sport. Leisure and popular sport also count as health-related physical activity.
The health-promoting effect of endurance training has been proved in numerous scientific studies and research programmes.

Endurance Training Has the Following Health-promoting Effects

- **Cardiovascular System**
  Most important are changes to the working muscles caused by load and the positive effect on the cardiovascular system and metabolism. As a result of peripheral and cardial adaptations, endurance training leads to economisation of the heart functions, i.e. heart rate, heart work and oxygen consumption of the heart muscle are reduced at rest and during submaximal physical activity. The heart works in low gear, so to speak. Through these functional changes, protective mechanisms against stress influences and cardiovascular diseases become effective. In patients suffering from coronary heart disease, haemodynamic adaptations lead to a reduction of the oxygen consumption of the heart muscle and in this way increase physical durability.

- **Flowing Properties of the Blood**
  The flowing properties of the blood are positively influenced by endurance training. The fibrinogen level decreases and fibrinolytic activity is increased, coupled with a simultaneous reduction in thrombocyte aggregation, i.e. coagulation of the blood is restricted physiologically and mechanisms to dissolve clots are increased. These effects are especially significant for sports participants with damaged vessels as the danger of blood clots is reduced.

- **Hormonal Regulation**
  A major effect of training is the reduction of the catecholamine level in the blood. Blood pressure, the heart function and the psychophysical processing of load are positively influenced by this changed adrenergic reactional situation. Hormonal changes are also reflected in the increase in endogenous insulin secretion, the improvement of glucose tolerance and the simultaneous raising of the insulin sensitivity of the muscle cells.

- **Fat Metabolism**
  A positive influence on fat metabolism through regular endurance training has also been established. This protective effect manifests itself in a reduction in cholesterol and in low density lipoproteins (LDL) with a simultaneous increase in high density lipoproteins (HDL) which protect the vessels.

- **Support Apparatus and Locomotor System**
  The support apparatus and locomotor system of the body profits from varied muscle training. As a result of increasing lack of movement, the locomotor system now takes first place in the illness statistics. A trained muscle system takes the pressure off joints and the spine. Bone metabolism is also positively influenced by physical activity, so that the development of continuous bone deterioration (osteoporosis) can be prevented. In Germany about four million people are currently affected by osteoporosis.

- **The Immune System**
  Moderate sporting activity strengthens the immune system and reduces proneness to infection (see chapter 4.6).

- **Performance Capacity**
  Endurance-oriented health training increases performance capacity and leads to improved handling of the demands of daily life. For older people in particular, the diverse adaptations of the body as well as improved fitness lead to an increase in the quality of life and verve and slow down the aging process. Retrospective studies have provided evidence of an increased life expectancy of about two years through regular endurance training.

- **Influencing of Risk Factors**
  A further major effect of regular endurance training lies in the influencing of risk factors. These lead to the development of arteriosclerosis with the typical illnesses caused by civilisation, such as heart attacks, high blood pressure, strokes and kidney diseases. Regular endurance training prevents the arisal and further development of risk factors such as fat metabolism disturbances, high blood pressure, excessive weight and diabetes mellitus. Endurance training is a natural compensation for increasing daily stress and can eliminate stress influences or reduce their effect on the body.

In the final analysis, lack of movement is itself a risk factor. Physical inactivity doubles the risk of developing coronary heart disease. Lack of exercise as a risk factor can be reduced in a natural way with regular training. If several risk factors have been diagnosed, sporting activity is urgently needed as the health damaging effects of risk factors do not only add up but multiply.

Health Promoting Sports

The endurance sports are definitely included among the sports that promote good health. Within the framework of health sport, age, sex, personal interests and previous sporting experience should all play a major role in taking up training in a suitable sport. Running training is for example not very suitable for overweight people, for whom swimming is better because of the smaller amount of load on the support apparatus and locomotor system. Taking individual prerequisites into consideration, the following sports can be recommended for health sport: hiking, walking, fast walking, running, cycling, swimming, cross-country skiing and triathlon (NEUMANN, 1991). Depending on the experience and sturdiness of the individual, sports such as tennis, golf, volleyball, soccer as well as the endurance sports rowing and canoeing are also suitable. Since 1992 roller blading has become a popular leisure sport for a wide age range in Germany (HOTTENROTT, 1996). In addition to the classical endurance sports, the modern offerings indicate a trend towards fun sports with an emphasis on risk, for middle-aged people as well.

The value for preventive purposes, a low level of injury and acceptable material and technical requirements are important factors for the choice of a suitable sport.

Intensity of Load

To achieve a training effect, the intensity of endurance training should reach a level of about 50 to 70% of maximum performance capacity. The basis for the individual target for weekly running velocity or ergometer performance are performance diagnostic tests or the training heart rate derived from these tests. In health sport a training heart rate of 180 minus age should be maintained.

In running training the training heart rate is on average ten to twenty beats higher than in cycling training. In the framework of health-oriented endurance training the intensity of exertion should be in the aerobic metabolism area. Lactate concentration in the blood should not be higher than 4 mmol/l.

Volume of Load

According to research by PAFFENBERGER et al. (1978), additional calorie usage through physical activity of 2000 to 3000 kcal/week or 300 to 400 kcal/day has proved to be effective in reducing the frequency and mortality rate of cardiovascular diseases. Even higher load volumes increase sporting performance capacity but in the illness prevention field do not lead to an improved effect. This fact points to an optimal level of preventive load through endurance training. For long-term illness prevention, three or four weekly running sessions of 45 to 60 minutes at a speed of about 10 km/h (6 min/km) for example would be ideal. In cycling the length of time required is higher because less energy is used. Taking the aspect of influencing fat metabolism (HDL increase) into consideration, the duration of a particular

Duration of load (Hours)	Walking (6 km/h or 10 min/km)	Running (12 km/h or 5 min/km)	Cycling 20 km/h or 3 min/km)	Swimming (12 km/h or 30 min/km)
1	600	870	400	680
2	1200	1740	800	1360
3	1800	2610	1200	2040
4	2400	3480	1600	2720
6	3600	5220	2400	4080
8	4800	6960	3200	5440

Table 1/1.2: Increased energy usage through leisure exertion level of a person weighing 70 kg (5 kg increase in mass increases energy use by c. 1 kcal/min)

training session should be at least 20-30 min (HASKELL, 1986). Table 1/1.2 (above) illustrates the additional energy usage in typical leisure sport activities in relation to the duration of load. Independent of prevention targets and individually strived for volumes to increase performance capacity, even one training session a week results in useful functional changes in the vegetative nervous system. Psychophysical well-being increases. In health sport the acceptance of a physiologically justifiable minimum is just as important as the orientation to the useful optimum level (ISRAEL, 1995).

Because the effects of endurance training cannot be stored by the body, lifelong physical activity is necessary.

Summary

The value of regular sporting training, especially endurance training, is undisputed. Endurance training improves performance capacity, increases the quality of life as well as general well-being and makes dealing with the demands of daily life more easy. Coupled with moderate eating habits, endurance training contributes to normalising blood pressure, blood fat levels and body weight. As a result of diverse cardial, hormonal and central nervous system effect mechanisms as well as the influence on risk factors and living habits, endurance training has an assured position in the prevention of illness. In the meantime it is indispensable in reducing complications after illness (secondary prevention) and for re-establishing performance capacity after illness (rehabilitation). The increased energy usage achieved through endurance training plays a key role in disease prevention. The optimal level of load is between 2000 and 3000 kcal/week. Depending on the sport, that corresponds to an average training volume of four to six hours per week at moderate speed. Low injury endurance load is a major component of health training.

2 Training Load and Demands on the Body

Sports training causes various reactions in the body which represent demands on it. Load can be seen as the sum of all external events affecting a person which change physical and psychological functions. Because of that the sporting load leads to an internal load of the total organism. The demands always have an individual dimension which depends on the extent of the disturbing stimulus and the current training state. An athlete's body does not immediately process loads, they linger on as tiredness remaining from the particular training session. Tiredness from training is a desired and normal state. The continuation of training always takes place on the basis of the remaining tiredness. The body has a constant interrelationship with its environment which is mainly self-regulating and relatively stable with regard to internal and external disturbances. The brain function is the self-regulating control centre. In this system the level of mental representation is the decisive leadership factor. The decision in favour of training load is made on the mental level and is the direct impetus for training.

In the information processing areas of the brain a movement plan is created which makes use of stable motor programmes. When the personal decision on the sport specific form of motor load is made, the cerebellum designs a motor programme which is the basis for its execution. The fast and slow twitch muscle fibres (FTF and STF) involved in the motor programme are stimulated via the nerves. The sport specific motor functions are supported by numerous functional systems, depending on the duration and intensity of load.

These systems influencing and securing performance include: the vegetative nervous system, the cardiovascular system, energy metabolism, the hormonal system, the immune system, temperature regulation, the water and electrolyte balance among others (Fig. 1/2, see p. 32).

All sport specific locomotion must first be supported fitnesswise by training before a particular distance can be covered at a desired speed.

Training-related muscle load is not felt as a demand on the body if it corresponds to the athlete's personal physical and psychological prerequisites. If the athlete loads himself too much, his demand tolerance is overstepped and he tires early. The increasing tiredness forces the release of performance reserves. The biological effort needed to deal with the load increases. Only by keeping up training higher demands can be met.

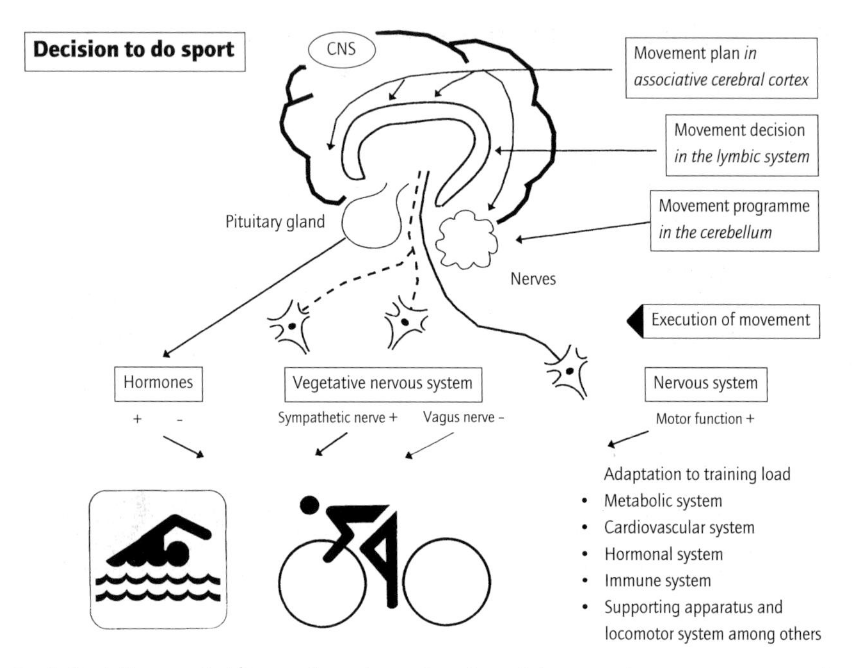

Fig. 1/2: Influence of the central regulatory function of the central nervous system on the functional systems called on in sport.

All high and repetitive psychophysical demands must be interrupted by breaks. The length of the break is determined by the amount of residual tiredness. The athlete himself decides on his ability to handle exertion and when he continues his training. Feeling good during training is not a reliable signal for recognising when periods of unloading are necessary.

Load and unloading (regeneration) are very complex in competitive sport. The successful handling of load always means an increase in the degree of load tolerance (Fig. 2/2, see p. 33). The deciding factor for higher load tolerance in sport is the adaptation achieved through training, which requires longer than generally thought. Before adaptation takes place (after four to six weeks) various phases of changed state in the body must be gone through. These three phases are:

- Current adjustment
- Regeneration (Restoration) and
- Adaptation

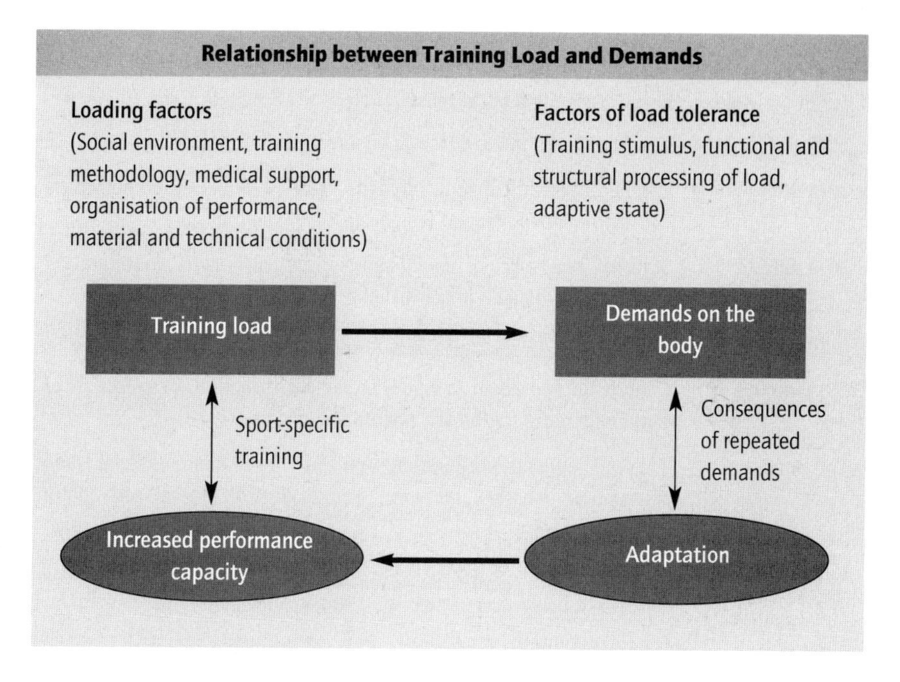

Fig. 2/2: Relationship between training load and demands on the body

Phase of Current Adjustment

Current adjustment is the organism's reaction to performance demands. In the adjustment situation, the organism's functional systems try to deal with the performance demands. The degree of functional adjustment varies and depends on the type, intensity and duration of the performance demands or the stimulus effect of training loads. The constant repetition of the catabolic (breaking down) processes triggered by training influence the organism's counter-reaction. In the end the strength of this counterreaction determines the degree of adaptation achieved. Before there can be adaptation, however, the organism has to process load stimuli and effect functional adjustments and structural changes.

Regenerational Phase (Recovery or Restoration)

In the regenerational phase the state of equilibrium (homeostasis) of the bodily functions disturbed by load and demand regulation is restored. Regeneration occurs at differing speeds in

Chronological Sequence of Regeneration in Sport*	
4th-6th minute:	Complete refilling of the muscular creatine phosphate stores.
20th minute:	Return of heart rate and blood pressure to starting values.
20th-30th minute:	Compensation of drop in blood sugar level; after carbohydrate consumption beginning of temporary rise in blood glucose.
30th minute:	State of acid/alkaline equilibrium is reached, lactate concentration goes down to under 3 mmol/l.
60th minute:	Inhibition of protein synthesis in muscles used declines.
90th minute:	Change from catabolic to mainly anabolic metabolism, increased use of protein for regeneration and adaptation.
2nd hour:	Almost complete restoration in the tired neuromuscular and sensomotor muscle functions (first stage of redeveloped motor exertability).
6th hour-1st day:	Evening out of liquid balance, normalisation of the relationship between solid and liquid blood components (haematocrit).
1st day:	Refilling of liver glycogen.
2nd-7th day:	Refilling of muscle glycogen in intensely used muscles.
3rd-5th day:	Refilling of the muscular fat stores (triglycerides).
3rd-10th day:	Regeneration of partially destroyed contractile proteins (actin, myosin, troponin) in muscle fibres. Return of submaximal endurance and strength performance capacity.
7th-14th day:	Structural build-up in functionally disturbed mitochondria (gradual regaining of full muscular, sport-specific and aerobic performance capacity).
1st-3rd week:	Psychological recovery from stress of exertion on the whole system and return to availability of sport-specific complex performance in short, medium and long duration endurance sports (LDE) I and II (not yet in LDE III and IV: marathon, 100 km run).

* *Average values, individually greatly influenced by duration and intensity of load and performance capacity.*

Table 1.2: Chronological sequence of regeneration in sport

the various systems (see Table 1.2). In the regenerative period (recovery) the anabolic (building up) processes begin again. Used-up energy stores are refilled, worn out cell components are restructured, the immune system regains full functional readiness, psychological relaxation begins, etc. During regeneration the body reaches a state which allows it to continue training without damage. With regard to duration and intensity the muscles are again ready to continue training. Not achieving greater training velocities is always a sign that regeneration is not yet sufficient. Seen this way it becomes clear that the continuing effects of residual tiredness are a permanent component of performance training. Continuing loading after regeneration that is too brief slows down the process of adaptation. The body is more occupied with overcoming tiredness than with processing the new training stimuli.

Adaptation Phase

As a result of regular training over a number of weeks a higher level of load and demands is reached. This takes place in several stages. It is characteristic of performance training that functional adjustments as a result of loading always take place on the foundation of regenerative processes still in progress as well as gradually increasing adaptation. During training there is thus an overlapping of regenerative processes in progress and the handling of disruptive factors, which together characterise the developing adaptation. The adaptive process in the organs and functional systems lessens the intensity of the training stimuli being applied and is thus the foundation for greater physical performance capacity.

Summary

Sporting training leads to demands on the human organism. The organism thus taxed changes its state, it reacts to the exertion in the regulatory area of its functional systems and recovers within certain periods. Repeated taxing leads to a lessening of the disruptive stimuli. Adaptation occurs in the course of load and demand regulation. Once it has adapted to the load the body can deal better with the disruptive stimuli set in motion by sport.

3 Adaptation to Training Load

Occasional loading or training is not enough to motivate the body to adapt. It has a number of options to compensate brief disruptive influences through sport. Each functional system has a certain regulative breadth which can be taken advantage of by sporting load. Exhausting the regulative breadth of functional systems is not yet adaptation but only represents the adjustment situation in the taxed systems. Under load the heart rate, for example, with and without the characteristics of an athlete's heart, can rise to up to 200 beats per min (bpm). The functional reserve of the high heart rate can be used by both trained and untrained persons. During physical or sporting load the functional systems being taxed adjust themselves to the necessary level of exertion. Because all psychophysical loads affecting the organism are stimuli that disrupt the resting state, it tries to reduce its reaction when the stimulus effect is repeated. It begins to prepare itself for a new functional state. In doing so it reorganises its functions and structures in a self-regulating manner in such a way that the effort required to deal with repeated disruptive effects drops. A familiar example for adaptation in sport is the increase in the size of the heart, known as an "athlete's heart". When required, the athlete's larger heart transports more blood to the loaded muscles and in addition it is able to function at a lower rate when he is at rest. The athlete's heart rate (HR) at rest is considerably lowered. The lowered resting HR is not only an expression of the development of an athlete's heart but also of the

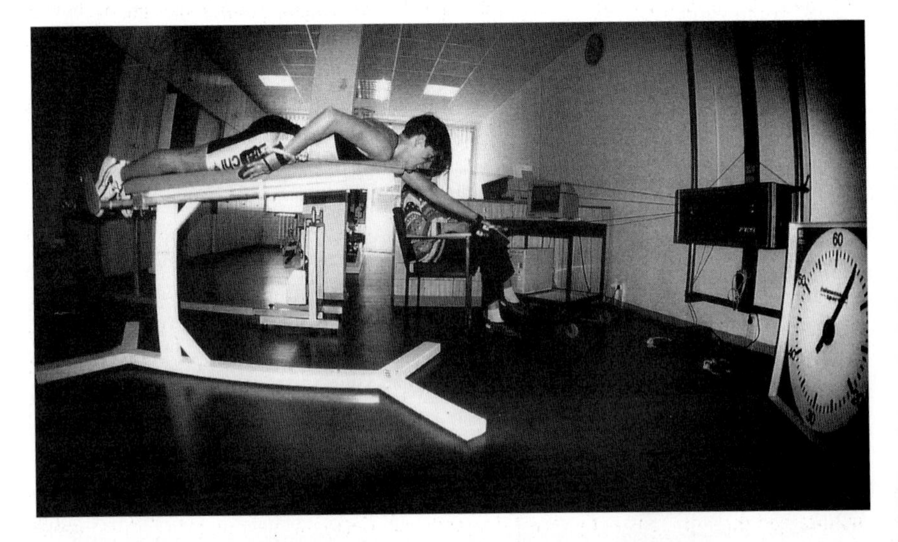

Measuring station training with the rope pulling ergometer (Photo: Arndt Pfützner, Leipzig)

adjustment of functioning in the vegetative nervous system. The vegetative nervous system has a braking part (vagus nerve) and a stimulating part (sympathetic nerve). The vagus leads to a lowering of the resting HR. Even during load, at comparable performance (velocity) levels endurance-trained athletes regulate with a heart rate that is 10 to 20 bpm lower. The main reason is the reduced drive by the sympathetic nerve.

The aim of the organism's adaptation is to reduce internal taxing and to make use of the taxed functions to deal with load as economically as possible. Before adaptation can take place the organism has to be forced to make regular adjustments in its functional systems over longer periods of time. The structure which is most taxed in sport and also the first to adapt is the muscle. With a mass of 23 to 28 kg the muscular system is the largest organ. Training of biomotor abilities is directed to the muscular system first. According to current findings, adaptation takes place gradually and can be divided into four stages (NEUMANN/SCHÜLER, 1994):

1st Stage of Adaptation: Changes in the Movement Programme

In this first stage of adaptation there are mainly changes in the movement programme as a result of the repeated motor demands of training. The superfluous movements of a sport-specific load are increasingly reduced, as in running, swimming, skiing or cycling. Unnecessary associated movements are cut down. The fast and slow twitch muscle fibres (FT and ST fibres) involved in the sport-specific movement programme adapt to the demands placed on them. After 1-2 weeks of training the athlete himself notices that sport-specific movement feels easier and more flowing. In running alone an improvement in running style can save 2 to 5 ml/kg.min of oxygen consumption. The system that reacts to training most quickly is the HR. It can sink significantly after eight days of training already (Fig. 1/3, see p. 38).

The result of the first stage of adaptation is that the state of equilibrium (homeostasis) between the organs becomes more stable; the motor regulatory programme adjusts itself to effective handling of loading. The increase in the activity of the muscle enzyme glycogensynthetase enables the glycogen stores to increase their size. With larger glycogen reserves the quality of load or velocity can be maintained longer. The lower energy deficit shortens recovery time. The first stage of adaptation requires about a week to ten days (Fig. 2/3, see p. 39).

The development of adaptations is a temporary state; motor adaptation is only maintained through constantly raised demands and decreases very quickly if the stimulus stops.

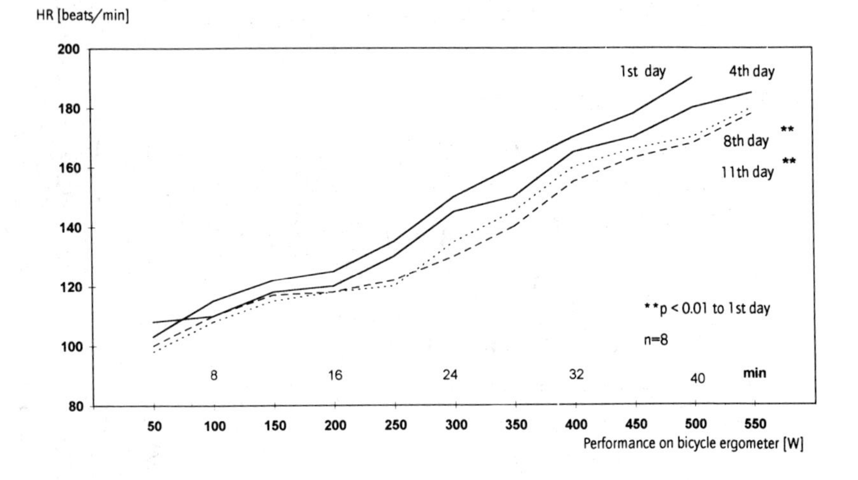

Fig. 1/3: Changes in heart rate (HR) of eight cyclists who carried out a standard level of load on an ergometer for eleven days. On the 8th day of load the heart rate was lower than the starting value for the first time.

2nd Stage of Adaptation: Increase in Size of the Energy Stores

In the second stage of adaptation there is a marked increase in the size of the creatine phosphate and the glycogen stores. After brief intensive (alactic) training stimulus the creatine phosphate stores (CP) grow and after longer anaerobic-aerobic training the muscle glycogen content rises. The energy stores can only increase in size if they have been practically used up by sport-specific load. The constant energy deficit forces the organism to increase the size of the stores.

Typical training loads for increasing the CP stores are repeated intensive sessions of only 6 s duration. Expansion of the glycogen stores on the other hand requires aerobic-anaerobic loads of over 60 min or aerobic loads of over 120 min duration. All forms of loads under 60 min duration lead to a low increase in the glycogen stores. Sprint training with single loads over 10 s duration in series is no longer a typical alactic load for increasing the CP stores; the duration of load is already too long.

The other energy storage form in the muscles, the triglycerides, need extreme forms of long lasting load in order to increase their size. Only aerobic endurance loads lasting many hours lead to an expansion of the intramuscular fat stores (triglycerides). Enlarging the energy reserves makes it possible to maintain sport-specific velocity longer. The form the load takes, i.e. the main type of stimulus applied and the training methodology selected in the sport, has a decisive influence on the changes in the energy stores.

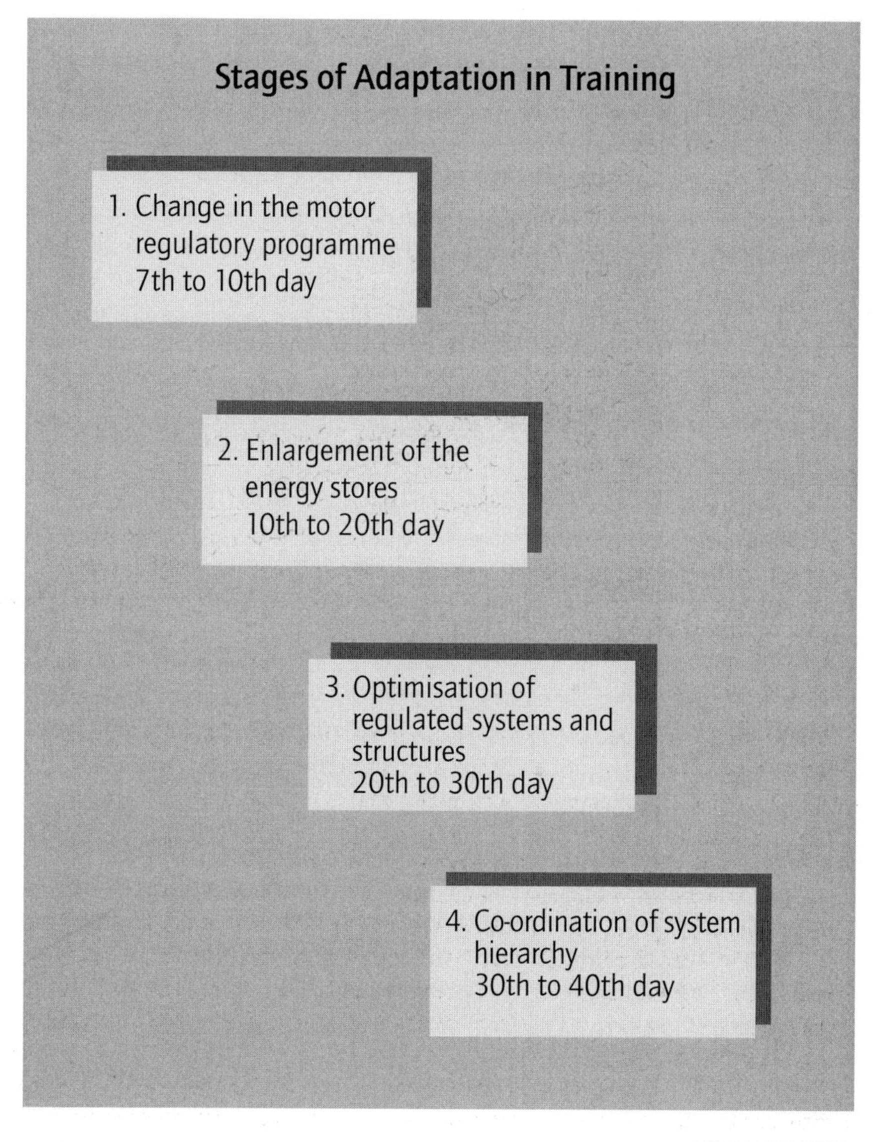

NEUMANN 1993

Fig. 2/3: Progression of adaptation in endurance performance training. Only after 4-6 weeks of training are structures and functions really changed and elevated to a higher level.

In this stage of adaptation the thickness of the muscle fibres changes if the training stimuli are resistance-based. If the muscle is also subjected to strength stimuli (increased resistance) it is forced to increase its reaction space for the contractile structures, it becomes stronger or hypertrophied.

The proteins involved in the contraction process (actin, myosin, troponin) are restructured according to the strength and the resistance so that they are better suited to the sport-specific strength endurance requirements. The reconstruction of these muscle proteins is determined by the amount of old proteins removed and worn out by training. Thus in the second stage of adaptation the main load stimuli are the repeated energy deficit and the wear on muscular structures.

3rd Stage of Adaptation: Optimisation of Regulated Systems and Structures

In this third stage of adaptation a process of optimisation between the restructured and new muscle structures and the sport-specific demands takes place.

As a result of adjustment, regeneration and adaptation, the working conditions of the functional systems and the muscle structures used improve. The muscle system is more resilient and has an increased sport-specific performance capacity. It receives support from further organ systems, in particular energetically. Thanks to the experience of regulation, especially of the metabolism, the organism can adjust to demands sooner. The adaptation takes place independently of willpower (autonomously). The different way the fast and slow twitch muscle fibres (FT and ST fibres) work physiologically is expediently made use of for sport-specific movement.

The nervous steering characteristics of the FT and ST fibres are better adapted to the energetic possibilities of the loaded muscles. The adaptations in the muscle triggered by nervous steering take place mainly on the level of the contractile structures and the energy supplying systems. Depending on the main form of loading, training leads to an increase in the flow of aerobic and anaerobic energy. Structural change occurs in various muscle proteins, such as myofibrils, mitochondria, sarcoplasmic reticulum and microsomes.

In a situation of "recently" improved performance capacity, the functional optimisation of the muscle work is a state susceptible to disruption. This adaptation taking place between the third and fourth training weeks (20th to 30th day) should be supported by reduced total load and thus energetical unloading in order to ease functional optimisation (Fig. 3/3). Intensive shorter loads and competitions with longer recovery are certainly possible in this period. The reduction of total load for about a week is, however, decisive. The cyclisation of training takes this course in adaptive processes into consideration (see chapter 9).

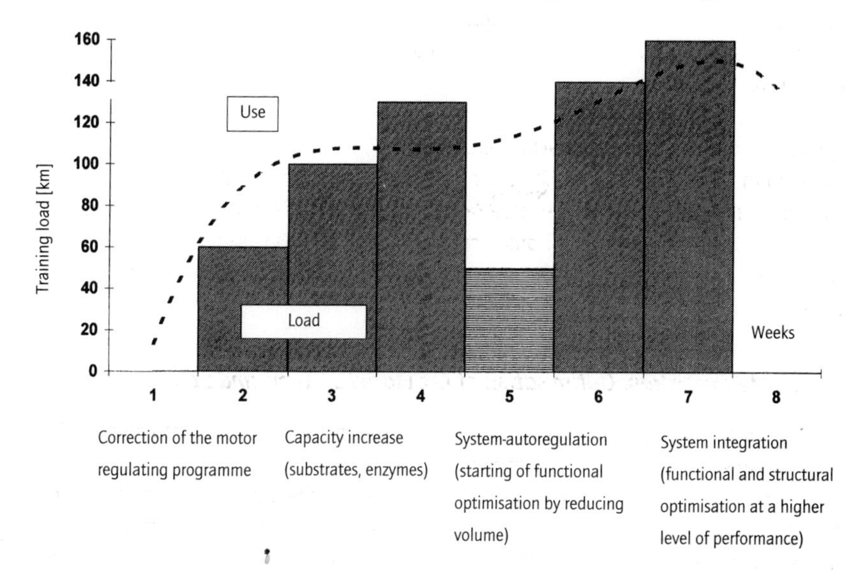

Fig. 3/3: Schematic course of adaptation in performance training. After about three weeks of increasing load a reduction of load is to be implemented so that performance physiologically a further increase in load is made possible.

4th Stage of Adaptation: Co-ordination of Systems Influencing Performance

There are also other functional systems involved in adaptation which have an influence on performance. Systems directly or indirectly influencing performance include the central nervous system, the vegetative nervous system, the cardiopulmonary system, metabolism, the hormonal system and the immune system among others. Adaptation is only complete when their functioning is matched. Adaptation is finished when the newly structured systems in the sport-specific muscle systems are in harmony with each other. The central nervous system regulatory programme affecting the muscles allows many degrees of freedom in response. This also explains why many sport-methodological loading variations can be individually successful. This fact is expressed in daily variations of form when the adaptive state is the same. The co-ordination of the regulatory systems with one another has the effect that if a muscle can no longer deal with a demand autoregulatively on its own, it receives activating support from the regulatory system above it. For activating states that can be adrenaline and the sympathetic nervous system and for economising processes it can be the vagus system and the hormonally supported supply of energy.

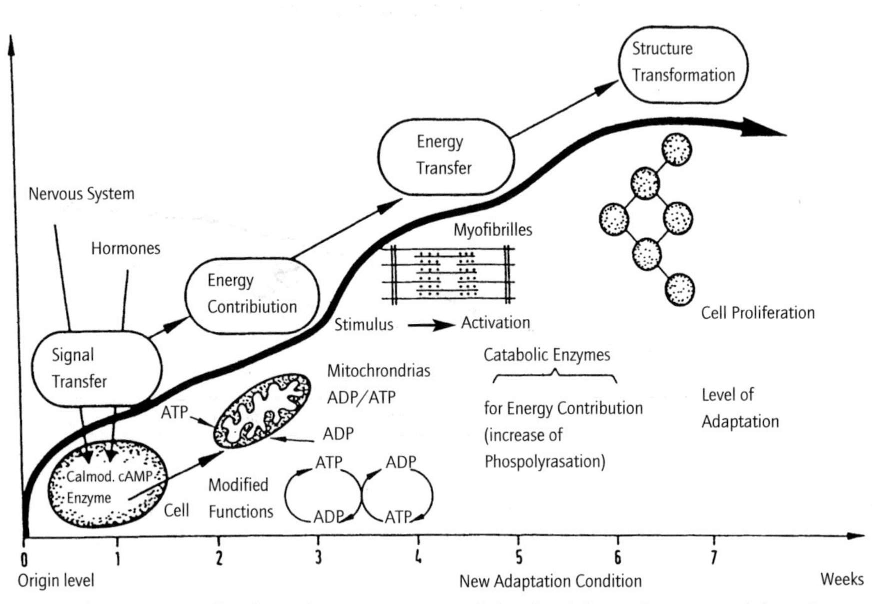

Fig. 4/3: Progress of adaptation on muscle cellular level in endurance training. From NEUMANN/BERBALK (1991)

Functional co-ordination between the central nervous system and the periphery is a process dependent on time which lasts about two weeks and takes place between the 30th and 40th day of adaptive training. The level of mental representation is also a part of the drawing together of the functional systems determining performance. The load must not only be processed morphologically and functionally, but also psychologically.

The adaptive systems shown overlap in training, but it must be taken into consideration that only after 4-6 weeks of performance training at the earliest can a new stage of adaptation be reached, which is expressed by the co-ordinated combination of function and structure (Fig. 4/3). The adaptation model shown is centrally valid for endurance-oriented training and not applicable to all sports (NEUMANN/BERBALK, 1991). The disregard of the time aspect of adaptation is one of the most common faults in training practice. Adaptation takes place in fixed time periods and cannot be accelerated by any methodical tricks. The development of maximum oxygen uptake from the fitness level to competitive sport level takes at least six months (Fig. 5/3). After that training load should be further increased. The level of adaptation is dependent on total training load.

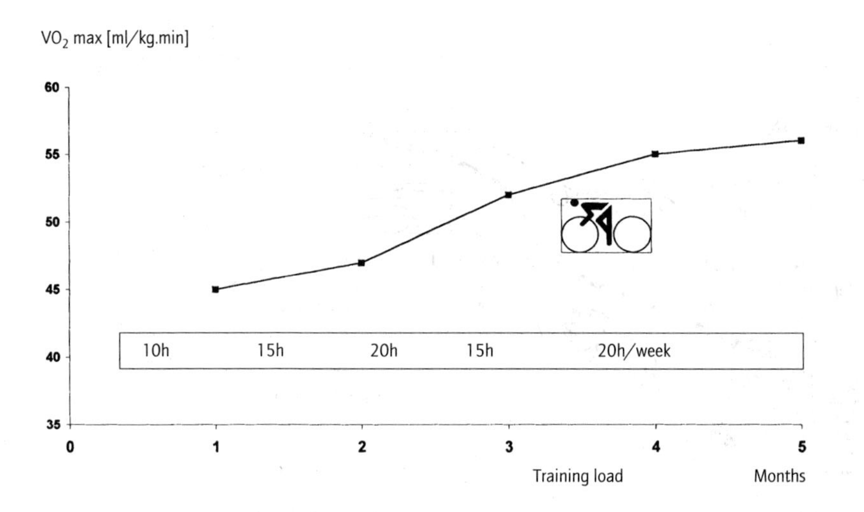

Fig. 5/3: Development of maximum oxygen uptake from fitness level by increasing weekly training load

If a certain stage of adaptation has been reached after about six weeks, then the load must be further increased either in total or in certain aspects. New stimuli are necessary for a higher level of adaptation to develop or to maintain an individually high level reached. The higher the adaptive state reached, the more quickly the athlete runs the risk of losing performance capacity if the loading stimuli are no longer applied. The build-up of aerobic performance foundations takes considerably longer than their reduction when loading stimuli are stopped or reduced.

Summary

If the current functional state of the body is to be changed in a stable manner, regular loading stimuli must be applied over a period of four to six weeks. Adaptation to training stimuli takes place in stages. After about ten days the motor regulatory programmes adjust themselves to effectively handle load.

The continuation of training load results in an increase in the size of the energy stores and thus in the length of time the body can handle demands placed on it. The content of training decides which stores increase most. Different types of loads are required for enlarging the stores of creatine phosphate, glycogen or triglycerides. Because the muscles cannot deal with demands of load autoregulatively on their own, they need support from other systems (central nervous system, hormones). Between the third and fourth week of loading the organism is in a delicate state which can be handled by reducing load (3:1 load-unloading rhythm). In the restructuring of performance the complex co-ordination of centrally regulating and comprehensive systems with the sport-specific movement programme takes about 30 to 40 days. If after reaching a certain stage of adaptation load is again increased, the organism processes the stimuli to an optimal level. In performance training there must be an ability to handle load over several years. Removal or reduction of load stimuli leads to a reduction in fitness within a short time which happens much more quickly than the build-up of performance through training.

4 Adaptation in Functional Systems

4.1 Heart and Training Load

Endurance load places great demands on the cardiovascular system. The increase in heart activity serves the increase in the output of the heart, i.e. during endurance load the heart volume per minute increases in relation to energetic requirements in order to ensure oxygen transport to the working muscles. During load the rise in the heart rate (HR) and the stroke volume lead to an increase in output. The HR is a practical measuring indicator for assessing cardiac demands during endurance training. The demands placed on the cardiovascular system vary depending on the performance structure of the particular endurance sports (see chapter 7).

Regular endurance training leads to morphological and functional adaptations of the heart, collectively known as **athlete's heart** (REINDELL et al., 1967; ROST, 1990).

The extent of adaptation depends on age, sex, amount of load, intensity of training and years of training experience. The adaptation of the athlete's heart is, however, also determined by individual factors.

The athlete's heart displays a physiological enlargement of the ventricles and the vestibules while at the same time the walls of the heart get thicker. In contrast to morbid enlargement of the heart, e.g. after a heart attack, in the case of valvular heart defects or forms of morbid myocardial hypertrophy, athlete's heart adaptation is characterised by a harmonious increase in the volume of the ventricles and hypertrophy of the heart muscle.

In order to monitor the development of athlete's heart, competitive athletes regularly undergo echo-cardiographic examinations as part of health diagnostics and as evidence of the adaptations caused by training. Sport cardiological diagnostics is an obligatory component of sports medicine examinations for squad athletes in endurance sports. As no sports medicine suitability examination is required of fitness athletes, medical observation is dependent on the commitment of the individual athlete. A survey amongst participants in the Roth Ironman indicated that less than half of the athletes regularly undergo a sports medical examination.

Adaptation of the Heart Function

As a result of endurance training a heart adapted to performance is developed. As the size of the endurance athlete's heart increases, an economising of the heart function takes place. In a resting state this adaptation is expressed in an increase in the stroke volume with a simultaneous decrease in the HR, the output of the heart is not much different from that of an untrained person. At low intensities of load the endurance-trained person has more effective circulatory regulation with a lower heart rate and greater stroke volume regulation.

Endurance athletes thus handle submaximal load with lower cardiac demand, i.e. with lower oxygen consumption of the heart muscle.

Cardiac economisation is a significant mechanism in the adaptation of functional systems relevant to performance. The extent of adaptation of the heart function can be seen from a longitudinal examination of the HR of a successful cyclist (Fig. 1/4.1).

In addition to optimisation of the functions, in endurance athletes the maximum output of the athlete's heart increases. The increase in the heart volume per minute results from the higher stroke volume of the enlarged athlete's heart, whereby the output of top athletes

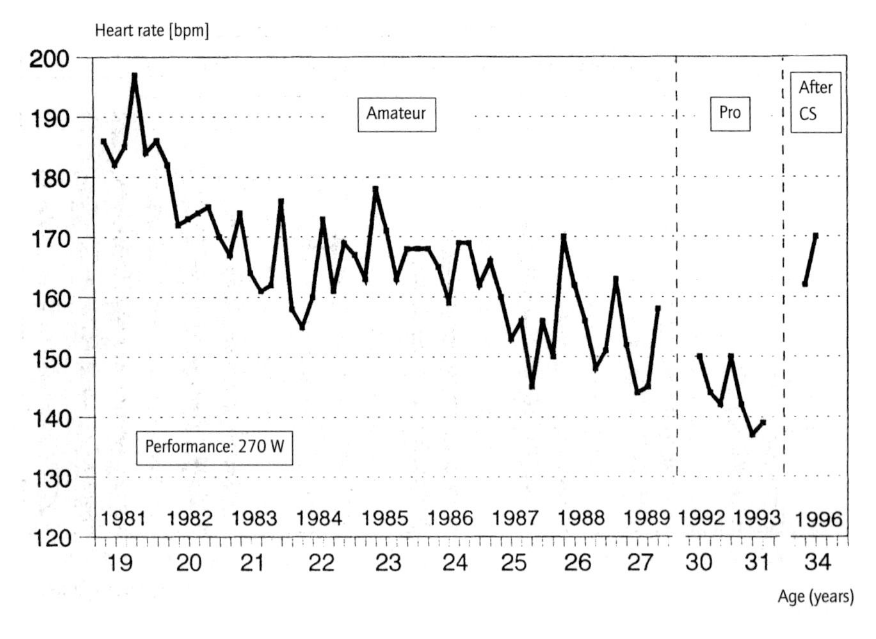

Fig. 1/4.1: Economisation of the heart rate (HR) of a successful cyclist in a longitudinal section over 15 years. At a constant ergometer performance the HR decreases by 60 bpm in this period. After discontinuing competitive sport the HR rises again.

can reach up to 40 l/min, i.e. nearly twice as much as untrained persons. The increase in cardiac output is a major factor in increasing the cardiovascular system's oxygen transporting capacity. The aim of cardiovascular training is on the one hand functional optimisation with reduced oxygen consumption of the heart muscle and on the other hand increased oxygen transport capacity. This results in economisation and functional maximisation of the heart's work.

Adaptation of the Athlete's Heart

In principle adaptation of the heart can be ascertained in all age-groups, from children to adults, if they train several times a week in an endurance-sport for a period of at least six months. An increase in heart size (heart volume) and maximum oxygen uptake was recorded in 8- to 10-year-old children after regular swimming training (ROST et al., 1985). In the children's basic training already adaptations take place in the organs and functional systems used (see

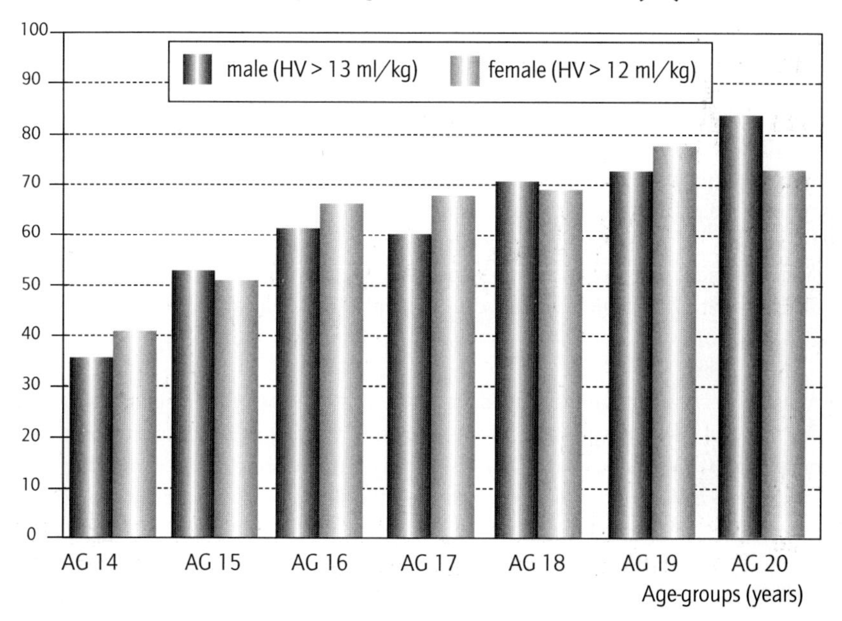

Fig. 2/4.1: Frequency of development of athlete's heart in 14- to 20-year-old endurance athletes of both sexes. For male athletes a lower limit of 13 ml/kg and for females of 12 ml/kg was assumed.

chapter 8). The training stages of build-up training and follow-up training which follow basic training display an especially marked influence on the young body. At this developmental age organ changes determined by growth and morphological and functional adaptations caused by training overlap. The hearts of endurance athletes increase in size. An athlete's heart has developed when male athletes have a heart volume of 13 ml/kg and females have a volume of 12 ml/kg body mass. At the age of 14 to 15 an athlete's heart can be found in about 50 % of athletes after build-up training already, and after follow-up training, 70 to 80 % of the 18- to 19-year-old athletes demonstrate athlete's heart adaptation (Fig. 2/4.1, see p. 47). 60 % of the young athletes' increase in heart size results from endurance training and 40 % from normal growth development (BERBALK, 1997). Despite a considerable increase in heart size in young athletes no indications of overloading of the cardiovascular system have been found in this age-group.

After completion of youth training, the heart can continue to adapt by means of increasing load over a number of years (Fig. 3/4.1, see p. 49). Top male athletes reach a relative heart volume of 17 to 19 ml/kg and top females of 15 to 17 ml/kg body mass. The largest athlete's heart we have found in a man was 19 ml/kg in a cyclist and the largest in a woman was 18.2 ml/kg in a long-distance runner (Table 1/4.1, see p. 49). Similarly large hearts in male and female athletes have already been described by REINDELL et al. (1967) and MEDVED et al. (1975). Despite considerable development in endurance performances in the last 20 to 30 years the upper levels of adaptation of athlete's hearts have not changed significantly. The conclusion is that athlete's heart adaptation has physiological limits which presumably have to do with the securing of sufficient blood circulation and the necessary oxygen supply to the heart muscle. The development of an athlete's heart can be divided into four areas of adaptation (Table 2/4.1, p. 50).

Athlete's heart adaptation is dependent on the total volume of training, intensity of load and years of training experience. If the volume of training is less than six hours weekly, morphological adaptation of the heart is unlikely. With ten to fifteen training hours weekly, competitive athletes achieve a small degree of athlete's heart adaptation. Owing to the large volumes of training they undertake, triathletes and cyclists have the largest athlete's hearts (DOUGLAS, 1989; REGUERO et al., 1995). To reach heart sizes of 17 to 18 ml/kg body mass, many years of intensive training with volumes of 25 to 35 training hours per week are necessary.

In all age and performance areas, female athletes show a lesser degree of athlete's heart. Heart volume and weight are considerably below the corresponding values for male athletes (Table

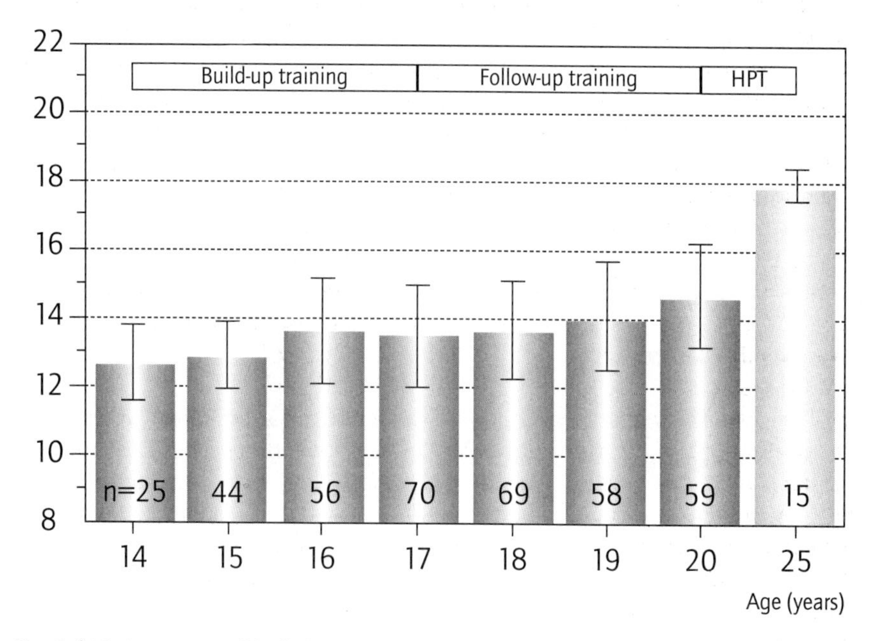

Fig. 3/4.1: Long-term athlete's heart adaptation from youth to top athletes (HPT = high performance training)

Sport	Heart volume (ml)		Heart volume (ml/kg)	
	Male	Female	Male	Female
Triathlon	1416	1010	18.5	16.4
Cycling	1436	960	19.0	15.4
Running	1321	941	18.7	18.2
Swimming	1405	1164	16.9	16.1

Table 1/4.1: Overview of the largest athlete's hearts amongst a surveyed athlete population (1500 endurance athletes)

Adaptation areas	Relative heart size (ml/kg)		
	Male athletes	Female athletes	Training volume (hours/week)
Low degree of athlete's heart adaptation	13-14	12 - 13	10 - 15
Medium degree of athlete's heart adaptation	15 - 16	14 - 15	15 - 25
Large degree of athlete's heart adaptation	17 - 18	16 - 17	25 - 35
Border area of athlete's heart adaptation	19 - 20	18 - 19	25 - 45

Table 2/4.1: Adaptation areas of athlete's heart (BERBALK, 1997)

3/4.1, see p. 51 and 4/4.1, see p. 52). Analogous to the markedness of the skeletal muscular system these findings clearly show a low morphological adaptation potential of the hearts of training women. This is mainly a result of hormonal, genetic and social factors.

In principle a healthy heart cannot be overloaded or pathologically damaged by intensive training. Tests with well-trained triathletes who already displayed major athlete's heart adaptation showed an increase in heart size of 10 to 15 % with simultaneous optimisation of the heart function after a further increase in load over a period of three months with 35 to 45 h/week. If the total volume of load is reduced or if the athlete has to take a break of several weeks because of injury, heart volume goes down again. Within a training year load-conditioned dynamics of regulative heart size adaptation can be shown.

The size of the athlete's heart is in direct relationship to the development of endurance performance capacity. In triathletes a close connection was found between relative heart volume and competitive performance in short triathlons (Fig. 4/4.1, see p. 53) as well as with performance diagnostical functional factors of cycle and treadmill ergometry.

The heart volume determined using echo-cardiography is a reliable parameter in performance diagnostics for endurance sports.

In the case of extreme athlete's heart adaptation, partial dimensions of the heart determined by echo-cardiography, such as heart wall thickness, the diameter of the ventricles and vestibules and heart muscle mass, can be well over the usual standard values found in clinical medicine (Table 5/4.1, see p. 53). The decisive criterion for physiological development of the heart is a harmonious forming of the heart muscle mass in relation to total heart volume.

Age-group	Absolute heart volume (ml)*		Absolute heart weight (g)*	
n = (male/female)	Male athlete	Female	Male athlete	Female
AG 14 (25/32)	793 ± 95	669 ± 104	332 ± 39	261 ± 41
AG 15 (44/32)	867 ± 112	728 ± 110	358 ± 47	296 ± 52
AG 16 (56/44)	943 ± 117	731 ± 90	393 ± 55	292 ± 45
AG 17 (70/39)	952 ± 126	745 ± 93	400 ± 59	302 ± 46
AG 18 (69/29)	997 ± 133	767 ± 137	421± 60	307 ± 64
AG 19 (58/30)	1028 ± 155	776 ± 116	431 ± 71	312 ± 57
AG 20 (59/25)	1075 ± 125	784 ± 122	442 ± 60	325 ± 61
Top athletes (15/15)	1224 ± 98	875 ± 67	533 ± 49	355 ± 35

**Determination method according to DICKHUTH et al., 1990*

Tab. 3/4.1: Absolute heart volume and weight in youth and top athletes (BERBALK, 1996)

Continuing training or competition participation when suffering infections is a health risk in competitive sport. One of the possible consequences is inflammation of the heart muscle because of impairment to the immune system. In its early stages this is difficult to diagnose. In the long-term, heart muscle inflammation can lead to serious health problems, especially if it is not recognised.

When training for competitive sport is ceased, it should be systematically reduced according to a plan running over at least six months. If "de-training" is not done, vegetatively caused disturbances of the heart function can occur and impair general well-being (unloading syndrome). If heart sensations or inexplicable problems occur after a sudden, long lasting training stop, an improvement can quickly be achieved through running load. After a training break of six to eight weeks the heart volume can already go down by 100 to 150 ml. If regular sporting activity is carried on after competitive training a slight heart size increase of 12 to 13 ml/kg body mass remains.

Age-group	Relative heart volume (ml)*		Relative heart weight (g)*	
n = (male/female)	Male athlete	Female	Male athlete	Female
AG 14 (25/32)	12.7 ± 1.1	11.9 ± 1.3	5.38 ± 0.61	4.68 ± 0.62
AG 15 (44/32)	12.9 ± 1.0	12.3 ± 1.0	5.25 ± 0.55	4.97 ± 0.55
AG 16 (56/44)	13.7 ± 1.6	12.4 ± 1.0	5.72 ± 0.80	4.97 ± 0.52
AG 17 (70/39)	13.5 ± 1.5	12,6 ± 1,2	5.65 ± 0.71	5.10 ± 0.57
AG 18 (69/29)	13.7 ± 1.5	12.6 ± 1.3	5.79 ± 0.74	5.04 ± 0.66
AG 19 (58/30)	14.0 ± 1.6	13.1 ± 1.4	5.86 ± 0.84	5.24± 0.68
AG 20 (59/25)	14.7 ± 1.6	13.0 ± 1.4	6.06 ± 0.77	5.38± 0.77
Top Athletes (15/15)	17.9 ± 0.5	15.3 ± 0.5	7.79 ± 0.50	6.22 ± 0.41

** Determination method according to DICKHUTH et al., 1990*

Table 4/4.1: Relative heart volume and weight in youth and top athletes (BERBALK, 1996)

Resting Heart Rate and Heart Rate Variability

The heart rate is a central measurement factor for assessing the cardiovascular function at rest and under load. At rest the HR of endurance-trained persons goes down. Depending on the volume of training, the resting HR goes down to values between 40 and 60 bpm, with about 10 % of top athletes HR values of even under 40 bpm are reached. The lowest HR in a resting ECG we found was of a runner with 25 bpm and a female triathlete with 30 bpm. The extremely low heart rates are not pathological findings, they are usually related to training.

The HR during body rest is a very sensitive indicator for changes in the activity of the vegetative nervous system. Endurance training leads to adjustments and adaptations in the vegetative state. The activity of the parasympathetic nervous system increases (increased vagotonia) and causes a decrease in frequency at the sinus node, the pacemaker of the heart. In addition to the vegetative nervous system the HR is influenced by a number of other cardiac, central and peripheral factors.

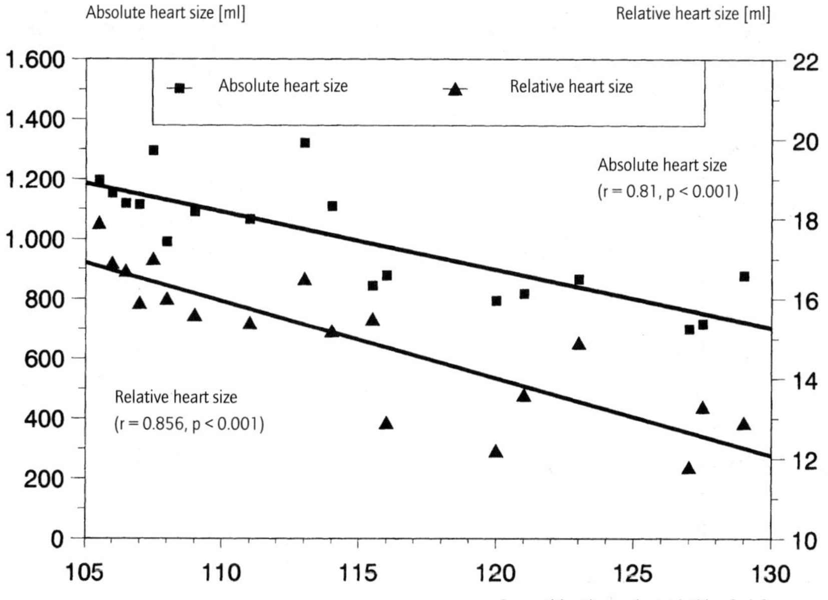

Fig. 4/4.1: Relationship of absolute and relative heart size to competition time in short triathlon

Echo-cardiographic parameter	Male endurance athlete	Female endurance athlete
Heart wall thickness (mm)	14	11
Left ventricle (mm)	65	58
Right ventricle (mm)	35	28
Left vestibule (mm)	48	44
Aorta diameter (mm)	40	35
Absolute heart volume (ml)	1450	1150
Relative heart volume (ml/kg)	20	18
LVMM (g)	300	200
LVMM (g/kg)	4.2	3.5

Table 5/4.1: Extreme values or echocardiographic findings regarding athlete's heart (LVMM = left ventricular muscle mass)

Endurance athletes should regularly measure their resting HR in the morning in order to recognise early any changes in the heart function. Measuring the resting HR has special significance for monitoring load tolerance and one's state of health. If regeneration is insufficient after great training and competition load, the resting HR can be up by more than five bpm. Furthermore, the HR is a sensitive indicator when there are health disturbances. If the HR is up by more than ten beats when there is an infection, training should be interrupted or only done in the compensation field and a doctor should be seen.

In addition to the HR, the rhythm of the heart beats can be used to assess the heart function. Fluctuations in the frequency of heart beats in sequence are a normal physiological phenomenon of heart activity. This variability of the heart rate is influenced by the vegetative nervous system. When there is high activity of the parasympathicotonia, heart rate variability (HRV) increases, i.e. the sequence of heartbeats becomes less rhythmic. When the sympathetic

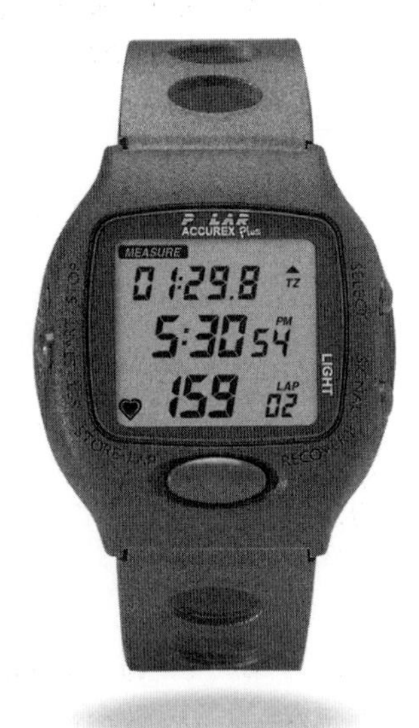

Polar Accurex Plus

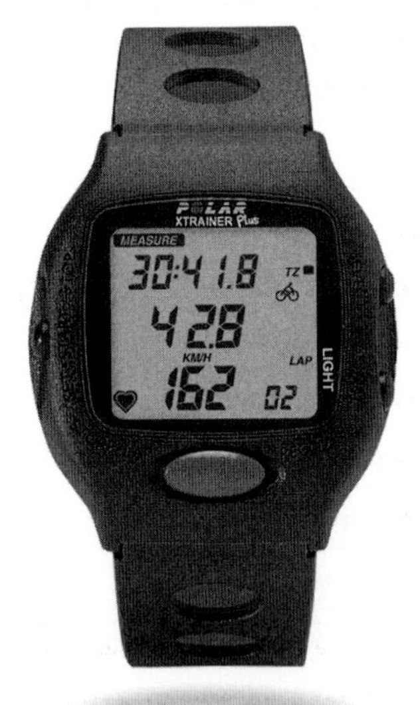

Polar XTrainer Plus

Fig. 5/4.1: Display of the POLAR watch with instant information on heart rate (HR) and heart rate variability (HRV)

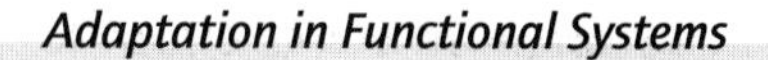

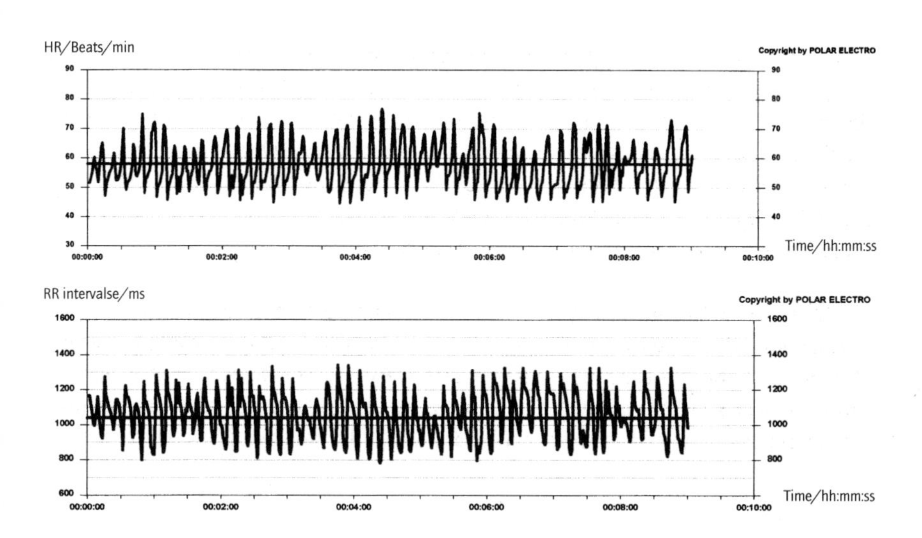

Fig. 6/4.1: Heart rate (HR) upper curve and heart time intervals (RR intervals) lower curve of an endurance athlete. The curves show clearly the fluctuations in the HR when this is measured from beat to beat.

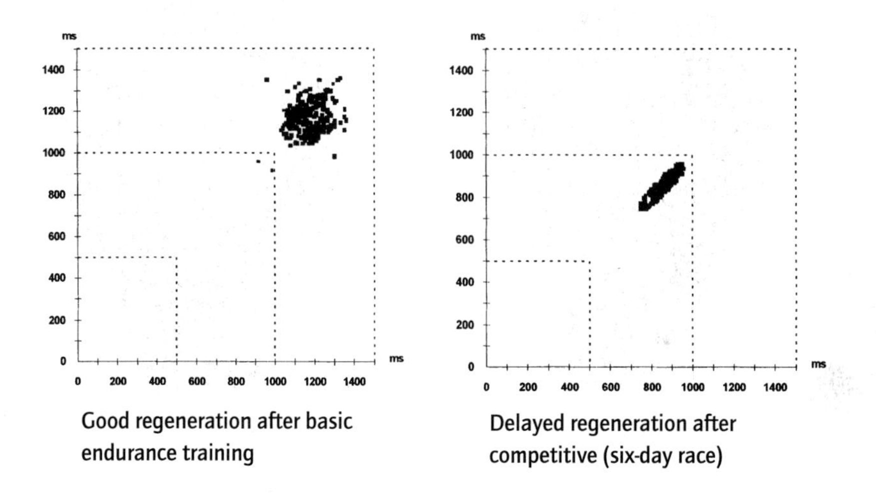

Fig. 7/4.1: Scatter diagram of the heart time intervals (RR intervals) of a cyclist after varying exertion the day before the examination. Left, normal heart rate variability (HRV). Right, reduced HRV after high psychophysical competitive exertion.

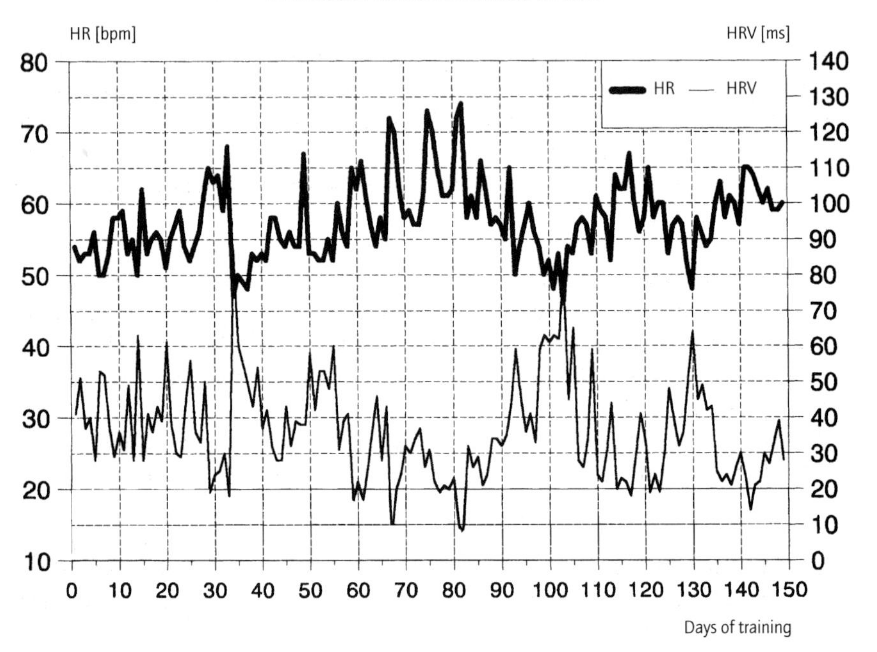

Fig. 8/4.1: Dynamics of resting heart rate (HR) and heart rate variability (HRV) of a successful cyclist over 150 training days. After high training and competitive loads the HRV falls considerably, with simultaneously increasing HR. During several six-day races the borderline area was crossed. (e.g. 65th - 85th day). This regulation is an expression of maximum psychophysical summation of load, during the whole period of research no state of overtraining occurred.

influences predominate, HRV goes down, i.e. the heart beat sequence becomes "rigidly frequent" and no longer shows any rhythmical fluctuations. At rest, because of the high parasympathicotonia, athletes display a marked HRV which increases further with reduction of the heart rate in general.

Thanks to new technological developments in heart rate monitors (VANTAGE NV from manufacturer POLAR), heart rate variability can be determined simply. The HRV appears as immediate information on the display of the POLAR watch. Here the HRV represents the current fluctuation of the heart rate as a time value in ms and takes every single heart beat into consideration in determining the value (Fig. 5/4.1, see p. 54).

The heart rate monitors have automatic storage functions for a total of 4000 heart beats. Using the analysing software the heart rate variability can be quantitatively recorded from these stored heart actions. Fig. 6/4.1 (see p. 55) shows the curve progression of the HR and the heart time intervals (RR intervals) of an endurance athlete. These curves illustrate marked time fluctuations of the heart rate sequence under resting conditions. The variability of the heart rate can also be depicted as a HR scatter diagram. Here all heart rate time intervals (RR intervals) are entered in the co-ordinate system as pairs. The size of the ellipse characterises the extent of the heart rate variability (Fig. 7/4.1, see p. 55).

By regularly monitoring the resting HR and the HRV, changes in the athlete's vegetative state can be registered and the physical demands in the training process observed. From the reading a clear dynamic can be recognised. Every athlete has an individual regulation area of heart rate variability. After high training load a decrease in the HRV can point to insufficient regeneration (Fig. 8/4.1, see p. 56). If the HRV shows considerably reduced values several days in a row, combined with a decrease in performance capacity and reduced willingness to perform, then the beginnings of a state of overtraining should be stopped and corrections to training load made.

After high psychophysical demand there are brief changes in the HRV which require no training methodological measures. A constant increase in HRV points to positive processing of load and adaptation of the vegetative state.

Summary

The athlete's heart is a heart adapted to performance with a high maximum output together with simultaneous optimisation of the heart function at rest and during submaximal demands through load. The extent of morphological and functional adaptation depends to a large degree on the total amount of training. Top male athletes reach an athlete's heart of 17 to 19 ml/kg and females of 15 to 17 ml/kg body mass. Heart volume stands in direct relationship to competition-specific endurance performance capacity and is a meaningful performance control factor. A decrease in the resting heart rate (HR) to 40 bpm and lower is an expression of functional adaptation in connection with a high vagotonia. Regular checking of the resting HR should be used increasingly by endurance athletes for load tolerance diagnostics in the framework of training regulation. Through the determination of heart rate variability with a heart rate monitor a new diagnostic option for the assessment of the vegetative state of athletes has become available. In this connection the decrease in heart rate variability can be an indicator for insufficient regeneration or for the beginning of overtraining.

4.2 Breathing and Training Load

Breathing ensures that the body gets the oxygen it needs when it needs it. This takes place in the form of external and internal breathing. Breathing involves subsystems for the intake, transport and processing of oxygen. These include:

- The intake of oxygen with air breathed in
- The exchange of gases in the lungs
- The binding of oxygen to the erythrocytes
- The transport of oxygen with the blood and
- The delivery and energetic using of oxygen in the tissue.

The proportion of oxygen uptake and oxygen transport as a percentage of the total system is estimated at about 50 % (HOLLOSZY, 1975).

The performance capacity of the total oxygen transport chain is, finally, the criterion for assessing the efficiency of the breathing system of endurance athletes. The breathing system and the cardiovascular system are closely linked. This is expressed in the complex term cardiopulmonary system.

Breathing in (respiration) is an active process in which the rib muscles (chest breathing) and the diaphragm (abdominal breathing) are mainly involved. Breathing out happens passively. The volume ventilated in one breath is the breath volume (BV) and is about 500 ml at rest. The BV only partially serves the exchange of gases in the lungs. The proportion of air remaining in the upper respiratory tracts, the windpipe and the bronchial tubes is called dead space. In the dead space the air is moistened, warmed and cleaned. When breathing through the nose these mechanisms are particularly effective. At low loads one should therefore breathe through the nose for as long as possible.

With increasing intensity of load, breathing is experienced as an impediment because the flow resistance for the air breathed is two to three times higher in comparison to breathing through the mouth. Under high load voluntary control over breathing is lost and inspiration takes place exclusively through the mouth.

Under intensive brief load the oxygen requirements of the breathing muscles can make up 10 to 15 % of maximum oxygen uptake. Endurance training strengthens the breathing muscles and also increases the aerobic metabolism potential of the breathing muscles. The breathing system of endurance-trained athletes demonstrates an increase in functioning along with performance. The reserves of gas exchange in the lungs are generally so high that breathing is not a performance limiting factor for endurance athletes.

Endurance athletes	Vital capacity		One second capacity	
	VC (l)	% Target	FEV 1 (l)	% Target
Male triathletes (n = 26)	6.05 ± 0.92	114	4.87 ± 0.54	110
Female triathletes (n = 16)	4.74 ± 0.45	116	3.78 ± 0.53	108
Male swimmers (n = 58)	6.70 ± 1.04	113	5.39 ± 0.88	111
Female swimmers (n = 72)	4.73 ± 0.79	112	4.62 ± 0.64	112

Table 1/4.2: Lung function values of male and female endurance athletes

Spirometry

Spirometry registers static and dynamic lung function values. In comparison to untrained persons, athletes have higher lung function measurements. Fit endurance athletes' vital capacity (VC) is 10 to 15 % above the norm (Table 1/4.2, see above). In swimming the maximum VC-reading is up to nine litres. The VC is very much influenced by constitutional factors, so that no certain conclusions about endurance performance capacity are possible. The dynamic lung function parameters of endurance athletes reflect the higher flowing speeds in the respiratory tracts. The maximum amount of air breathed out per second (one second capacity or FEV 1) and the maximum speed of expiration (PEF) are higher in endurance athletes.

Spirometry shows a higher lung capacity or functional dynamics in most athletes. It also makes it possible to eliminate ventilation disruptions. Even in competitive sport, ventilation disruptions (narrowing of the respiratory tracts) triggered by training load are not uncommon. When using therapeutical medications that expand the bronchial tubes of athletes, doping regulations must be taken into consideration (see chapter 14.2).

Spiroergometry

Spiroergometry is used to determine the lung function parameters during sport-specific load.

- ***Breath Volume per Minute***

The breath volume per minute (BVM) is the decisive functional value for oxygen uptake. BVM is the product of the breathing rate (BR) and breath volume (BV). At rest the BVM is 8 to 12 l/min. The BVM of untrained persons rises to about 100 l/min under maximum performance demands. Endurance athletes reach average values of 150 to 200 l/min. Top cyclists have had maximum BVM of 250 l/min measured. The rise in BVM is a result of increased BV and BR. Depth of breathing and breathing rate have a major influence on breathing. When the BVM remains constant, more frequent breathing is less economical; the breathing muscles consume more oxygen. Endurance-trained athletes have greater breathing economy than untrained persons, i.e. where the BVM is the same, BV is higher and BR is lower. Under submaximal load breathing can be influenced subjectively.

By consciously regulating breathing depth and breathing rate, more economical breathing can be trained. The economisation of breathing found in endurance athletes reflects the adaptations of the breathing muscles and the vegetative nervous system. The working muscles placed under load by a particular sport benefit from the reduced oxygen consumption of the breathing muscles of the person training. The effectiveness of muscle work increases.

- ***Respiratory equivalent***

The relationship between breathing volume per minute and oxygen uptake can change under load within certain limits. This relationship between BVM and O_2 intake is called the Respiratory equivalent (RE). The RE shows how many litres of breathed air are necessary for the intake of one litre of oxygen. The smaller the RE, the more effective breathing is with regard to oxygen uptake. Under similar load, athletes have a lower respiratory equivalent than untrained persons. Because of the non-linear dynamics of the BVM under increasing intensity of load, the RE can be used to determine the anaerobic threshold (see chapters 4.4 and 10.5).

- ***Respiratory Quotient***

In spiroergometric tests, in addition to O_2 intake, CO_2 expulsion is also constantly measured. Using CO_2 expulsion and O_2 intake, the respiratory quotient (RQ) is calculated. The RQ is used as a criterion for assessing whether more load can be handled ($RQ > 1$). A rise above 1 explains compensation mechanisms of the acid-alkali balance (see chapter 4.1). At constant intensity of load the RQ can be used to estimate the share of carbohydrate and fat metabolism in energy provision (see chapter 4.5).

Breathing and Movement Structure

In a number of sports the coupling of breathing rhythm and sport-specific movement plays an important role. A swimmer must sensibly co-ordinate his breathing rhythm with the rate of movement. The correct breathing rhythm also influences performance in rowing and canoeing. In these sports the thorax muscles are simultaneously part of the muscle system involved in movement and an influencing factor of breathing. In rowing a close coupling between rowing movement and breathing cycles has been found. As a result of high resistance in the respiratory tract, a high rate of breathing regulation with breathing rates of 70 to 100/min reduces the inspiratory flow (STEINACKER et al., 1994). Only in extreme situations can the breathing system have a limiting effect on endurance performance capacity.

Summary

In athletes the breathing system undergoes complex adaptations as a result of training. Endurance training strengthens the breathing muscles and raises ventilatory capacity as a major prerequisite for increasing maximum oxygen uptake. Through training, maximum breathing volume per minute (BVM) can be doubled. Endurance training improves breathing economy. Trained athletes breathe more deeply and less frequently than untrained persons and thus use oxygen more economically. Normally the breathing system does not limit endurance performance capacity. A high rate of breathing (hyperventilation) raises the oxygen requirements of the breathing muscles and thus also the energy requirements. Only deep, infrequent breathing is economical. If breathing goes above 70 % of maximum possible BVM it can no longer be influenced subjectively.

4.3 Blood and Training Load

Through the system of blood vessels the blood reaches all areas of the body and because of its composition and constant circulation it links the system of organs to make a functional unit.

The main tasks of the blood are its transport, buffer and defence functions (Fig. 1/4.3, see p. 62).

Components of the Blood and Haematological Parameters

Blood consists of two main components, the blood liquid (plasma) and corpuscular parts, consisting in turn of erythrocytes, leucocytes and thrombocytes. The relationship between the corpuscular and the liquid proportions is on average 45 %, i.e. there is more blood plasma. Plasma separated from the coagulation protein fibrinogen is called serum.

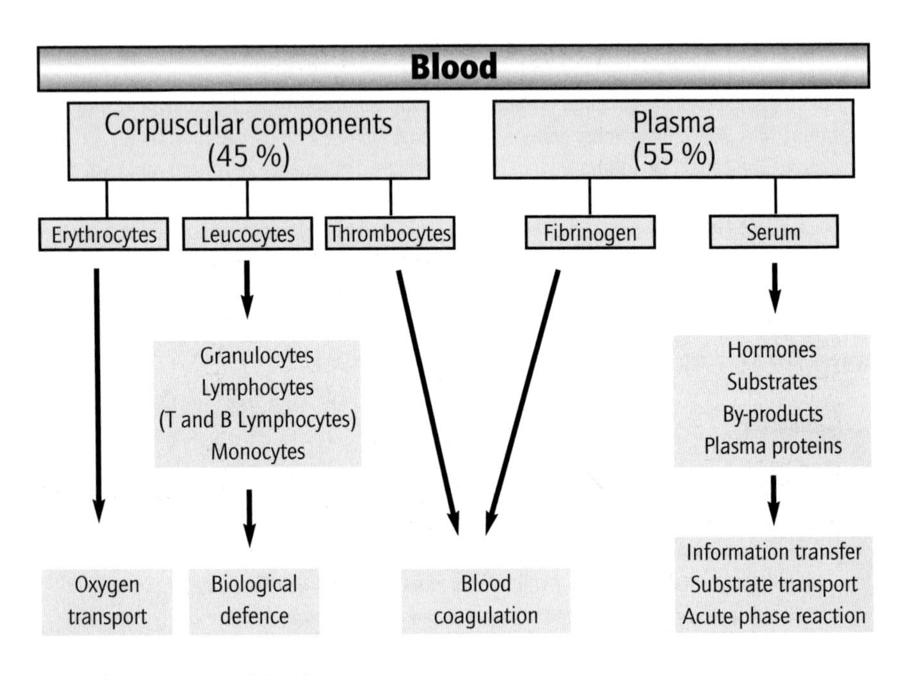

Fig. 1/4.3: Functions of the blood

In order to understand the flowing properties from a physical point of view, the components and contents of the blood and their soluble behaviour must be observed. In blood plasma, salts and low molecular substances (glucose, free fatty acids, creatine, urea among others) are dissolved. There are high and low molecular proteins (globulins and albumins) in the form of a colloidal solution which serve the maintenance of colloidal osmotic pressure in the blood. The osmotic effect, in particular of the lower molecular proteins, prevents the exit of water from the blood into the tissue when flowing through the capillary system. Drops of fat in the blood after a meal also give the blood the property of an emulsion. Because of its composition, in particular through the proportion of blood corpuscles and proteins, the viscosity of blood is four to five times higher than that of water.

Haematocrit

The flowing property of blood (viscosity) is expressed in the haemocrit (HC). The HC is the relationship between the solid and fluid elements of the blood. The average HC of men is 45 % (40 to 52 %). Women's HC is somewhat lower at 41 % (37 to 47 %). The corpuscular and fluid proportions of the blood can be changed as a result of water loss or endurance load.

Effect of Training on the Blood

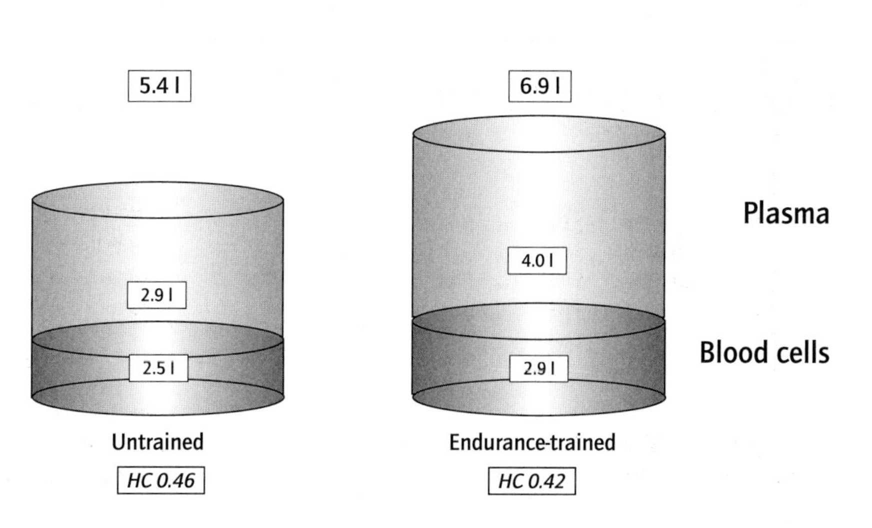

Fig. 2/4.3: Effect of training on solid and fluid blood components

The flowing properties of the blood are influenced. Endurance athletes often have reduced haematocrit values, their blood is thinner. Especially after extensive endurance load the HC goes down in the sense of a dilution of the blood (haemodilution). Lower HC values are favourable to capillary gas exchange and provision of oxygen to the muscles. As a result of sporting load, however, sweat loss and insufficient fluid intake can also cause the HC concentration to rise. In a state of dehydration, HC values of over 50 % are reached. Above an HC of 53 % unfavourable influencing of maximum heart volume per minute and a reduction in oxygen transporting capacity must be reckoned with as a result of increased viscosity (THOMSON et al., 1982; SPRIET et al., 1986). If the HC goes up further, health risks cannot be discounted (danger of embolism).

Erythrocytes and Blood Volume

The blood contains approx. five million erythrocytes per μ/l. The most important component for oxygen transportation is the haemoglobin (Hb), the red blood colouring. Through a reversible coupling with iron the Hb allows rapid O_2 intake in the lungs and CO_2 expulsion in the tissue.

Laboratory chemical parameters/norm	Male endurance athletes (n = 120)	Female endurance athletes (n = 103)
Erythrocytes m: 4.5 - 6.0 mill/ µl w: 4.0 - 5.5 mill/µl	5.21 ± 0.46	4.61 ± 0.39
Haemoglobin m: 14 - 18 g/dl f: 12 - 16 g/dl	16.1 ± 1.4	13.8 ± 1.3
Haematocrit m: 40 - 52% f: 37 - 47%	0.47 ± 0.04	0.42 ± 0.04
MCV m/f: 83 - 93 fl	88.6 ± 3.0	89.1 ± 4.3
MCH m/f: 1.55 - 1.90 fmol	1.81 ± 0.10	1.82 ± 0.08
MCHC m/f: 20 - 22 mmol/l	21.1 ± 1.3	20.5 ± 1.2
Iron m: 14.3 - 26.9 µmol/l f: 10.7 - 25.1 µmol/l	18.1 ± 7.1	17.5 ± 6.2
Ferritin m: 40 - 440 ng/ml f: 30 - 300 ng/ml (Limit: 15 ng/ml)	66.2 ± 31.2	36.6 ± 22.7

MCV = Median Corpuscular Volume
MCH = Median Corpuscular Haemoglobin
MCHC = Median Corpuscular Haemoglobin Concentration

Table 1/4.3: Haematological parameters and iron values of male and female endurance athletes

Sufficient availability of iron is a prerequisite for the development of sufficient haemoglobin. The average Hb value of men is 15.5 g/dl (14 to 18 g/dl) and of women 13.8 g/dl (12 to 16 d/gl). The total volume depends on body weight and is about 75 to 80 ml/kg. As a result of endurance training the total volume of the blood increases, whereby the proportion of corpuscular and fluid components remains relatively constant or tends to change in favour of the blood plasma (decrease in HC) (Fig. 2/4.3, see p. 63). In this way total haemoglobin increases without major changes in the erythrocyte or Hb concentration in the blood being found.

Checks on the haematological values, including iron metabolism parameters, should be part of athletes' regular sport medical check-ups. Table 1/4.3 (see p. 64) summarises the haematological results of top endurance athletes, including iron values.

Transport Function of the Blood

Through the blood the provision of oxygen and nutrients to the body and at the same time the removal of metabolism by-products and carbon dioxide take place. For endurance athletes the decisive factor here is the oxygen transporting capacity of the blood. For every gram of haemoglobin, 1.34 ml of O_2 can be absorbed. Changes in the Hb in the blood have a considerable influence on oxygen transporting capacity. This physiological background is the basis for unnatural manipulation of the Hb (see chapter 14.2). The mediating function of the blood is supported to a large extent by the effect of hormones circulating in the blood, which ensure a quick combination of the activities of the organs and the functional systems in relationship to current load demands.

At the same time the bloodstream takes heat released by the working muscles to the skin and thus has an important function in removing heat. The blood helps to regulate body temperature. This necessary increased blood flow to the skin as part of heat regulation takes place at the expense of the blood flow to the muscles, so that in extreme exposure to heat in endurance sports performance capacity decreases (see chapter 15.1).

Buffer Function of the Blood

The blood's buffer systems are of great significance for the acidity arising through lactate production during intensive load. The measurement of blood acidity is the concentration of hydrogen ions, the pH. Normally the pH level of the blood is 7.4 and is thus in the slightly alkaline area. Even slight changes in the concentration of hydrogen ions can unfavourably influence metabolism, in particular the effectiveness of enzymes. As a measure of the proportion of non-volatile acids in the blood, in addition to the pH level the base excess

(BEX) is determined. Of all the buffer systems of the blood, the carbonic acid hydrogen carbonate system (bicarbonate buffer) plays the most important role. The buffer properties occur in that the carbon dioxide can escape as CO_2. The body compensates the overacidity of the blood (metabolic acidosis) caused by the rise in lactate first of all through breathing. As a result of harder breathing (hyperventilation) a greater expulsion of CO_2 with exhaled air occurs, the CO_2 partial pressure in the blood goes down, leading to a compensatory balancing of the acidosis and stabilisation of the pH level. In spiroergometric tests the greater increase in CO_2 in exhaled air in comparison to O_2 intake during intensive load is reflected in the increase in the RQ to levels of 1.2 to 1.3. The RQ over 1.0 is an expression of respiratory compensation of metabolic acidosis. In addition to the bicarbonate, Hb, plasma proteins and phosphates are also involved in the buffer effect of the blood. If during intensive performance demands the body is no longer able to regulate the acid-base balance (e.g. at pH levels below 7.2, a BEX of -15 to -20 and $pCO_2 < 30$ Torr), then load is reduced or ended.

Defence Function of the Blood

The blood fulfils an important protective function against pathogenes and foreign bodies. First a cellular defence of the blood is started by the leucocytes. Acute or chronic states of inflammation are coupled with an increase of leucocytes in the blood to more than 10,000 per µl (leucocytosis). The differentiation between the various types of leucocytes (granulocytes, lymphocytes and monocytes) through the so-called differential blood picture provides diagnostical indications of the course of the illness. As further components of the blood the lymphocytes, in particular the T and B lymphocytes, are significant for immunological reactions. Independent of these biological defence functions the white corpuscles react to stress from sporting load. Especially after long periods of endurance load the leucocytes are released from the bone marrow in greater numbers and increase up to more than 25,000 per µl. After marathon runs a reactive leucocytosis of over 15,000 per µl is almost normal. The lymphocytes also show a temporary increase after load (lymphocytosis). In addition to the biological protection provided cellularly there are other defence mechanisms active in the blood, such as special plasma proteins (e.g. acute phase proteins) and immune globulins. Moderate endurance training stimulates the immune system and raises cellular and humoral defence potential. Chronic overuse in training can have an immune depressive effect (see chapter 4.6). By determining the immune globulins the defence function of the blood can be monitored.

Athlete's Anaemia

A decrease in the Hb concentration in the blood reduces the oxygen transporting capacity and endurance performance capacity. In endurance athletes low Hb levels without an obvious cause are often observed. This state has been explained as athlete's anaemia. This athlete's anaemia is based on the dilution of the blood (haemodilution). The HC falls and with it the Hb concentration. The volume of erythrocytes, however, remains unaffected.

Haemodilution is caused hormonally. After strenuous endurance load there is an increase in aldosterone and adiuritin. These two hormones hold back water and sodium in the blood. Their effect lasts for up to two days after load, when the hormone concentration goes down on the third day after load there is a rise in HC and a considerable increase in urination. The regulation in the fluid balance described here has its physiological reason: it protects the body from losing too much water.

Real athlete's anaemia based on a lack of iron in the haemoglobin can greatly influence performance capacity. On average a decrease in haemoglobin of 0.1 % means a reduction of VO_2 max. of 1 %. A reduction of the Hb in an endurance athlete from 15.5 to 14.0 g/dl can lead to a decrease in O_2 intake and to a loss of performance of about 5 % (GLEDHILL, 1993). This fact underlines the necessity for regular laboratory chemical tests for endurance athletes. When assessing the haematological parameters (number of erythrocytes, Hb and haematocrit), however, it must always be considered that one is looking at concentrations and that a possible increase in total blood volume or total haemoglobin cannot be registered using the blood picture. As haemoglobin synthesis depends on sufficient availability of iron, the parameters of iron metabolism (serum iron, ferritin, transferrin and potentially the capacity to absorb serum iron) are also of diagnostic significance.

Using these factors it is possible to register disturbances in the blood picture due to insufficient iron supply. In a sample of highly-trained endurance athletes, reduced haemoglobin levels were found in 3 % of the males and 6 % of the females, while 5 % of the males and 18 % of the females had subnormal ferritin levels (below 15ng/l).

In competitive sport training, increasing tiredness, early drops in performance and disturbances of one's general state should always be cause to think of the iron supply and to have the storing iron ferritin checked. Regular taking of iron supplements should only be done on medical advice. The medicinal compensation of iron deficiency takes several weeks.

Summary

The blood has the function of a link between the organs. Adaptations of the blood to sports training include an increase in blood volume, a tendency for the haematocrit to go down, an increase in the amount of haemoglobin and the buffer capacity as well as an increase in immunological defence potential. Regular checks on haematological levels and iron metabolism serve the indirect monitoring of the oxygen transporting capacity of the blood in competitive sports training and are necessary for ensuring ability to handle load.

4.4 Oxygen Uptake and Training Load

Constant oxygen uptake is vitally necessary for the body.

The obtaining of energy can take place with and without oxygen, i.e. aerobically and anaerobically. The brain cannot function without oxygen and can only stand a lack of oxygen for a very short time. The situation for the muscles is similar. When muscle work begins, the oxygen requirement immediately jumps. To nevertheless maintain muscle work the anaerobic mechanisms for obtaining energy are involved. The muscles gain energy for 10-20 s through creatine phosphate (CP) without developing lactate. At the start of load anaerobic energy production must compensate for not yet fully functioning aerobic energy metabolism. The degree to which anaerobic metabolism is used depends on the intensity of load. Anaerobic energy production is always before aerobic production or takes place together with it if intensive load continues. Maximum oxygen uptake can only be fully utilised with a delay of one or two minutes at the beginning of load. The "oxygen debt" at the beginning of every load is compensated for in sporting practice by "cranking up" aerobic metabolism with various forms of "pre-start warming-up". This is significant before intensive short-time loads.

The greatly increased oxygen requirement at the start of load or when intensity is increased stimulates breathing. Parallel to the increasing oxygen requirement, breathing volume per minute increases.

As long as the athlete can still hold a conversation during load, the supply of oxygen to the muscles is sufficient. If oxygen uptake rises to over 70 % of the individually possible maximum, then breathing work is so great that talking becomes increasingly difficult and finally stops.

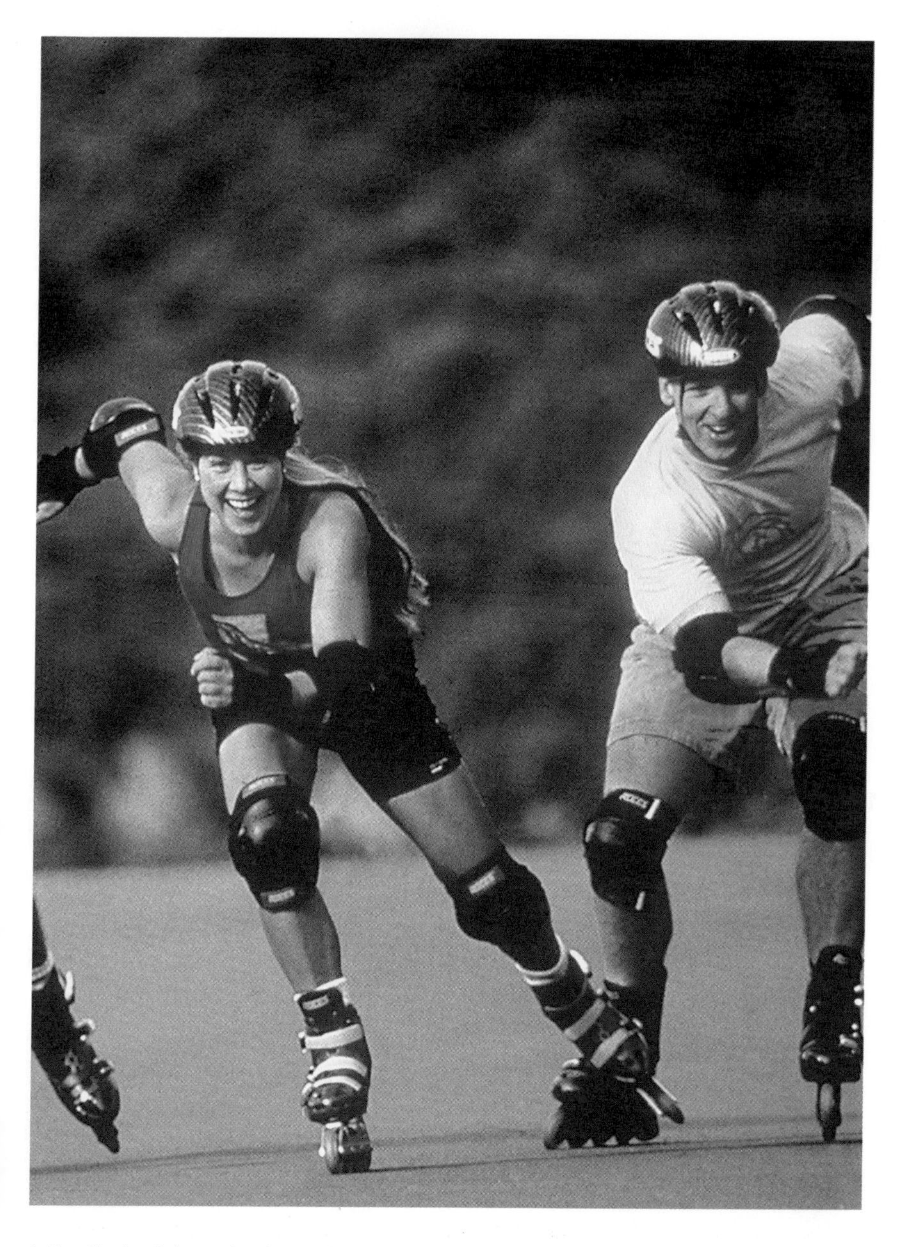

Inline Skating is becoming increasingly popular. (Photo: Raquel Goldmann, Constance)

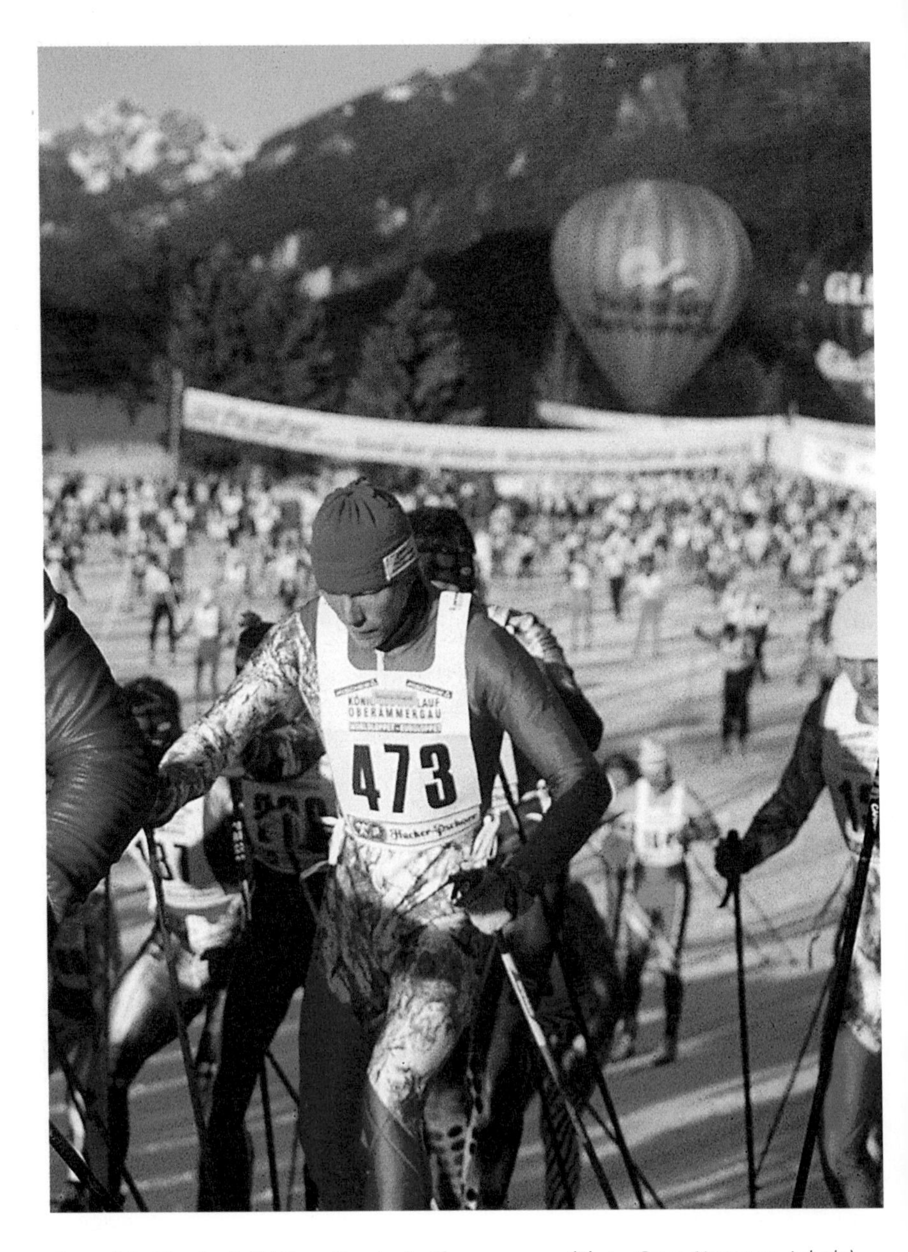

Start of the King Louis Ski Cross-Country in Oberammergau (Photo: Georg Neumann, Leipzig)

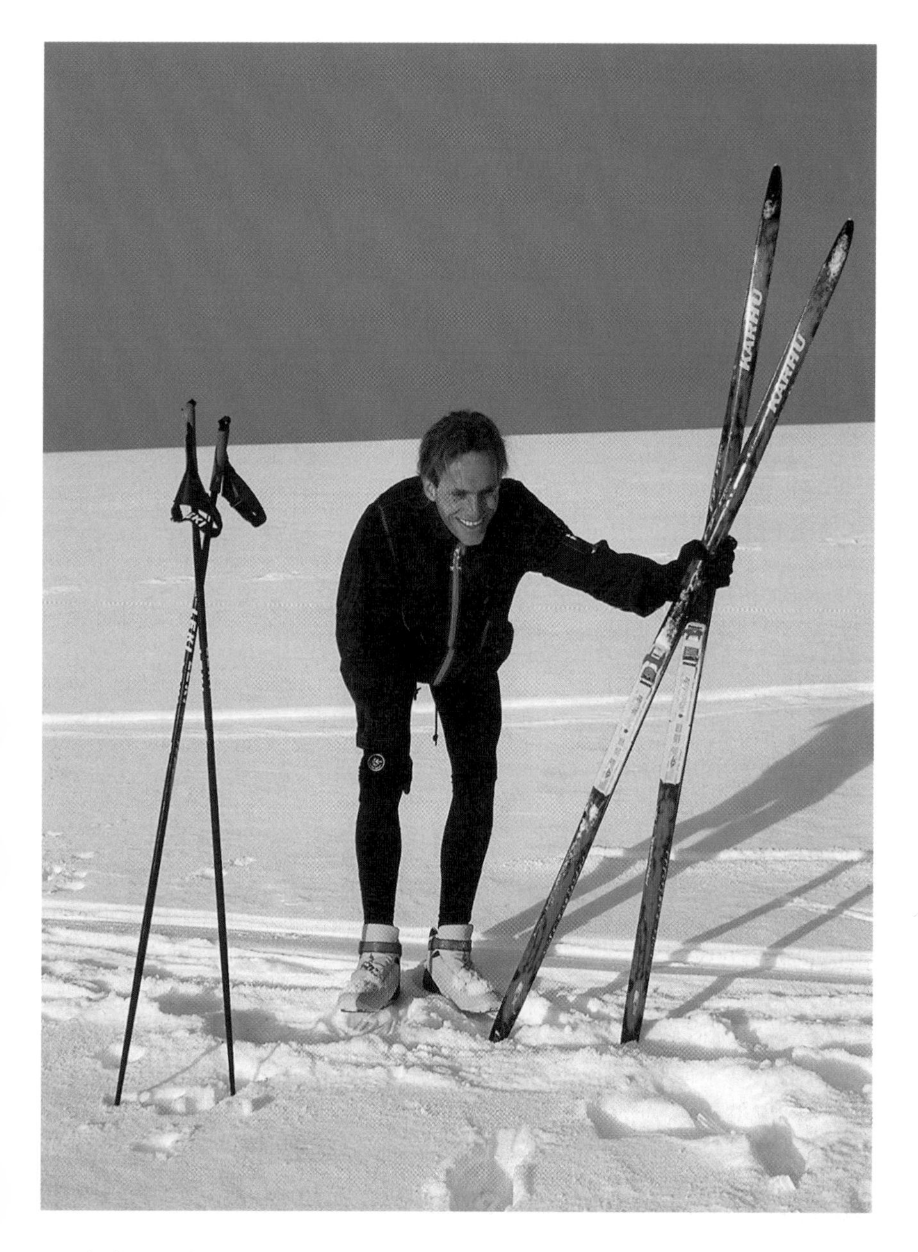

WAG's Photo and Text Agency, Freiburg (Photo: Armin Schirmaier, Freiburg)

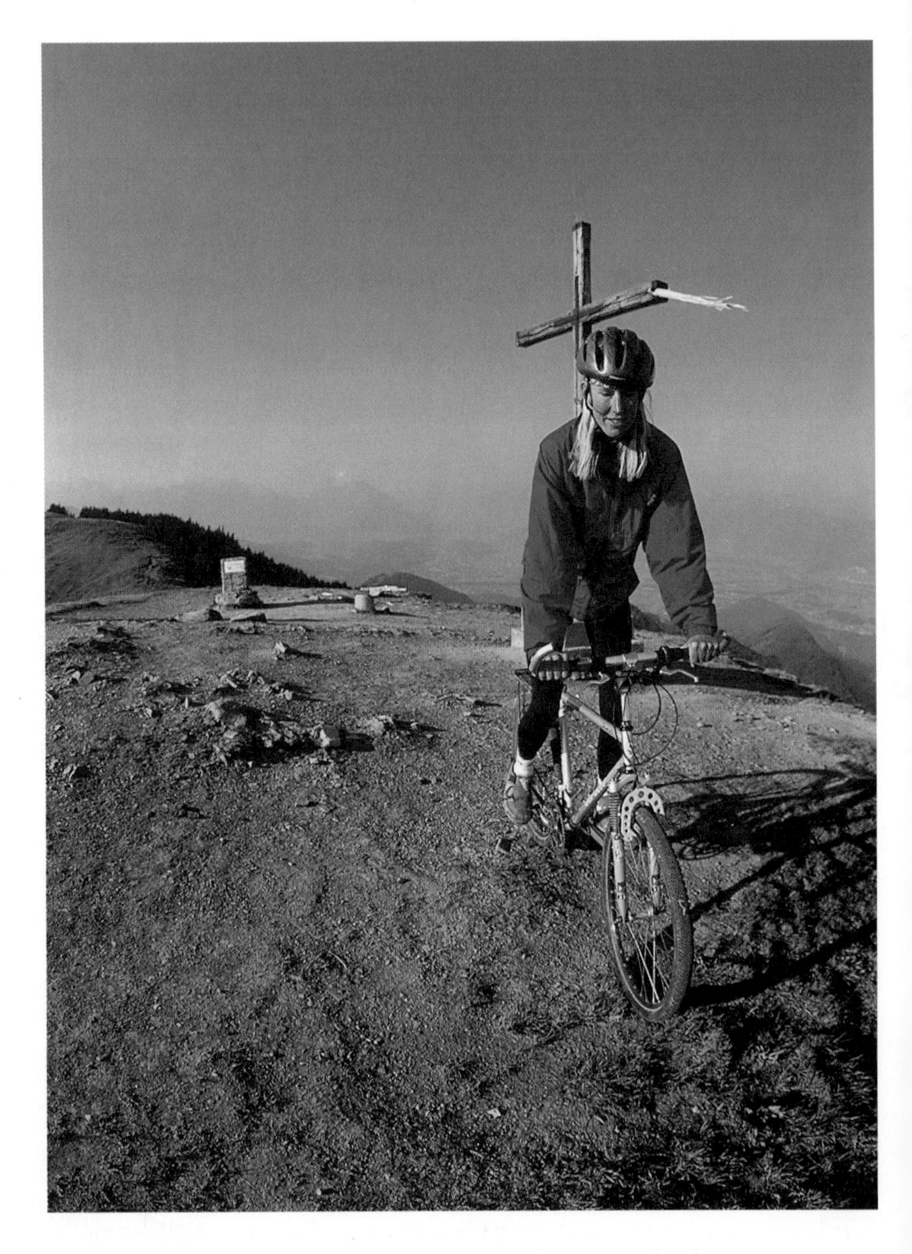

WAG's Photo and Text Agency, Freiburg (Photo: Armin Schirmaier, Freiburg)

Maximum oxygen uptake (VO_2 max) represents the performance capacity of the oxygen uptake, transporting and processing subsystems of the body. Thus the VO_2 max is the result of the oxygen diffusion of the lungs, oxygen transport in the blood and oxygen uptake in the loaded muscles. Through oxygen uptake the aerobic energy flow in the body is represented. For this the VO_2 max is the major measuring factor.

VO_2 max is an individually limited factor. Internationally it is considered a reliable measure of maximum aerobic performance capacity and is also described, not quite correctly in a physical and energetic sense, as a measure of aerobic capacity.

The relationship between oxygen uptake and breathing volume per minute has performance diagnostical significance and is expressed in the quotient: breathing volume per minute/oxygen uptake (respiratory equivalent).

The respiratory equivalent (RE) on the other hand expresses the effectiveness of breathing under load and shows how much oxygen is taken in with the air inhaled. Energy metabolism leaves the steady state when under increasing load, in relation to the increased breathing volume per minute, less and less oxygen is taken in. Under normal load the RE is 25 to 27 and indicates a stable metabolic situation. If during load the RE rises to over 29, breathing is considerably more difficult and the anaerobic proportion of energy transformation increases. The regulated steady state of metabolism is left, the proportion of glycolysis rises. A B E over 29 shows the clear exceeding of aerobic performance capacity and is an indication of insufficient supply of oxygen under load. The oxygen taken in through breathing is no longer enough for performance; anaerobic metabolism must be increasingly made use of.

Aerobic performance capacity indicates the sport-specific performance or speed reached at defined submaximal and maximal levels of load. oxygen uptake is often placed in relationship to certain metabolic measurement factors (e.g. lactate). An improvement in aerobic performance capacity is characterised by increased metabolism and circulation economy at submaximal levels of load. Thus oxygen uptake, heart rate and/or lactate concentration can decrease.

Optimal endurance training can lead to both an increase in submaximal and maximal aerobic performance capacity. To a large extent the training content in the practised sport determines the direction the change in aerobic performance foundations takes.

With an increase in training load over longer periods (months), aerobic performance capacity rises. The raising of the level of aerobic performance capacity is a necessary prerequisite for raising VO_2 max which serious intensity training requires.

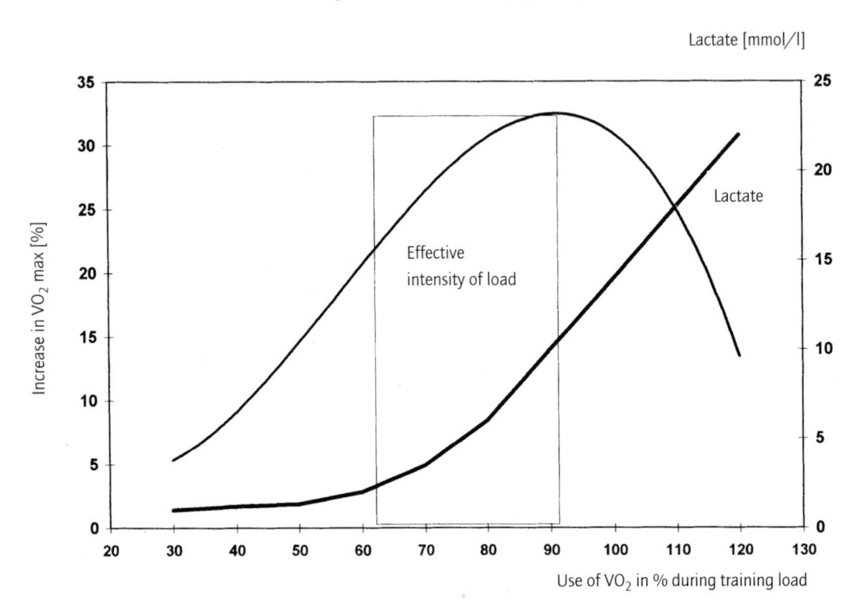

Fig. 1/4.4: Training intensity necessary for the development of maximum oxygen uptake

In order for an increase in maximum oxygen uptake to take place, several months of training with intensive content are necessary (Fig. 1/44, see above). The decisive physiological foundation for an increase in VO_2 max is an increase in the processing of oxygen by the muscles (increased activity of the enzymes of aerobic energy metabolism) in the slow twitch muscles (STF) and an increase in oxygen transporting capacity.

Maximum oxygen uptake and submaximal aerobic performance capacity together represent the aerobic foundations of performance.

Maximum oxygen uptake increases when the sport-specific load is so intensive (strenuous) that the current aerobic muscular performance level is exceeded and anaerobic metabolism is also partially made use of. The first indication that the aerobic performance capacity level has been exceeded is the rise in the blood lactate concentration to over 2 mmol/l (Fig. 2/4.4, see p. 75). Training VO_2 max requires more intense training stimuli than the development of aerobic performance foundations. Only after longer load in an aerobic-anaerobic metabolism situation (lactate above 6 mmol/l) are the stimuli required for the development of maximum oxygen uptake intense enough. 100 % exploitation of the individual VO_2 max is only possible for a few minutes. Highly-trained athletes can manage it for four to seven minutes. Longer lasting performances can only be achieved with incomplete exploitation of VO_2 max The range

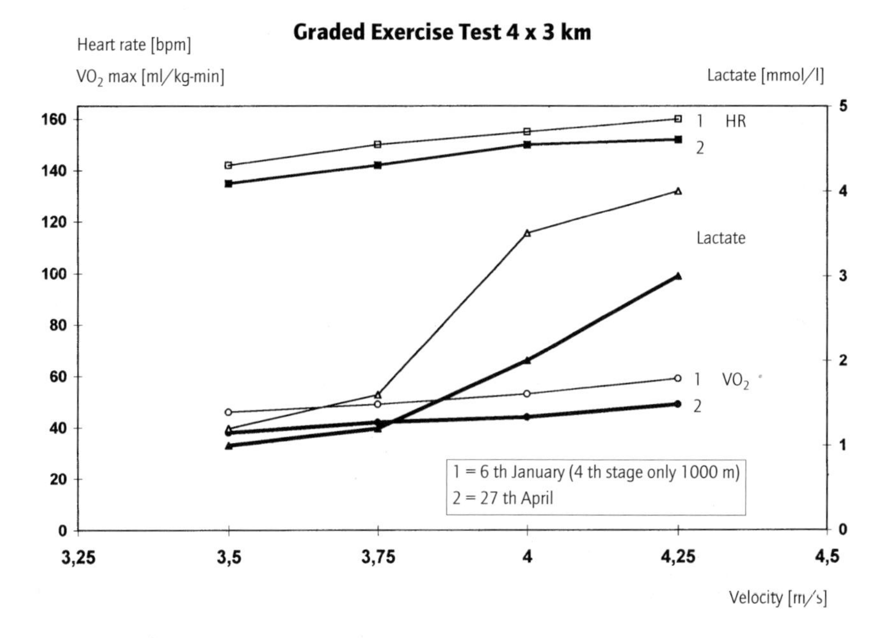

Fig. 2/4.4: Behaviour of heart rate, lactate and maximum oxygen uptake during a performance diagnostics test on the treadmill. Between the first and the second test there is a drop in all factors; that indicates an economisation of these systems.

of exploitation of VO_2 max then lies between 85 and 98 % and is dependent on the duration of load which can still be handled sport-specifically at highest possible intensity.

In order to develop maximum sport-specific aerobic performance capacity, at least 10% of total training load must be trained aerobic-anaerobically.

The aerobic performance capacity of top athletes is expressed in their ability to handle high velocities or performance levels in a situation of aerobic metabolism. Thus world-class runners can cover longer distances at 19.8 km/h (5.50 m/s) using aerobic metabolism (< lactate 2 mmol/l) (Fig. 3/4.4, see p. 76). An average runner either does not reach this velocity, or if he does, then only with a high anaerobic metabolism proportion.

When endurance-trained athletes consume less oxygen than untrained persons at submaximal levels of load it is an expression of the higher effectiveness of their muscle work. This statement also applies to differences in the state of training between more and less well-trained people in a particular sport. At similar sport-specific performance levels the effectiveness of the muscle work of the better trained person is higher.

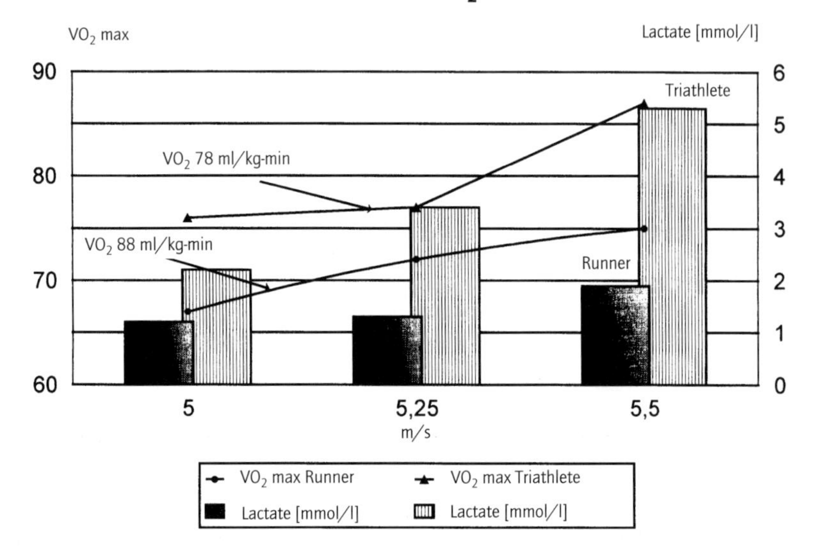

Fig. 3/4.4: Comparison of oxygen uptake and lactate concentration between a long-distance runner and a triathlete. The runner has a considerably higher oxygen uptake (VO_2 max) and lower lactate concentration than the triathlete at similar velocities. The percentage use made of VO_2 max is also lower for the runner.

The increase in the degree of effectiveness of the muscle work is expressed in the declining calorie equivalent, i.e. at a certain submaximal performance level the amount of energy expended is less for the better trained person. The increased effectiveness is not only recognisable in lower oxygen uptake and the lower respiratory quotient (RQ) but also in the regulatory behaviour of the breathing, cardiovascular and metabolism systems (see chapters 4.1, 4.2 and 10.4). When effectiveness is improved the more performance capable athlete uses more fatty acids, develops less lactate, regulates with a lower HR and breathing rate and has a lower oxygen uptake at the same performance level. In relation to performance (velocities) at 2 mmol/l lactate the better trained athlete uses less of his VO_2 max. In addition, the better training state is not only noticeable in the economisation of submaximal performance capacity but also in the increase in maximum aerobic performance capacity. Thus under optimal competitive training conditions the higher aerobic performance foundations are expressed both in an increase in effectiveness under submaximal load and in improved functioning under maximum load (increase in VO_2 max).

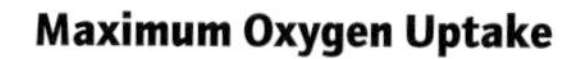

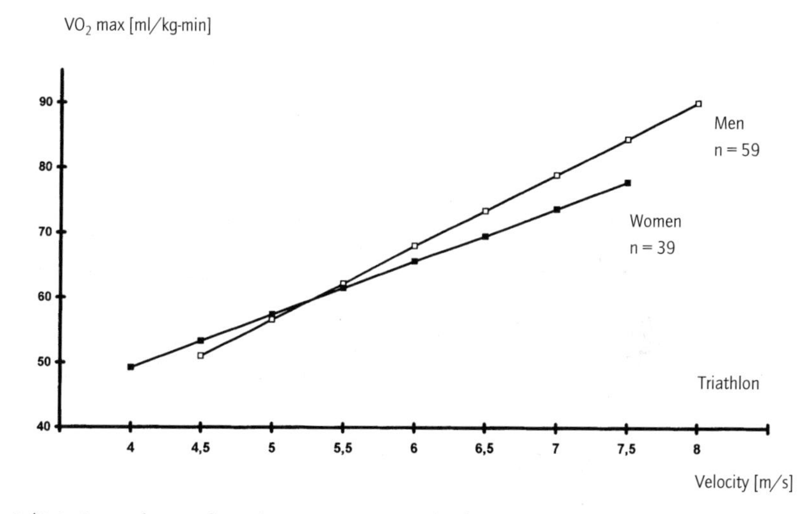

Fig. 4/4.4: Dependence of maximum oxygen uptake (VO_2 max) on running speed on the treadmill (short-graded exercise test)

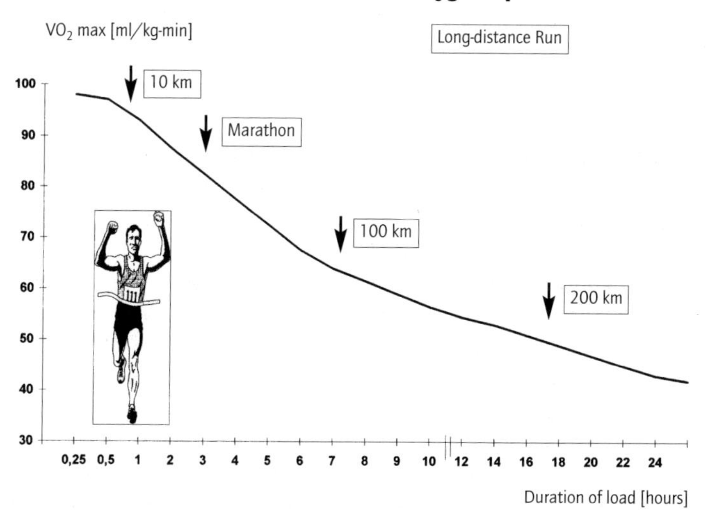

Fig. 5/4.4: With increasing distance the possible use made of maximum oxygen uptake (VO_2 max) decreases. During load over long running distances the VO_2 max is less developed.

If maximum oxygen uptake is determined in a laboratory it is dependent on the basic motor performance capacity when running (treadmill) or the maximum strength endurance on the bike (cycle ergometer test) (Fig. 4/4.4, see p. 77).

If in training the athlete does not strive for or achieve higher velocity or more intensive strength endurance performance then his maximum oxygen uptake will only develop slightly. Often the increase in aerobic performance capacity does not take place in even proportions. Its development is greatly dependent on training methodology (see chapter 6). Frequently only the development of one aerobic performance component is evident. This leads to the conclusion that the simultaneous sport-methodological development of maximum oxygen uptake and aerobic performance capacity is not so simple. This is because of the sport-methodological problem of the disruptive influence of high total load on the implementation of high quality training content (velocities, strength endurance). The residual tiredness resulting from large amounts of training hinders the release of motor speed or speed endurance (see chapters 8, 9 and 10).

Although the phenomenon of uneven development of the aerobic performance foundations is known, it cannot always be optimally solved through training methodology. Aerobic performance capacity can be easily trained by increasing training distances (distance mean) with a high total volume of training. In doing so, however, usually unintentionally a decrease in velocity or performance occurs because the proportions of intensive training are too low.

Using the example of running it becomes clear that with increasing duration of running there is increasingly lower percentage use made of VO_2 max (Fig. 5/4.4, see p. 77). Through aerobic basic training mainly metabolic economy (fat metabolism) is trained and not the high use of energy necessary for the development of VO_2 max.

Even in the border area of current performance capacity, when duration of load is too long, training stimulation is too low for the development of VO_2 max. Long races also do not provide sufficiently strong stimuli to affect development of maximum oxygen uptake as they only make use of 50 to 70 % of maximum oxygen uptake (see Fig. 5/4.4).

A correction of the intensity deficit afterwards is possible. By reducing total load, capacity is created for more intensive training. Intensity training requires longer recovery periods than volume training.

The prerequisite for the development of VO_2 max is training in the individual motor borderline area. In order for the intensive training sessions to have an effect, a certain proportion of total load must be attained. 5 to 15 % of total load as intensive training with crossing of the upper aerobic capacity limit is considered to have a stimulating effect. The longer the race distances are, the greater the proportion of intensive training sessions can be, corresponding to performance structure.

Sport type groups	Men	Women
Endurance sports	75 - 80	65 - 70
Game sports	55 - 60	45 - 52
Duelling sports	60 - 65	50 - 53
Speed-strength	50 - 55	45 - 50
Technical sports	50 - 60	45 - 50

Table 1/4.4: Maximum oxygen uptake (in ml/kg.min) in the sport type groups

	Top sport 20-35 h/week	Competitive sport 15-25 h/week	Fitness sport 4-12 h/week
Long-distance runners	83 - 88	75 - 80	55 - 65
Cross-country skiiers	85 - 90	77 - 82	53 - 63
Triathletes	78 - 83	70 - 78	55 - 65
Cyclists	82 - 86	70 - 78	50 - 60
Swimmers	70 - 75	67 - 72	45 - 50
Walkers	65 - 70	55 - 63	45 - 50

Table 2/4.4: Dependence of maximum oxygen uptake (ml/kg.min) on training load in the endurance sports

Through regular training with intensive contents competitive and top category training differentiate themselves clearly from fitness sport. In fitness sport, basic endurance training is given preference. Intensive proportions of training occur either by chance or are determined by the frequency of competition participation.

In order to compare the stage of development of athlete's VO_2 max, this is related to body weight. Depending on the sport or sport group, relative VO_2 max varies (Table 1/4.4). Sport-specific performance in competitions is not directly dependent on VO_2 max the athlete has access to further compensatory possibilities such as sporting technique, racing technique, racing experience etc. In sporting practice the higher use made of anaerobic metabolism is the usual compensation variation used when VO_2 max is too low. In endurance sports the level of VO_2 max is a measure of the amount of load reached in the sport (Fig. 6/4.4, see p. 80).

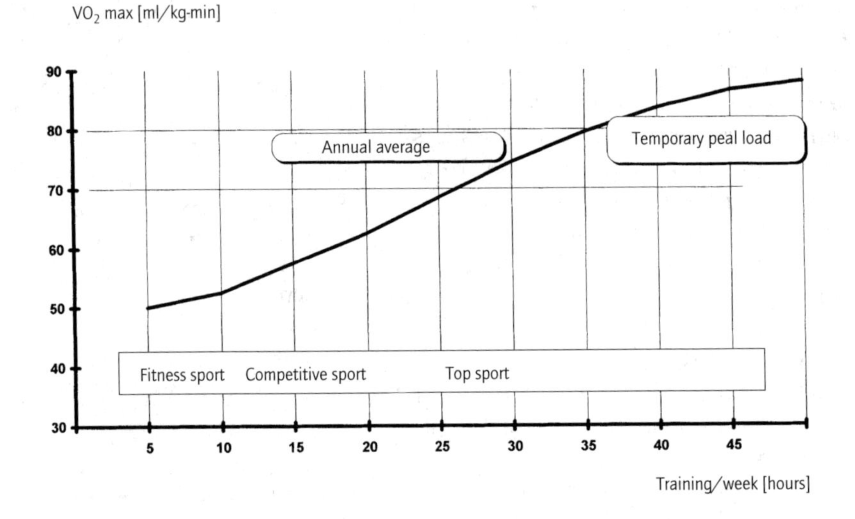

Fig. 6/4.4: Dependence of the development of maximum oxygen uptake (VO_2 max) on average training load per week

The top performance in a sport is dependent on the athlete reaching a certain reference level of VO_2 max (Table 2/4.4, see p. 79). The more clearly performance in the sport is influenced by the biomotor ability endurance, the higher the reference value in VO_2 max must be. The endurance sports running, cycling and cross-country skiing differ for example from game sports and duelling sports in the use made of endurance ability in carrying out performance, they require higher VO_2 max. For carrying out non-endurance sports different motor and co-ordinative demands must be met than for the endurance sports.

Summary

The increase in maximum oxygen uptake (VO_2 max) is advantageous for numerous sports, in particular for endurance sports. VO_2 max and aerobic performance capacity at submaximal levels of loads (e.g. performance or velocity at lactate 2 mmol/l) are the two main characteristics of aerobic performance foundations for sport-specific endurance performances.

4.6 Immune System and Training Load

There is a close relationship between the level of adaptation achieved through training and the state of health. Among the central functional systems affecting health in a major way is the immune system; it is right in the middle of the field of tension between aerobic basic training, aerobic-anaerobic training, competitions and summation loads (Fig. 1/4.6, see p. 108). The greatest immunological tolerance is achieved through aerobic basic endurance training (BE). BE training makes up 60 to 75 % of total load in endurance training. The involvement of the immune system in the load-stress reaction is a normal accompanying reaction, the degree of which is dependent on the total level of exertion. The increased accompanying reaction of the immune system during training is also a protective measure against pathogenes entering the system.

The accompanying reaction of the immune system consists of an immune specific and an unspecific part. It is a normal physiological reaction in competitive training, just like the increase in lactate during intensive load or the increase in serum urea during protein breakdown.

It has been scientifically proved that moderate aerobic training leads to a strengthening of immunological defence and thus increases health stability. According to research by NIEMAN (1994) the influence of training on health risk can be shown in the form of a-curve (Fig. 2/4.6, see p. 109). The amount of training load in aerobic metabolism is not necessarily a risk element for the immune system. Rather the risk lies in the intensive load stimuli in anaerobic metabolism situations and the high psychophysical pressure to perform.

Currently it is not yet possible to ascertain an individually bearable level of exertion which is good for health and at the same time increases performance capacity in individual borderline areas. The immune system measuring factors available in practice allow no quantifiable statements on the state of health and sporting load tolerance. That does not mean that the immunological basic state is not assessable.

The immunological process is very complex. The defence weakness observable after a high level of sporting effort is not the same as an illness. After a high level of psychophysical exertion there is a so-called "open window" for about four to eight hours. This term describes the increased vulnerability of the person involved to pathogenes entering the system (PEDERSEN et al., 1989). This is not identical with an illness. An illness involves the attachment of pathogenic germs, usually in a state of reduced defence. The assumed health instability of competitive athletes in comparison with untrained persons with regard to colds and related illnesses are probably connected with the reduction in immune defence through load. The illnesses among athletes are mainly limited to the upper respiratory tracts.

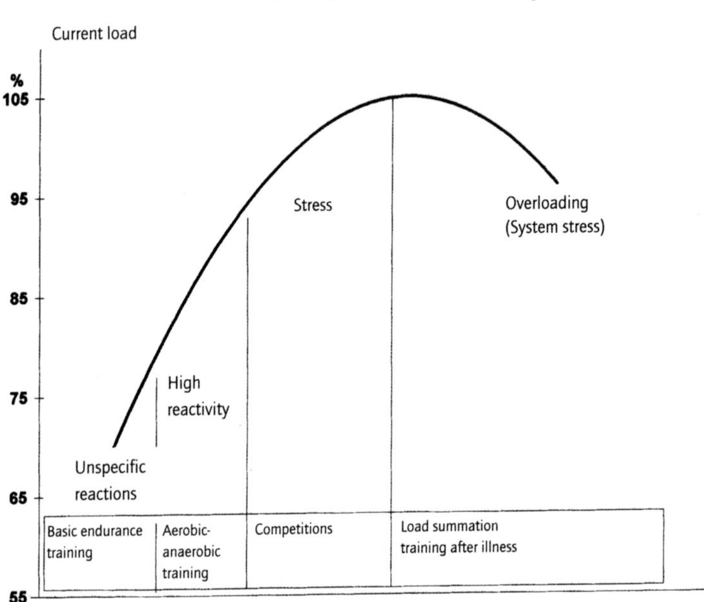

Fig. 1/4.6: Schematic presentation of the possible load tolerance of the immune system through training

The peaks of infection frequency are in spring and winter and affect up to 19 % of competitive athletes (WEISS, 1994). If the annual average of infection of the upper respiratory tracts is 5 %, then it can be estimated that competitive athletes have twice the rate of infection of untrained persons. This is also related to the fact that in competitive sport, training takes place regardless of weather conditions. The only remedy is close-meshed medical care, training based on scientific criteria and keeping to immune-prophylactic measures.

Surveys and observation of top athletes showed that they only suffer infections about once every two years. They are more careful about their state of health and avoid disruptive factors in training (Table 1/4.6, see p. 110).

The difficulty in objectively registering the immunological state of athletes is that the numbers of cells (lymphocyte and leucocyte subpopulations), plasma protein concentrations, mediator substances (interleucine), antibodies (immunoglobulins) etc that can be determined in the blood only represent a "snapshot" and do not sufficiently represent the quickly changing immunological process.

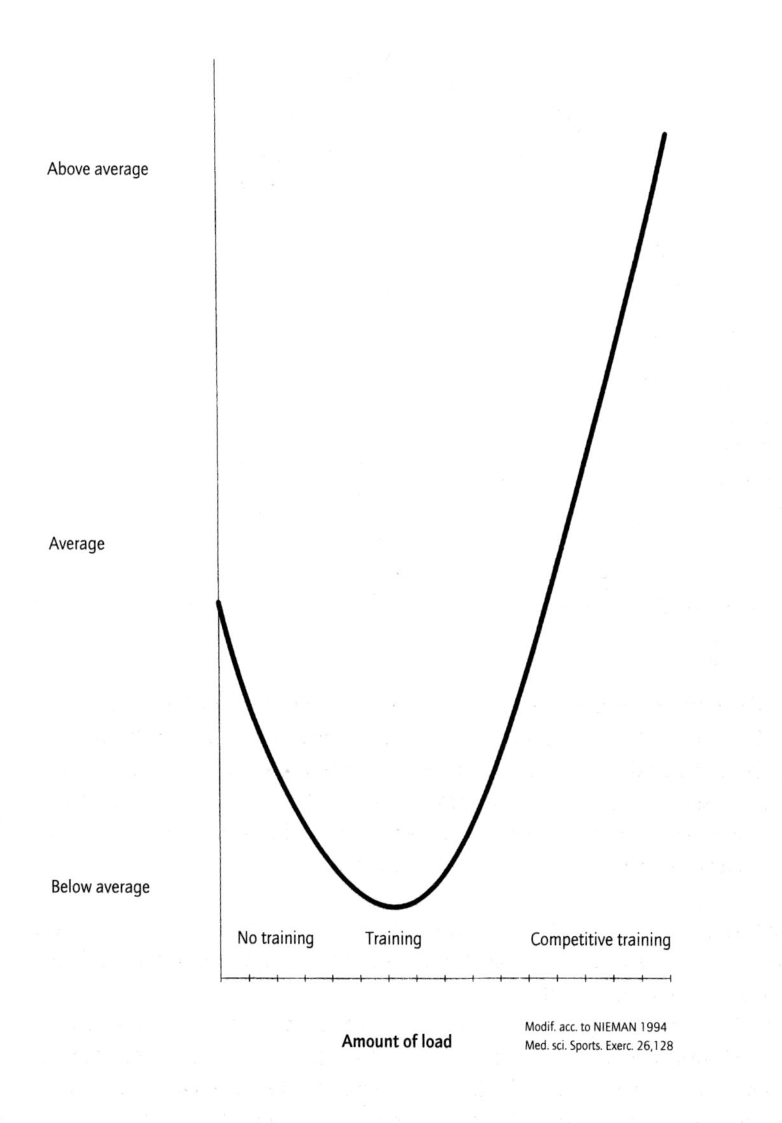

Fig. 2/4.6: Relationship between amount of load and risk of illness. The so-called J-phenomenon according to NIEMAN (1994)

Possibilities for Infection Prophylaxis in Top Competitive Sport
• Exclusion of standard risk situations arising from general and local chilling due to wet and sweaty clothing. (Preplanning of clothing change, head protection and maintenance of body warmth).
• Avoidance of stress situations not related to sport (psychological stress influences).
• Reduction of drastic time zone and climatic changes (deliberate planning of travel in connection with competitions).
• Avoidance of contact with unknown and potential infection sources (public transport, large gatherings of people in closed spaces, presentations).
• Recommendation of infection prophylaxis also to direct contact persons in the family.
• Strict keeping to unloading periods (psychophysical regeneration, sleep).
• Deliberate supplementation with vitamins, minerals and immune stimulants. Physio-prophylaxis (sauna).
• Appropriately timed addressing of focuses of inflammation.

Table 1/4.6: Possibilities for infection prophylaxis in top competitive sport

Immune System in Competitive Sport
• The close functional and morphological connection of the immune system with the central nervous system leads to a joint reaction to stress.
• High load stress can depress the immune system for several days.
• In competitive training phases of planned unloading are necessary to maintain the functionality and stability of the immune system. A rhythm of load and unloading of 3:1 (days, weeks) is necessary.
• Regular sports training adapts the immune system and improves the immunological functional state. Individual load limits cannot be registered with measurement factors of the immune system.
• In comparison to load duration, load intensity has a greater influence on activating the humoral and especially the cellular immune system.
• If during competitive training infections are developing, load must be considerably reduced or stopped altogether. Unloading from training can have a positive effect on the defensive performance of the immune system.

Table 2/4.6: Immune system in competitive sport

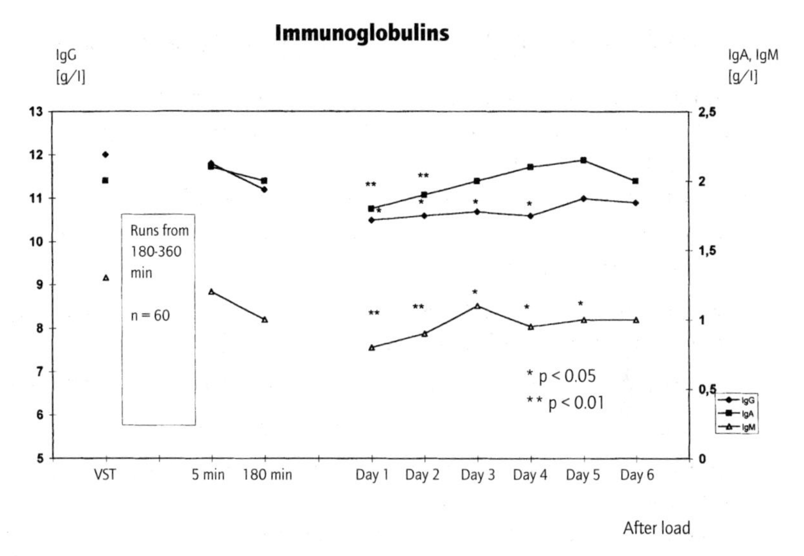

Fig. 3/4.6: Changes in the immunoglobulin concentration (IgG, IgA and IgM) after long duration endurance runs. In the first days of recovery there is a decrease in immunoglobulin concentration which shows a state of reduced defence.

The ongoing effects in the immune system are less after moderate training than after personal extreme performances. Regular reduction of load in competitive training is of great significance with regard to strengthening natural immunological defence.

Another significant job of the immune system should be pointed out. This applies to the training-affected structural destruction in the muscle which in its mild form is known as aching or strained muscles. The protein fragments released when the muscle is overloaded cause an aseptic inflammation and must be identified by the immune system as internal ("self") or external ("not self") and neutralised. The immune system "fights" the products of cell decay and cell breakdown with the same means as penetrated foreign substances (DUFAUX, 1989). Thus the immune system of athletes is in constant training of the breakdown of muscle decay products. The capacities used for clearing-up work are of course not available for defence as a whole. Very strong defence work of "muscle remnants" means that the biological defence potential against penetrating germs can be weakened (Table 2/4.6, see p. 110). Stimuli which are especially disruptive to the muscle function include eccentric load (running down hill) and all forms of unaccustomed brief duration high intensity loads.

The activation of the humoral and cellular immune system is dependent more on the level of the intensive exertion stimuli than on the duration of load. Aerobic endurance training is immunologically easier to deal with than forms of aerobic-anaerobic load.

Summarising the complicated accompanying reaction of the immune system during training it can be concluded that with a high degree of probability, after great psychophysical demands in the form of competitions, competition series, training camps etc, in the two days following there will be a weak point for the gathering of pathogenes. This is also comprehensible from the decrease in concentration of the immunoglobulins (specific antibodies) (Fig. 3/4.6, see p. 111).

Summary

The immune system is closely linked to the central nervous system and can therefore jointly defend against stress effects with this. High sporting load stress reduces immunological defence potential for several days. Therefore preventive measures through unloading take on increasing significance. To maintain functional performance capacity of the immune system, regular unloading is necessary in competitive training. In comparison to the duration of load, the intensity of load has a greater influence on the activation of parts of the immune system. Individual limits of load tolerance cannot be registered with certainty using the measurement factors of the immune system.

If infections begin to develop during competitive training the most effective measure is to reduce load or take a break. Unloading from training ensures the integrity of the immune system and assists immunological defence performance.

4.7 Muscle and Training Load

Because of their structure, the muscles must be constantly loaded. Lack of use leads to muscular atrophy with considerable loss of strength. This was especially noticeable amongst astronauts in weightlessness in space. Staying in the Skylab for 28 days resulted in the same degree of loss of leg extension strength (20 %) as 30 days in bed (CONVERTINO, 1991). Muscle atrophy is known from rest periods due to injury, longer periods of being bedridden and lack of movement and often affects athletes more than untrained persons. The greater potential to build up and restructure trained muscles is linked with a greater deterioration potential through lack of use or considerable reduction of load. Even load breaks of ten days are the absolute limit for trained muscles to maintain their state.

Of all the organs, the muscle system is the largest at 23 to 28 kg in mass. The muscle system is the organ which is mainly used to assess or measure the effects of training. The changes in function and structure of the muscle are the orientation factor for adaptations in competitive training.

Depending on the particular training stimuli, the muscles react to speed, strength and endurance demands in a specific way. Muscle performance can be trained in speed, precision and reliability (endurance). This requires not only training of energy metabolism, but also of the steering of the muscles through the nervous system. Adaptations take place with regard to both the motor co-ordinative functions and the energy potential of the muscle. IKAI (1967) developed a diagram in which the independence of the development of the biomotor abilities strength, speed and endurance in the individual sports is demonstrated. The varying use made of these abilities in the individual sports was emphasised. These considerations were later confirmed muscle-bioptically by PIEPER/SCHARSCHMIDT (1981) (Fig. 1/4.7, see p. 114). For the endurance sports a model of the varying demands of strength endurance and speed abilities during short, medium and long-term load in competitive situations was developed (NEUMANN, 1991; see chapter 7).

The introduction of needle biopsy of the muscle system by BERGSTRÖM (1962) was a pioneering development for assessing changes to the muscles as a result of training. This research technology made it possible to get a detailed idea of muscle fibre distribution, muscle fibre area, capillarisation, metabolism behaviour, substrate balance, enzyme activity and ultra-structure in the muscles in relation to training.

Muscle Fibre Distribution

Using histochemical colouring methods the muscle fibres can be divided into fast and slow twitch fibres. The fast twitch fibres are called FTF and the slow twitch fibres STF. Muscle fibre distribution can be determined for three muscle groups. These are the delta muscle (M. deltoideus), the side thigh muscle (m. vastus lateralis) and the calf muscle (m. gastrocnemius). Muscle fibre distribution is individually predetermined, i.e. hereditary, and cannot be changed by training. For comparisons of muscle fibre distribution between the sports the side thigh muscle is preferred (Fig. 2/4.7, see p. 115).

The majority of untrained persons show a balanced relationship between STF and FTF. The muscle fibre situation plays a role in determining in which sport a young person will later be successful. Generally, sprinters have a high proportion of FTF and endurance athletes of STF.

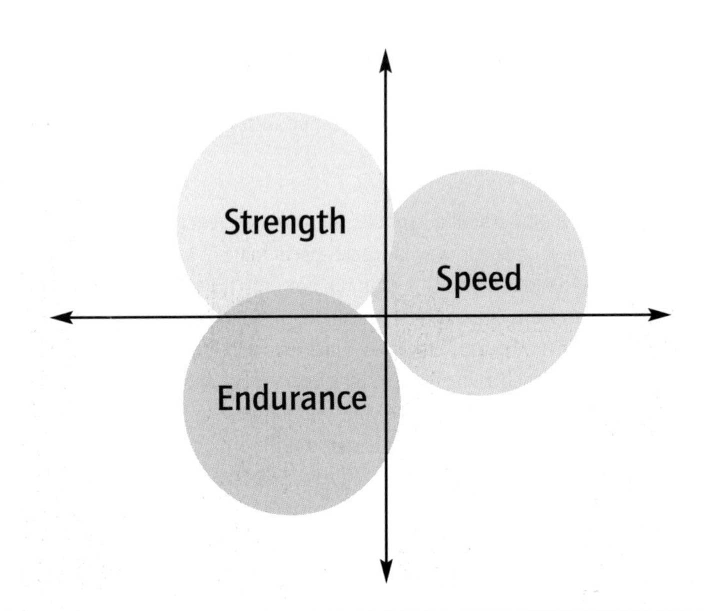

Characteristic	Speed-dominated athlete (n = 50)	Strength-dominated athlete (n = 96)	Endurance-dominated athlete (n = 124)
Body weight (kg)	65	79	65
VO_2max (l/min)	3.3	4.5	4.2
ST Fibres (μm^2)	6500	7000	6700
FT Fibres (μm^2)	7600	8600	7100
STF Area (%)	51	53	72
Citrate synthetase (µmol/s.kg MW)	340	475	430
Phosphoglycerate kinase (mmol/s.kg MW)	4.5	4.1	2.1

Fig. 1/4.7: Illustration of the biomotor abilities strength, speed and endurance and their relationship to the biological foundations body mass, oxygen uptake, muscle fibre area and enzymes of aerobic and anaerobic metabolism per kg wet weight (WW). According to PIEPER/SCHARSCHMIDT (1981)

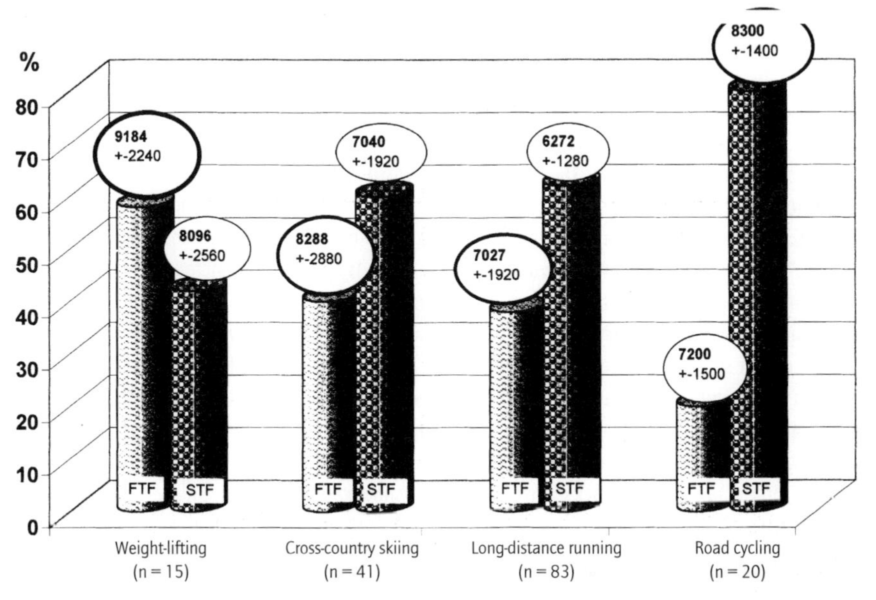

Fig. 2/4.7: Distribution of fast and slow twitch muscle fibres (STF and FTF) and the fibre area of top athletes of the GDR

Endurance athletes have an average of 65 to 85 % STF and sprinters as well as speed-strength-dominated athletes have 60 to 70 % FTF (COSTILL et al., 1976). Although in principle the presence of a high proportion of FTF predestines athletes for speed, that is no guarantee for top performances. This always requires deliberate sport-specific speed training with high FT muscle fibre presence.

Muscle Fibre Area

Through training that emphasises resistance, i.e. strength and strength endurance training, the muscle fibre can increase in strength, it hypertrophies. If the resistance stimulus is left out and only endurance capacity is trained, then fibre volume decreases. This state can be useful from a training-methodological point of view because it allows a better exchange of energy. The endurance load cannot be increased to extremes because the athletes become too slow as a result of speed monotony. For endurance sports the development of aerobic strength endurance is a performance reserve, for only this guarantees an increase in forward propulsion performance (Fig. 3/4.7). In comparison to untrained persons, athletes generally have a larger muscle fibre area; this is the main prerequisite for increasing strength ability. It is also the lower muscle fibre area of women which determines the average 20 % lower strength ability of women compared to men.

The muscle fibre strength (area) of the STF and FTF differs. The fibre volume of the FTF is usually larger than that of the STF, in competitive training the optimal relationship is 1.3 to 1.0. A decrease in the area of the FTF means a loss of strength. The main forms of training influence the development of muscle fibre strength through the central nervous regulation system. As a result of strength training the FTF increase more and through endurance training the STF increase more. Hypertrophy of the muscle fibres is based on an increase in the amount of contraction proteins (actine, myosine, troponine). Increased muscle strength is not necessarily seen in the form of externally larger muscles. With increasing strength training in the particular sport the FTF area increases (Table 1/4.7, see p. 117). If the training resistance stimulus to the muscle is reduced, then the fibre hypertrophy and with it strength ability rapidly deteriorates again. This also applies to a change in training content of the sport. If a track cyclist changes to road cycling, the specific strength potential he needs for acceleration will regress. On the other hand, track cyclists use road cycling to develop their endurance capability.

Muscle Fibre Capillarisation

Training increases the supply of blood to the muscles. The prerequisite for this is that the number of capillaries surrounding a muscle fibre increase. Through endurance but also through strength training, muscle blood supply increases. The improved blood supply is necessary to increase the stability of endurance performance capacity. On average the FTF are supplied by four and the STF by three capillaries. Endurance training leads to an increase in the degree of capillarisation by 40 %. Under the physiological conditions of training it is probable that the reserve capillaries are opened and no new capillaries developed. Under load the trained muscle receives more blood. The triggering stimulus for the improved blood supply to the muscle is the energy deficit caused by load.

Enzyme Activities in the Muscle Fibres

As a result of training, the metabolism characteristics in the muscle fibres change. The hereditary distribution of STF and FTF, however, remains uninfluenced. Depending on training content, the anaerobic breakdown of glycogen (glycolysis) or aerobic carbohydrate and fat metabolism can change greatly. The prerequisite here is that the key enzymes of these metabolism forms adapt to the appropriate training stimuli. Clearly targeted training load leads to more lasting metabolism changes in the muscles than mediocre mixed training.

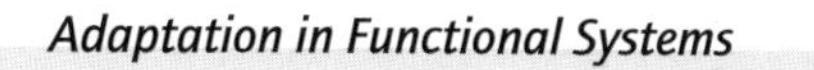

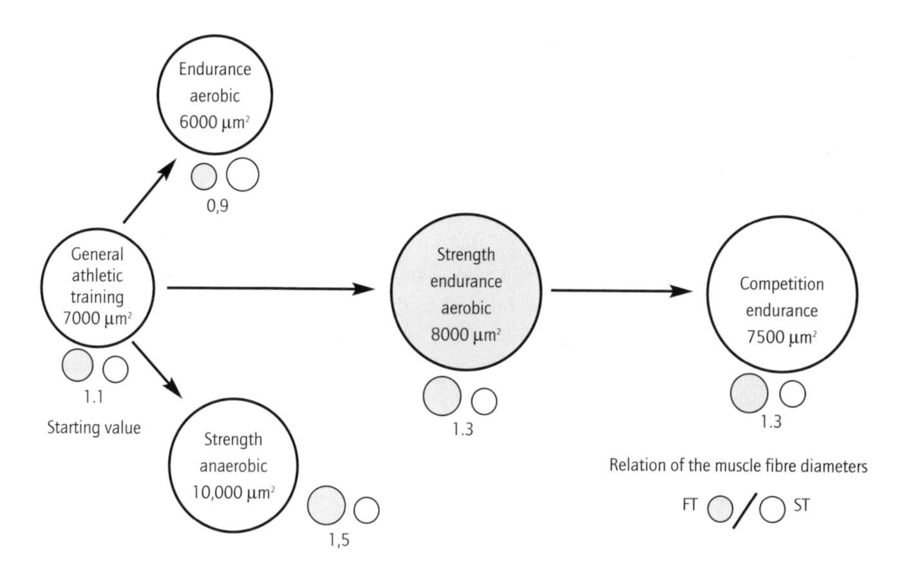

Fig. 3/4.7: Model derived from real muscle bioptic findings demonstrating the necessity of training lasting adaptation of strength abiliy before endurance competitions.

Maximum oxygen uptake, Muscle Fibre Distribution and Muscle Fibre Areas of Elite Cyclists in the GDR 1988						
Sport	Number	VO_2max (ml/kg.min	ST fibres (%)	FT-fibres (%)	Fibre area STF (µm²)	Fibre area FTF (µm²)
Sprinter/ Track	5	64	65	35	9000	13,500
1000 m Track cyclist	5	66	72	28	8500	12,000
4000 m Track cyclist	10	76	78	22	8000	10,000
Road cyclist	20	78	80	20	7000	8000

Table 1/4.7: Maximum oxygen uptake and muscle fibre distribution of Elite cyclists

Enzyme Activity in Cycling					
Enzymes μmol/kg FG	Road cyclists n = 19		Track cyclists n = 12		Significance p <
	x	± s	x	±s	
Glycogen synthetase	**127**	23	68	35	0.002
Phosphoglycerate kinase x 1000	2.90	0.80	**4.27**	1.0	0.001
Pyruvate kinase x 1000	1.72	0.36	**2.88**	0.8	0.001
Lactate dehydrogenase	3.82	1.20	**6.50**	1.90	0.001
Citrate synthetase	**717**	189	488	169	0.005

Table 2/4.7: Enzyme activities in cycling

For example, intensity-oriented track cycling leads to different enzyme changes on the muscle cell level than endurance-oriented road cycling training (Table 2/4.7). In Table 2/4.7 it can be seen clearly that in road cyclists the enzymes of aerobic metabolism (citrate synthetase) and in track cyclists those of anaerobic metabolism (phosphoglycerate kinase, lactate dehydrogenase) have increased considerably. The increase in lactate development is only possible if the glycolytic key enzyme phosphoglycerate kinase (PGK) increases. On the other hand, as a result of training the activity of the PGK decreases and with it lactate development. Balance is achieved through the increase in aerobic energy metabolism, recognisable e.g. by the increase in citrate synthetase (CS). CS in endurance-trained athletes can double in comparison to untrained persons.

Maximum oxygen uptake can only increase if the key enzymes of aerobic metabolism (CS, succinate dehydrogenase) increase their activity and thus cause increased processing in the cells of the oxygen brought by the blood. The determination of maximum oxygen uptake is a repeatable measurement for the assessment of muscle cell aerobic adaptation potential or aerobic enzyme capacity.

Energy Reserves

On the muscle level there are three forms of energy reserves, not counting the small reserves of ATP, ADP and AMP. Creatine phosphate serves to secure immediate performance of the muscles (see chapter 4.5.1). With this reserve the muscle can work for a maximum of 6 to 10 s.

Energy Stores at 70 kg Body Weight				
Carbohydrates				
	Untrained		Trained	
Liver glycogen	80 g	328 kcal	120 g	492 kcal
Muscle glycogen	250 g	1025 kcal	400 g	1640 kcal
Glucose (body fluids)	15 g	62 kcal	18 g	74 kcal
		Fats		
Subcutaneous fat	8000 g	74,400 kcal	6000 g	55,800 kcal
Intramuscular	50 g	465 kcal	200 - 300 g	1860 - 2790 kcal
		Proteins		
Amino acid pool	100 g	410 kcal	110 g	451 kcal
Structural proteins (muscle)	6000 g		7000 g	

Table 3/4.7: Energy stores at 70 kg body weight

The creatine phosphate store is trainable, in sprinters it is larger than in endurance athletes. The increase through training is 20 %. The most significant energy store of the muscle is glycogen. Through endurance training this store can be almost doubled. At rest the glycogen content of the muscle is 1.5 to 2.0 g/100 g muscle moist weight (MW). That corresponds to 15-20 g/kg MW or 150 to 200 g of 10 kg muscle mass used.

At rest and through an emphasis on carbohydrate intake the glycogen store in the muscle can rise to 3 g/kg MW. The varying figures on the size of this store are a result of the estimate of the amount of muscle mass used in load. Glycogen only increases in muscle groups that have been trained. Altogether the glycogen stores in the trainable muscles increase from about 300 g to 500 g (Table 3/4.7). Under intensive load (competition) the glycogen stores are emptied earlier than under training load with 70 % of VO_2 max (see Fig. 5/4.5.2).

Glycogen overcompensation through high carbohydrate intake is only possible when the activity of the glycogen producing enzyme, glycogen synthetase, has been increased through training. In addition to creatine phosphate and glycogen the muscle system also has a third energy store. This is neutral fat (trigylcerides) which is stored next to the mitochondria. The information on this store varies greatly. Its size fluctuates from 50 g to 350 g. The greatest amounts of muscle triglyceride are found in extreme endurance athletes. The reason for these large fat energy reserves is extreme endurance training. The endurance-trained muscle thus has stable energy reserves directly next to the mitochondria. Theoretically 4500 kcal of energy can be generated from the muscle fat stores.

Ultra Structure

The structures in the muscle which actually create energy are the mitochondria. Evidence of them is given microscopically. Endurance training leads to an enlargement of the volume and density of the mitochondria as well as to an increase in the surface area of the folded inner mitochondria membrane. The increase in mitochondria volume is in close relationship to maximum oxygen uptake (HOPPELER et al., 1990). The inner surface of the mitochondria membrane increases from 1.88 m^2 in untrained persons to 2.77 m^2 in ultra distance runners (HOWALD, 1982). Thus the morphological basis for greater oxygen uptake and energy generation is assured.

Summary

The muscle fibres, nervous system steered by the sport-specific movement process, adapt to the requirements of energy generation, reliability of the working form (endurance), speed in the twitch sequence and overcoming resistance (use of strength). Sports training increases the twitch speed of the muscle groups involved in a programme of movement, the forward propulsion performance (strength and strength endurance) and the resistance to tiredness (capability of longer load tolerance). Linked with this are a greater use of energy, increase in the substrate stores, increased blood supply and enlargement of the working space (muscle fibre hypertrophy). Depending on training content, the proportions of aerobic and anaerobic energy generation at the muscle cell level can change. Muscle fibre distribution is hereditary and cannot be changed with training. Larger proportions of fast twitch muscle fibres (FTF) favour speed and strength performance, larger proportions of slow twitch muscle fibres (STF) on the other hand allow stable endurance performance capacity.

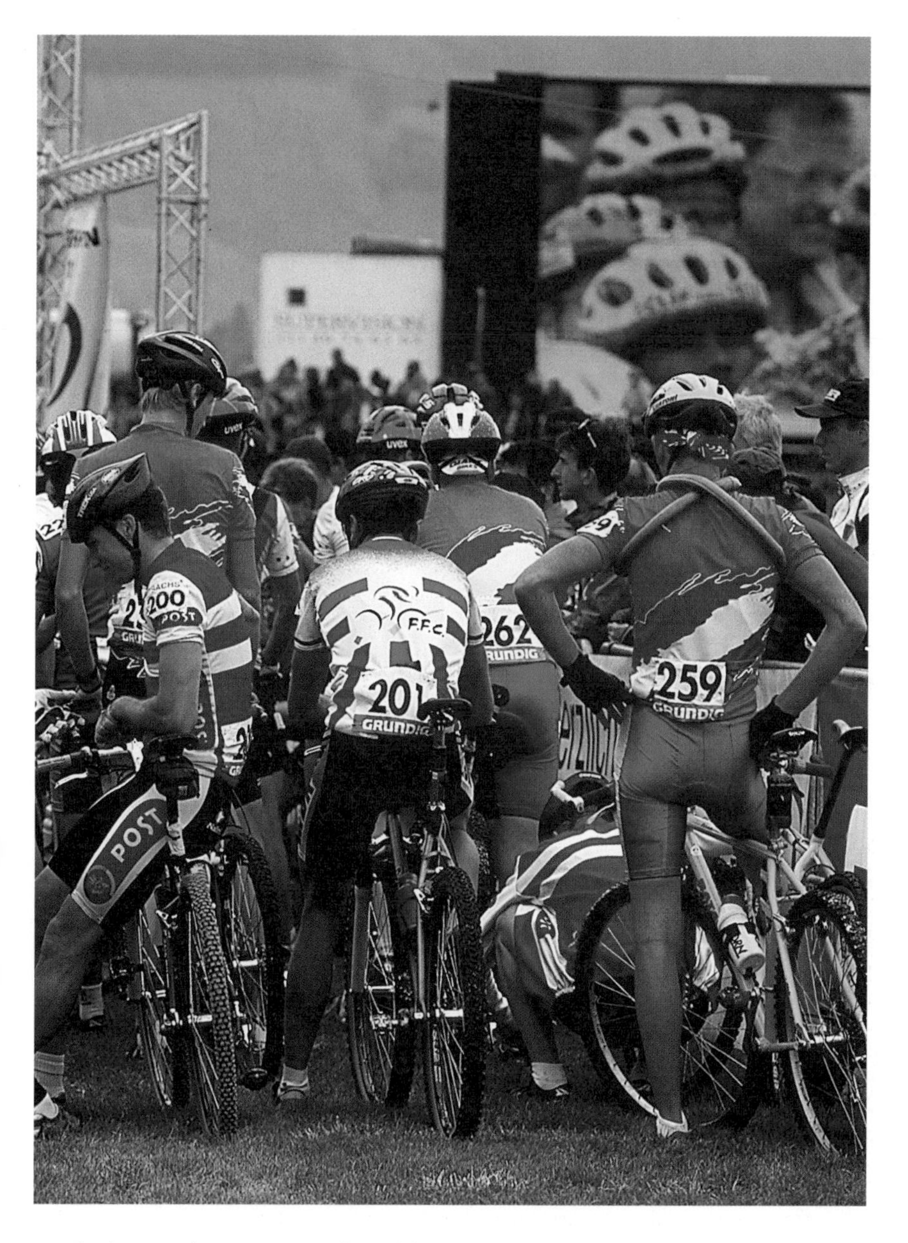

WAG's Picture and Text Agency, Freiburg (Photo: Armin Schirmaier, Freiburg)

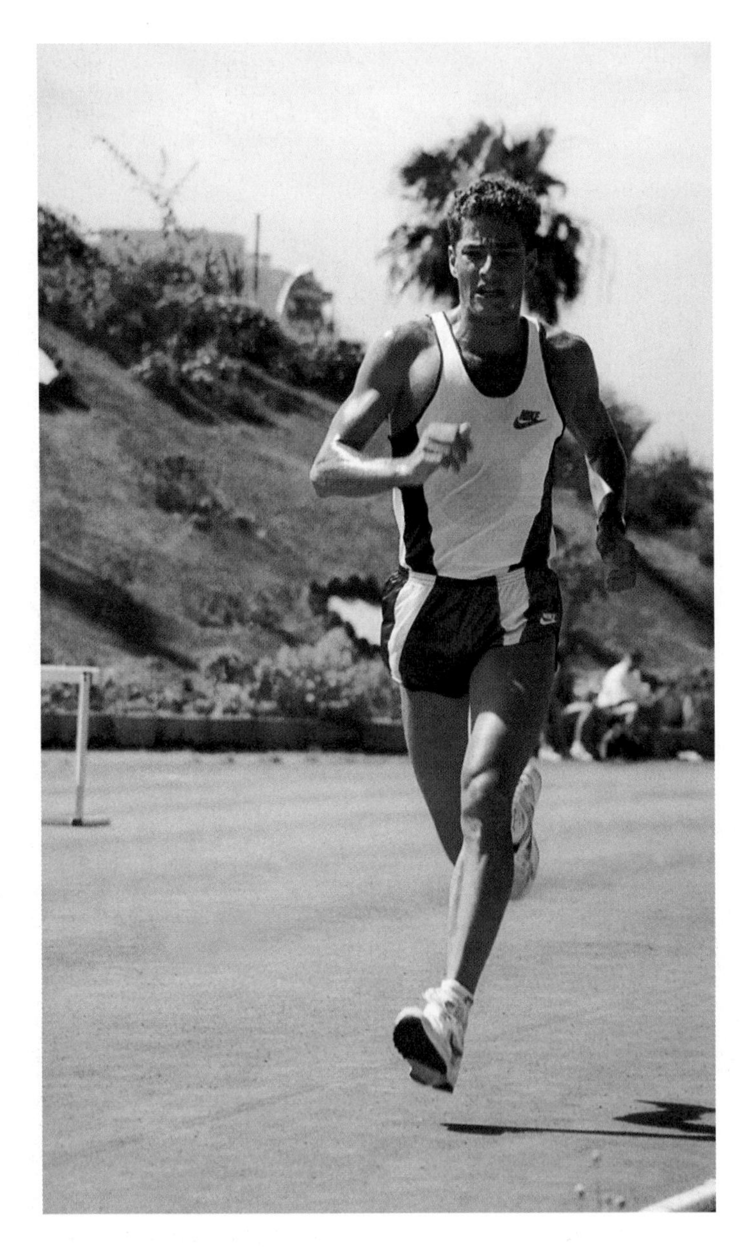

Top triathlete Lothar Leder doing interval training (Photo: Georg Neumann, Leipzig)

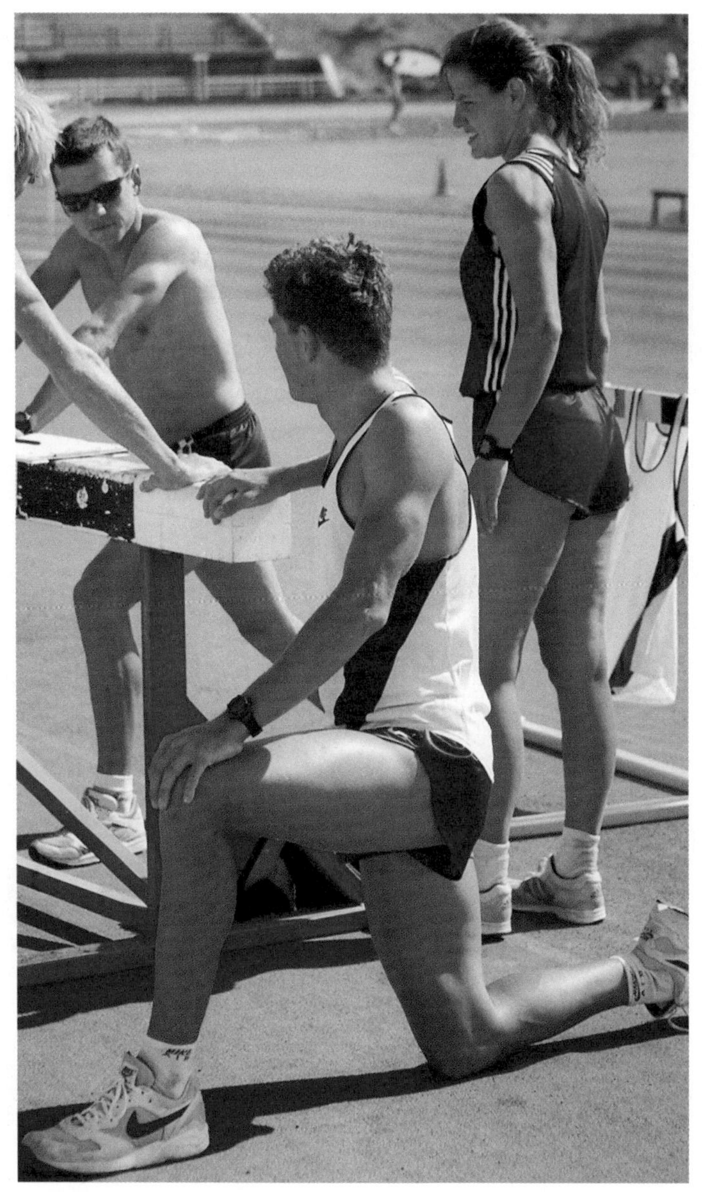

Top triathletes Lothar Leder, Thomas Hellriegel and Katja Meyer warming up before interval training (Photo: Georg Neumann, Leipzig)

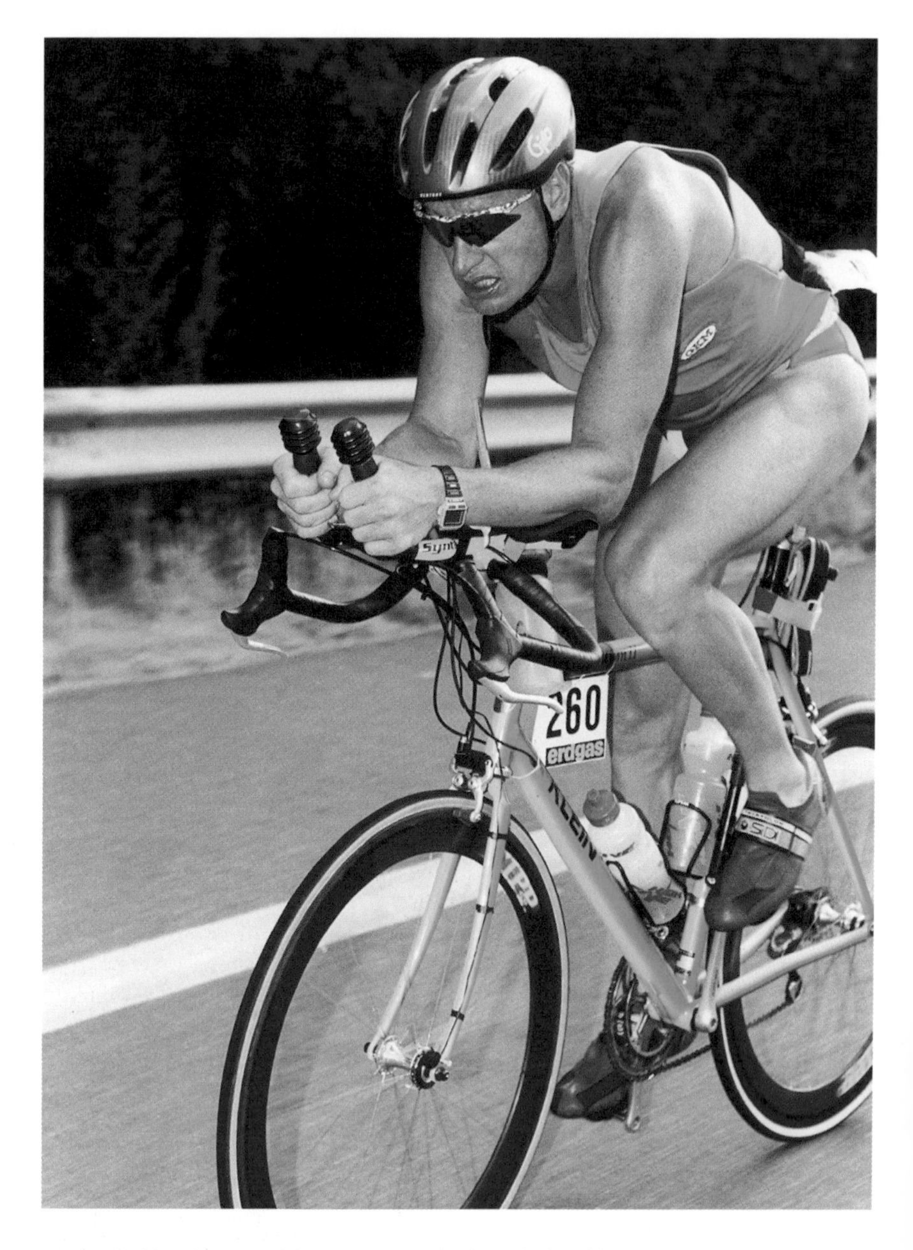

AK 30 triathlete in a race (Photo: Georg Rombach, Cadenburg)

5 Performance Goal and Training Load

The total degree of load in a year decides to a great degree whether or not the performance goal is achieved. Training by feeling is a thing of the past in all sports, especially when top performances are intended. To achieve international top performances and maintain them for longer periods of time, the use of scientifically based sport-specific training methodology cannot be done without. Training must be done professionally. Those athletes, however, who have lower performance goals, must also load themselves according to the basic principles of competitive training. Nevertheless, training in leisure or fitness sport at a lower level of load allows many variations in the structuring of load and unloading rhythms.

5.1 Performance Categories

In endurance sports three categories of athletes can be clearly differentiated according to performance goals and possible volume of training (Fig. 1/5.1, see p. 126).

Fitness Athletes (Leisure Athletes)

Fitness or leisure athletes usually practise several summer and/or winter sports. They are diverse in practising and training. The training motives are maintaining performance capacity (fitness) over longer periods of life and increasing performance capacity within the age category. The amount of training is under 300 hours per year, about four to six hours of load per week. Participation in competitions is not obligatory but is determined by the value of the experience to the individual. Maintaining health is a desirable side-effect of training.

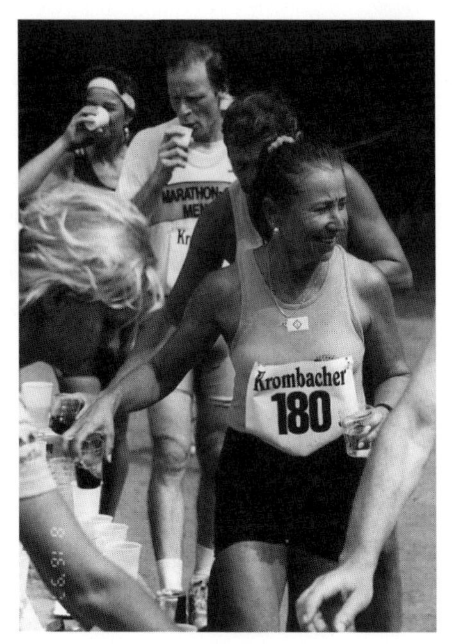

At the refreshment stop during a long- distance run (Photo: Georg Neumann, Leipzig)

Training Load in Fitness Sport (FSP), Competitive Sport (CSP) and Top Sport (TSP)

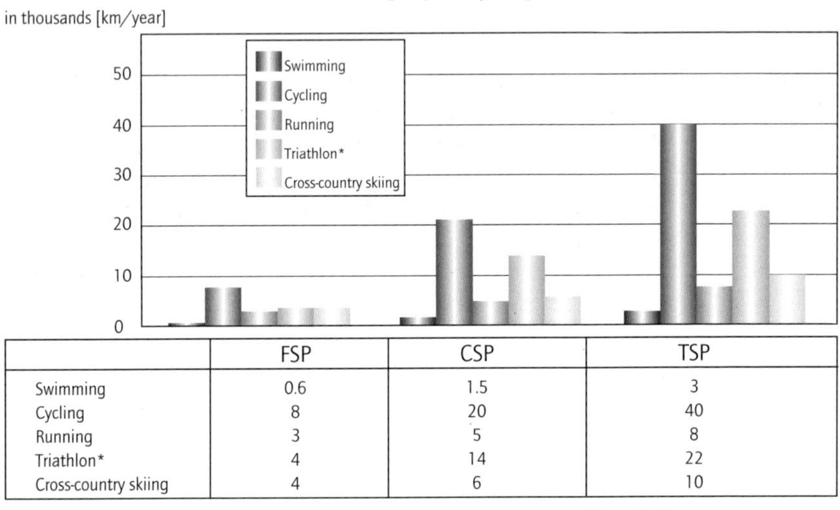

	FSP	CSP	TSP
Swimming	0.6	1.5	3
Cycling	8	20	40
Running	3	5	8
Triathlon*	4	14	22
Cross-country skiing	4	6	10

*Sum of all sports

Fig. 1/5.1: Comparison of training load in selected endurance sports during the year in the three categories of men practising sport

Competitive Athletes

These train in their spare time outside of their job and train more than 300 hours per year in one or related seasonal sport. They reach top training volumes of up to 1000 hours per year. Weekly training time is ten to fifteen hours and the volume is influenced at any particular time by preparations for selected competitions. For some athletes the loading border to top athletes is small when top performances in age categories are strived for. Increasing load is limited by occupational and social (family) influences. For short periods load of 20 hr/week while holding down a full time job is possible. Over longer periods of time the double strain causes conflicts and there is a reduction in one of the two spheres of activity. A lack of coaching increases the likelihood of incorrect load or overtraining.

Top Athletes

They train under professional conditions and reach loading levels of 1000 to 1600 hours per year. Training per week is 20 to 35 hours. Weeks of top levels of load of up to 50 hours are repeatedly possible. The foundation of top sport training is sporting talent and the possibility of social and material recognition of achievements. The rhythm of load is oriented to participation in international competitions.

Currently top performances have the following characteristics:

1. Training velocity was raised to a considerably higher level under aerobic and aerobic-anaerobic metabolism conditions and made use of accordingly in competitions.
2. The endurance and strength endurance potential of the muscles directly involved in forward propulsion was developed in such a way that a larger cycle results and was maintained in a stable manner in competitions.
3. Over the entire competition distance performance can be structured stably and variably and even when tiredness sets in, optimal movement technique is still possible.
4. The broadness of regulation of movement rates includes increases in pace according to the tactical requirements of all sections of the competition.

Summary

In relationship to the volume of training load, three groups of athletes can be characterised. These are fitness or leisure sport, competitive sport and top sport. The largest group is that of the fitness or leisure athletes. If high performances are strived for in the age categories, competitive sport begins at about 10-15 hr/week of load. If load regularly rises to over 20 hr/week then the prerequisites for top sport are created. Success is not decided by load alone, but also by talent.

5.2 Effectiveness of Training

The greatest influence on results in competitive and top sport comes from training systems. The optimisation of the training system determines the level of development in performance. Analyses of competitive training, expert judgements and athlete surveys have led to the following opinions with regard to the achievement of world-class performances in elite fields or in the age category:

- The central element in top sport is the increase in training load to at least 25-30 hr/week or 1000 to 1500 hours per year.

- Training load must be clearly oriented to a performance structure; the start in competitions takes place in fixed time periods. This means e.g. for running that training for personal top performances in a range from 5000 m to marathon distance is not likely to be very effective. This does not apply to fitness sport.

- The increase in load must always be combined with effective regenerative measures of a sports-methodological and sports medicine kind.

- The annual training structure must be concentrated on selected performance peaks. Through double periodisation two peaks are possible.

- Load tolerance for higher sport-specific training stimuli must be ensured through constant general athletic training, deliberate changes of sport, physiotherapy and other measures to encourage regeneration.

- Competitions are the most effective training means for the development of specific load stimuli.

- Individual development potential and the training methods, forms and means necessary for its realisation determine advances in performance more than ever.

In the training concepts of the world's best athletes the focus is on the optimisation of basic and strength endurance training. Training at medium altitudes is increasingly becoming a training element, especially in order to increase oxygen transport capacity.

Before the first competitions begin, the aerobic or aerobic-anaerobic performance foundations must be stably developed. Only they guarantee competition stability during the season. It is agreed that extraordinary performances and advances in performance also require extraordinary load stimuli. Training can be increased within a year and also in the course of several years. To achieve the goal it is necessary to keep up measures encouraging regeneration. One should not do without the stable accompaniment of an experienced counselling team. Often athletes who have given up constant management and had successes think they will again manage alone in future. In the long-term this behaviour is not very innovative. The potential top athlete must carry out his training and his management professionally; this does not exclude the possibility of changes to the team.

Factors favourable to performance include:
1. High level of training load at normal altitudes (below 1500 m)

2. Altitude training several times a year (altitude training chains).

3. Frequent climate changes, especially in the seasonal transitions.

4. Tight sequence of high level competitions in the season, the number of which, however, should be limited.

5. Load oriented diet and supplementation with physiological active substances.

6. Making full use of the possibilities for training control.

7. Regular sport medicine check-ups and carrying out of preventive measures to ensure load tolerance.

Summary

The effectiveness of training is based on a number of factors. The central element is the amount of regular training load. The training structure should be planned on the basis or findings of interdisciplinary sports science. For the realisation of individual potential, effective training methods, forms and means play a major role. Extraordinary performances and advances in performance call for extraordinary increases in loading. The effectiveness of increases in load depends on the use of physiological performance reserves.

5.3 Volume of Training

Analyses over several years of the development of performance and of the training of world-class athletes show that training load continues to be the central category in training and competition systems. On the basis of the performance structure of the sport, training parameters should be developed which allow an individual and effective level of total load in the annual and long-term training structure. In this way total load of up to 1500 hours per year are possible. Within the framework of this high degree of total load, up to 1000 hours per year can be trained in the sport itself. For world-class performances these high degrees of exertion are an absolute prerequisite. Talent and tactics then decide over victory or defeat in any case. The greatest talent fails if it is not prepared to accept the usual loading norm for the sport at world-class level.

Currently there are no limits to the increase in training load in sight. Problems arise in individual limiting of ability to sustain load. Increasing general and sport-specific load tolerance is a particular methodological category in the framework of increasing total load.

Athletes can only train hard if they have prepared their body over a longer period of time by means of suitable adaptation in the support apparatus and locomotor system, the central nervous system and in metabolism. The individual limiting of load tolerance usually has biological causes.

One can argue about the sense and nonsense of extreme load. Objectively, however, it must be stated that those persons who have raised the limits of their load tolerance very high have opened up new dimensions of load.

Again and again attempts are made in training practice to avoid or reduce the time consuming volume factor. Terms such as "intensification", "effectivisation" or "raising of quality" are used as arguments in favour of this. These concepts have seldom led to real advances in performance. Organisational pressures to carry out a progressive increase in load are not a licence for intensification and at the same time drastic reduction of volume. At the most they are a risky compromise.

When established findings and experience regarding the necessary total amount of training time are ignored, unstable performance characteristics are programmed.

Summary

The volume of training is the key link in competitive training in the endurance sports. The degree of training an individual can handle has meanwhile reached a level of about 1600 training hours per year in top-level sport. The longest lasting load levels are possible in combination sports, such as triathlon. Deliberately changing from one sport to another in the training year is the decisive door to increasing total load and handling regeneration.

5.4 Training Faults

Stagnation of performance capacity and decreases in performance often have complex causes. In most cases these are to be found in a lowering of performance and training standards as well as in unprofessional training organisation. The following are the causes or tendencies which result in not achieving training objectives or in insufficient performance growth rates:

- The volume of training is reduced to less than what has already been achieved.

- The intensification of training is carried out before a background of insufficient basic training.

- The necessary organisational and training methodological prerequisites for increasing the quality of training are not created.
- The frequency of competition participation is often far removed from the physiological possibilities to deal with them (too many competitions and competitions over periods that are too long).
- Training load is not systematically increased and periodised in the course of the training year.
- Load peaks in training are too close (1-2 weeks) or too long before the performance peak.
- There are individual deficits in the use of competition rules and in the active structuring of situational competition strategies.
- Insufficient mental preparation and adaptation to changed demands.
- Lack of ability to regulate load and training. Training recommendations are based on one-sided functional diagnostics which are also usually not sport-specific, and which do not sufficiently take into consideration real load in training.
- Insufficient training documentation hinders the assessment of success or failure.

Summary

Training faults often have complex causes and can rarely be explained without reliable documentation.

Increasing the intensive proportions of training load on the basis of insufficient aerobic sport-specific performance capacity or great reductions in total load are the main faults causing unstable performance. Failure to increase training load during the training year and gaps that are too long between load peaks and performance peaks hinder the development of personal top performances. Not observing load-unloading periods reduces the quality of training considerably and thus also the level of adaptation. Too many races too close together which cannot be coped with performance-physiologically shorten the individual periods of peak performance during the training year.

6 Training of Biomotor Abilities in Endurance Sport

In endurance sports longer training and competition performances are limited by increasing tiring processes. The capacity to carry out reliable ongoing usage of the body in a sport is called endurance. Endurance is always linked with concrete conditions of movements and with energetic performance prerequisites (SCHNABEL et al., 1995). Practising endurance sports requires a differentiated spectrum of biomotor abilities, which ranges from basic and strength endurance and competition-specific endurance to general prerequisites of performance (Table 1/6). For the most part endurance ability is determined by basic endurance ability, competition-specific endurance ability and the general foundations of performance. Within these trainable complexes the individual biomotor abilities endurance, strength, speed and co-ordination are included (Fig. 1/6 and 2/6).

6.1 Basic Endurance Ability

Basic endurance ability (BE ability) allows one to cover longer distances in aerobic metabolism. It is the main prerequisite for practising endurance sports. Increasing competition performance is in a proven relationship to the level of basic endurance ability (NEUMANN et al., 1995). In sports methodology the developmental level of BE ability is called Basic Endurance (BE).

Development of Abilities in Endurance Training		
Abilities	Training forms	Intensity area(%)
Competition endurance (CE)	Competition training	100
Speed endurance (SPE)	Speed endurance training	95-120
Strength endurance (SE)	Strength endurance training	85-95
Basic endurance 2 (BE2)	Basic endurance training 2	90-95
Basic endurance 1 (BE1)	Basic endurance training 1	75-90
(Compensation/regeneration)	*(Compensatory training)*	*< 70*

Table 1/6: Development of capacities in endurance training

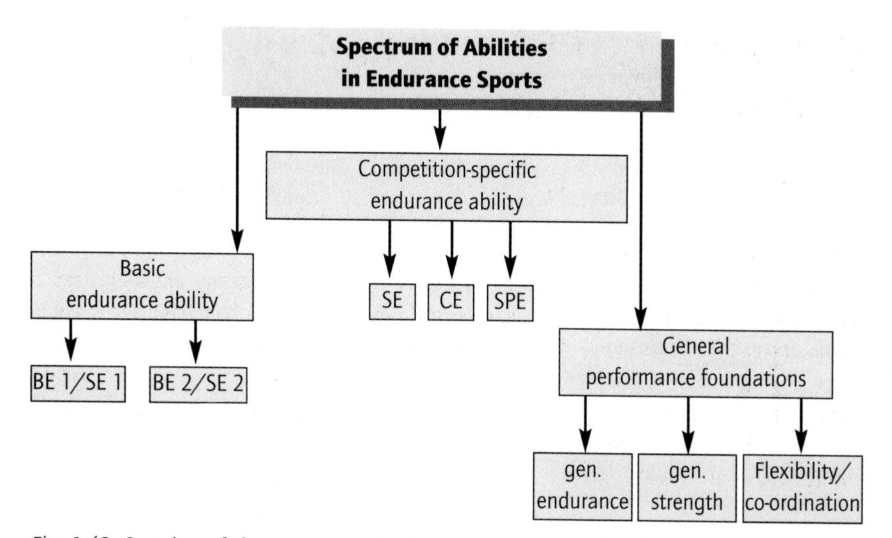

Fig. 1/6: Overview of the spectrum of endurance ability, of which the main components are basic endurance ability (BE), competition-specific endurance capacity (CE) and general performance foundations.

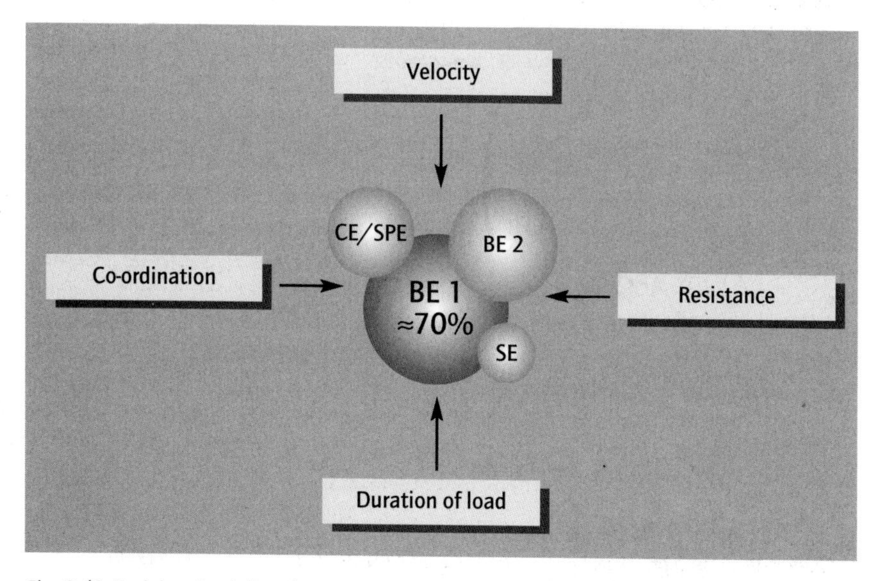

Fig. 2/6: Training, load duration, resistance, speed and sport-specific execution (co-ordination) have an effect on the muscle. No capacity is trainable in isolation.

The term basic endurance describes the adaptation of the body at the level of motor basic functions, energy transformation, substrate supply and also of mental stability to cope with endurance. The criterion for assessing BE is the velocity reached or performance in the area of submaximal load. Performance-physiologically, BE can also be characterised with regard to metabolism, breathing and cardiovascular (circulation) behaviour. The terms aerobic and anaerobic metabolism thresholds have become accepted, usually determined from lactate levels (NEUMANN/SCHÜLER, 1994). Basic endurance or basic endurance ability is developed using the variants of basic endurance training.

Basic Endurance Training

In the training process of endurance sports the development of basic endurance plays a key role. BE ability has a prerequisite function for coping with increasingly high velocities in competitions. With a percentage of 60-85% of the total training volume, BE training is the main focus which determines development.

BE training must have three key qualities:

1. BE training is oriented to **duration**.
2. BE training is oriented to **velocity**.
3. BE training is oriented to **resistance components**.

Basic Endurance 1 Training (BE 1)

BE 1 training calls for a large volume of training per week. Thus duration is the decisive loading stimulus. The training distance is chosen in such a way that load can be applied in a stable aerobic metabolism situation. Velocity during training is between 75-85% of individual performance capacity. Up to 80% of this training field is made use of in the methodological structuring of the prescribed distances (see chapter 6.5). The best method for BE 1 training is the continuous method. With this method both glycogen and fatty acids are used for energy generation in aerobic metabolism.

Basic Endurance 2 Training (BE 2)

BE 2 training calls for higher velocity and is not mainly duration-oriented. With the increase in velocity in BE 2 training it is intended to cross over current aerobic performance capacity limits. For this, relatively high velocities and short distances are always required. The volume of training in BE 2 should only make up 10-25% of the total volume of load.

Ability Spectrum Generally Used in Endurance Sports		
Abilities	Term	Metabolism
Basic endurance	BE 1	aerobic
Strength endurance	SE 1	aerobic
Basic endurance	BE 2	aerobic-anaerobic
Strength endurance	SE 2	aerobic-anaerobic
Competition-specific endurance	CE	anaerobic-aerobic
Speed endurance	SPE	anaerobic
Strength/speed	ST/SP	anaerobic
Compensation and regeneration	CO	aerobic

Table 1/6.1: Ability spectrum generally used in endurance sports

Because the distances are shorter than in BE 1 training, intensity must rise to 85-95% of individual performance. Higher speeds in BE 2 training prepare the way for competition-specific endurance ability.

Suitable methods for BE 2 training include intensive and variable continuous training as well as extensive forms of interval training.

Strength Endurance 1 and 2 (SE 1 and 2)

In endurance sports, strength training is primarily endurance training against increased resistance. The point of reference is the median degree of resistance required in competitions. The increases in resistance in the phases of start, course, intermediate and finishing sprints must be differentiated from this.

The prerequisites for SE 1 and SE 2 training are present when additional resistance demands are applied within the framework of BE 1 and BE 2 training (Table 1/6.1). Experience in endurance sports indicates that up to 50% of BE training should have an emphasis on resistance (REISS, 1992). In road cycling it is now normal to cycle for hours against resistance (e.g. alpine passes in high gears).

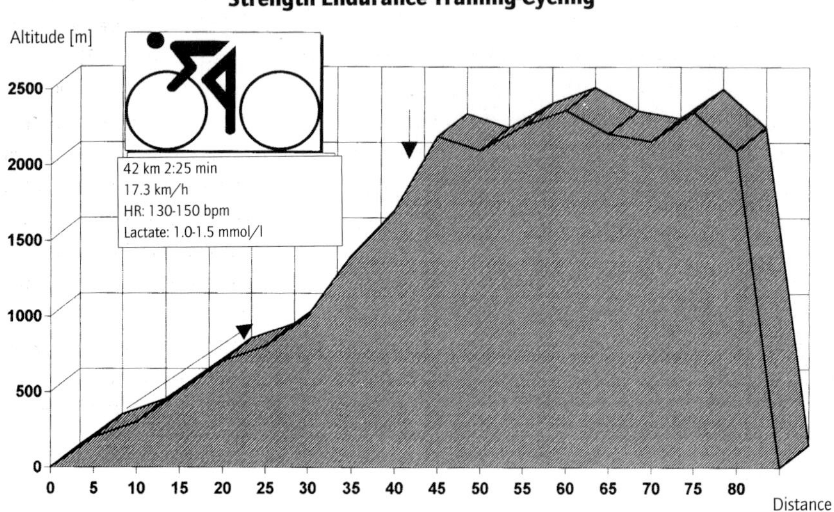

Fig. 1/6.1: Example of structuring of strength endurance training in cycling through long uphill climbs at low speed and in aerobic metabolism

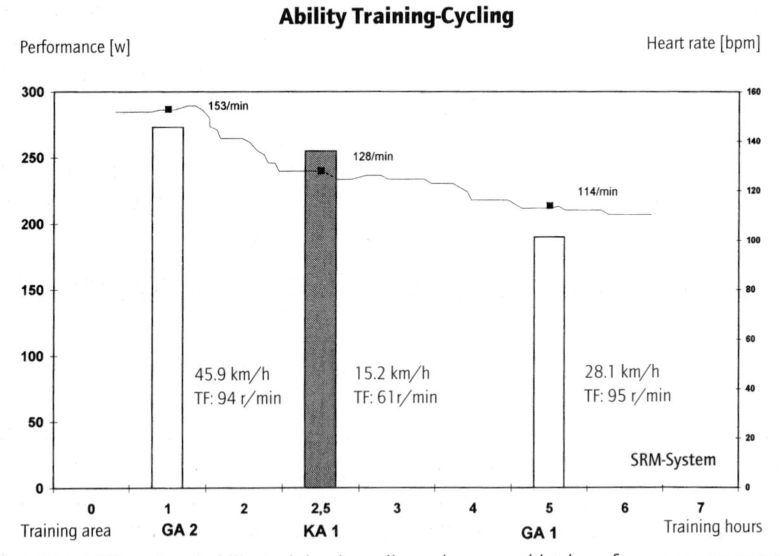

Fig. 2/6.1: Differentiated ability training in cycling, where an athlete's performance was measured using the SRM System (Schoberer Cycle Measuring System) directly attached to the racing bike.

Biologically, SE training generates a greater hypertrophy stimulus to the muscles than does BE training. This stimulus is necessary to create lasting adaptation, for under low resistance endurance load, the strength potential of sport-specific muscles hardly increases at all (see Fig. 3/4.7).

Duration-oriented SE training should include resistances which are greater than competition demands (Fig. 1/6.1, see p. 136). Longer distances are preferable, even when SE training takes place in the form of intervals. Metabolism should be aerobic. Studies involving runners showed that to maintain the training areas in SE training, tractive resistance of 2 kp requires a reduction in velocity of 0.25 to 0.5 m/s compared to the normal velocity programme without tractive resistance (CBE training). When this velocity reduction took place during tractive resistance training in running the stride rate did not change and it was possible to maintain the aerobic and the aerobic-anaerobic metabolism forms (REISS et al., 1994).

In SE training, the training distances (load duration) are shorter than in comparable endurance training (Fig. 2/6.1, see p. 136). Major muscle acidity should be avoided in SE training. If in doubt, extend the duration of load for the resistance stimulus so that the aerobic metabolism form is not departed from.

Summary

Basic endurance ability (BE ability) is the ability to cover a longer distance in the aerobic metabolism form. BE is the decisive prerequisite for endurance performance as 60-80 % of training is used to develop BE ability. BE consists of an extensive and an intensive component, BE 1 and BE 2. BE 1 is trained at 75-85 % of individual performance capacity, BE 2 at 85-95 %. Endurance training can also be carried out with increased resistance. The ability developed in this way is called strength endurance (SE). Analogous to BE ability, SE ability is developed in the form of SE 1 and SE 2 training. Endurance training with an emphasis on resistance can be up to 50 % of BE training and should be done in the aerobic metabolism area.

6.2 Competition-specific Endurance Ability

Competition specific endurance ability (CSE) ensures maximum race velocity over various distances. This occurs through the usage of aerobic-anaerobic energy metabolism and the inclusion of the fast twitch muscle fibres (FTF) in the programme of movement. Developing competition-specific endurance in training means that an increasingly greater cycle distance (propulsion) per time unit in the individual cycle of movement is achieved. In competitions this ability must be able to be called upon in a high band of variation of the cycle time (movement rate).

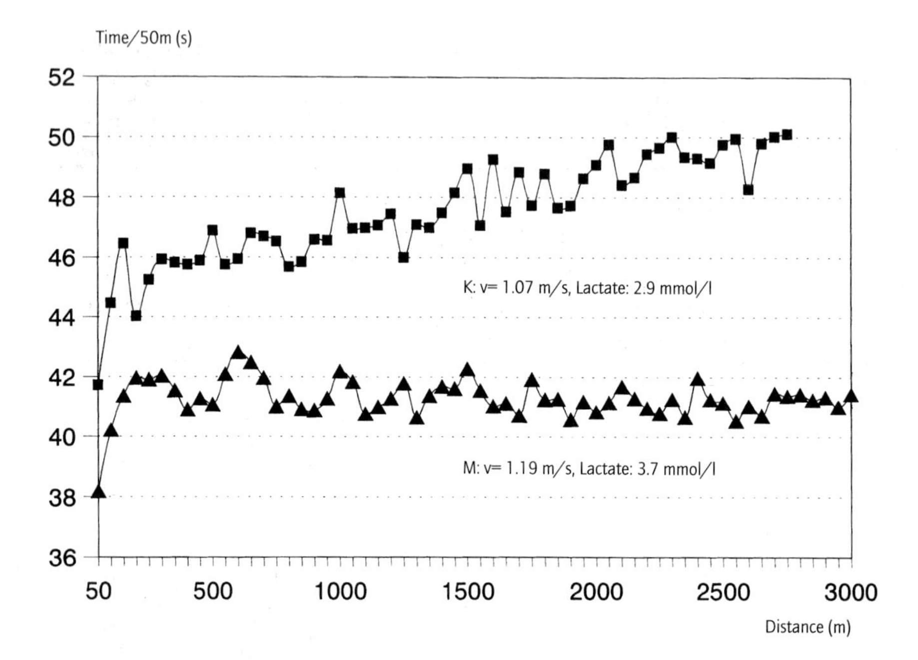

Fig. 1/6.2: Comparison of swimming performances over 3000m covered by two female triathletes in differing section times. K. initially overestimated her performance capacity and became increasingly slower and did not complete the distance.

From a metabolism point of view in the particular sports, this assumes high aerobic and anaerobic (glycolytical) energy flow rates. A characteristic of CSE is the increase in maximum oxygen intake (VO_2 max). The decisive link for the development of competition-specific endurance is the learning of new targeting patterns for the sport-specific propulsion muscles. The best training means for this are competitions themselves. From a sports-methodology point of view the repertoire for developing competition-specific endurance ability should include coping with starts, intermediate and finishing sprints, inclines and descents. The speed and strength training necessary for CSE derives from strength-time progressions, strength-distance progressions, the relationship between active and passive phases in the movement cycle, the variability in the use of technique and recovery capacity during competitions. The development of CSE is assessed using velocity progression in competitions and the structure of movement (Fig. 1/6.2).

Competition-specific endurance is developed analogous to BE ability using an appropriate training form. This training form is competition-specific endurance training, before which BE 1 and BE 2 training with time prognosis should be placed (Table 1/6.2).

		Basic endurance training		Competition-specific endurance training	
	Measurement factors	BE 1	BE 2	SPE 1	Prognosis CSE complex
Swimming	Distance (m) Time Velocity (m/s) Heart rate (bpm) Lactate (mmol/l)	3000 400 m in 4:56 min 1.35 140-150 3-4	5 x 400 400 m in 4:45 min 1.40 160-180 4-6	15 x 100 100 m in 1:02 min 1.6 180-190 6-9	1500 100 m in 1:08 min 1.47 170-180 5-7
Cycling	Distance (m) Time Velocity (m/s) Heart rate (bpm) Lactate (mmol/l)	150 5 h 31 120-140 1-2	4 x 10 10 km in 14:17 min 42 150-170 2,5-5	6 x 2 2 km in 2:30 min 48 160-180 5-8	40 10 km in 13:30 min 44.4 170-180 4-5
Running	Distance (m) Time Velocity (m/s) Heart rate (bpm) Lactate (mmol/l)	20 km 1000 m in 4:00 min 3.80 130-160 1.5-2.5	10 x 1000 m 1000 m in 3:16 min 5.10 170-180 3-4	20 x 400 m 400 m in 1:10 min 5.70 180-190 4-10	1000 m 1000 m in 3:05 min 5.38 170-190 5-7

Table 1/6.2: Prognosis-oriented training requirements Triathlon Olympic Distance/Men (selected training standards)

Competition-specific endurance training (CSE training) has several contents and represents a complex for the development of at least three capacities. The three main elements of CE training are:

1. Competition endurance (CE)
2. Sport-specific speed endurance (SPE)
3. Sport-specific strength endurance (SE)

Through training in the corresponding velocities and resistances the necessary variability for competitions is prepared. The training goal is the development of competition-specific performance ability in a wide spectrum. This spectrum is characterised by the ability to cope with underdistance and overdistance demands, related to the particular distance (REISS/ERNST/GOHLITZ, 1996).

This serves the competition pace over the preferred distance. The evidence of these methodological demands are the massive velocity increases in the range of 400 m to 1500 m or even over 5000 m e.g. during a 10,000 m run which led to new records.

The results of tests and experience of VERCHOSHANSKIJ (1992), MADER (1992), REISS et al. (1994) show that the effectiveness of CSE training depends on the level of BE, SE and SPE ability reached.

Competition endurance is differentiated into short, mid and long duration endurance (see chapter 7). Because of their biological foundations, these abilities function independent of the sport and are influenced by the interplay between duration and intensity of load.

Competition Endurance Training (CE)

The training competition itself is the best form of CE training. This sport-specific training form should be developed in the variation range of competition performances. Training is carried out according to the control and competition method with velocities and distances close to competition conditions. In CE training the amount of training is less than 5% of the total training volume. Depending on the distance, the velocity should be about 95-105 % of individual performance capacity.

Speed Endurance Training (SPE)

Speed endurance training is learning training for the development of competition endurance. With SPE motor training a lasting adaptation of individual speed is aimed for. The emphases of SPE training are oriented towards target pace in competition situations (prognosis performance), the movement rate to be calculated and the necessary forward propulsion. The methods used are intensive forms of interval training. The lactic proportion of energy generation is higher than in real competition situations. The amount of training in SPE training is only 2-3 % of the total training volume. The spectrum of training velocities ranges from 100-120 %, in relation to the targeted distance.

Strength Endurance Training (SE)

The typical strength training of the CSE is characterised by fast strength effort within a single movement cycle and its multiple repetition. In addition the mobilization ability for start-, intermediate- and final spurt situations is developed. The effect of this strength training is converted event-specific and developed by event-specific strength endurance, speed strength endurance and maximum strength training. Greater movement propulsion is only physiologically possible through a particular sport-specifically trained muscle fibre hypertrophy. The development of the necessary strength abilities varies from sport to sport, according to competition demands and specific aspects of the distance. The sport-specific forms of SE training, which take place under anaerobic-aerobic metabolism conditions, are structured according to the interval or competition method. The strength impulses in the single cycle should be above the average strength impulses of the single cycles of motion in competitions. SE training involves repetitions which correspond to the sections of a competition as well as to technical demands similar to competition conditions but with higher resistances. Training velocities are oriented to competition and speed endurance training. The volume of training in SE training is, as in SPE training, about 2-3% of the total training volume.

Summary

Competition-specific endurance ability (CSE) represents a complex of abilities which make it possible to cover distances in a sport at the highest possible velocity. From a physiological point of view, competition-specific endurance ability, corresponding to the requirements of performance structure, involves all metabolism forms, including the preferred targeting and using of high proportions of fast twitch muscle fibres (FTF) in the sport-specific programme of movement. The methods for developing this complex ability are the competition itself as well as speed and strength endurance training. In most endurance sports stable competition performances can only be achieved and repeated with high aerobic performance foundations.

6.3 Basic Prerequisites for Performance

The training of basic prerequisites for performance is necessary for the development of specific performance capacity and for a more stable level of aerobic endurance and strength abilities, speed capacities as well as technical and co-ordinative foundations.

Basic prerequisites for performance or the general state of being trained are significant for raising the load tolerance of the body and for optimising regeneration.

Through the application of general and semi-specific training means, the necessary effects for the sport (event) in the area of general endurance, strength and speed foundations are to be achieved. General endurance is linked to the extension of aerobic, aerobic-anaerobic and alactic energy potentials. The general strength foundations should be developed in the muscles most important to the particular event. Deliberate neuro-muscular targeting, demands on reaction ability and motor switching ability support the development of the general speed foundations. Furthermore, in the area of general agility, achieving the necessary flexibility, stretching and relaxing ability for sport-specific needs is important.

Therefore general performance foundations should constantly be raised to a new level in long-term and several year long building up of performance, and training with general means should be oriented to specific requirements.

Summary

The basic prerequisites for performance represent the general and diverse state of being trained. Agility, flexibility, stretching and relaxing abilities are important prerequisites for performance capacity in the sport and for load tolerance. These can be developed using unspecific and semi-specific training means and are a permanent component of basic performance ability at a level necessary for the sport.

6.4 Relationship between Strength Ability and Technique

An athlete's movement only happens as a result of the co-ordinated effect of the strength of muscles. It requires strength transmission in the form of braking and accelerating strength, static energy and lifting capacity. Inertia, friction and current energy also have an effect. There can be no technique without the use of energy and vice versa. Each sport-specific movement is linked to a typical power progression. The biomechanical model is oriented to the most effective use of energy in each case and can be objectivised with the aid of modern video technology. Currently energy use can only be assessed in connection with external effects. If there is a change in external conditions during a competition a certain degree of variability in technique becomes necessary. It must be variable in relation to the range of influences. Some sports, such as cross-country skiing, call for a constant repertoire of additional movement. The various course profiles call for these capacities and skills in order to be able to handle them.

In endurance sports, over most of each competition section the use of strength is dosed and adapted to the duration of movement.

The most important training means is the original competition or training close to competition conditions in the specific movement and the appropriate use of technique. In a state of tiredness the technical model of forward movement changes.

Summary

Sporting technique is linked to specific strength abilities. The use of strength or energy must always adapt to changes in technique. For the effective use of energy in the various sports, biomechanical models have been developed which can be objectivised and assessed with the aid of video technology. Mastery of sporting technique becomes obvious in competition and especially with increasing tiredness.

6.5 Training Areas

Training to develop the differentiated endurance abilities takes place in training areas (intensity areas). In training practice, six training areas are used (Table 1/6.5, see p. 144). For the complex development of abilities the following training areas are differentiated:

- Competition-specific endurance training (CSE training),
- Basic endurance training 2 (BE 2 training)
- Strength endurance training 2 (SE 2 training)
- Basic endurance training 1 (BE 1 training)
- Strength endurance training (SE 1 training)
- Compensatory training (CO training)

The terms for the training areas have developed historically in the individual sports and still vary (Table 2/6.5, see p. 145).

Uniformity of the training areas would be helpful for mutual understanding of athletes, coaches and sports scientists. There would be no difficulty in harmonising the terms because the physiological background for the different methodological terms in the sport functions independently of it (NEUMANN et al., 1995). In the endurance sports it is possible to agree on a generally necessary ability spectrum of which different proportions are made use of and which make use of metabolism to differing degrees. The intensity areas are velocity categories graded from competition performance (Table 3/6.5, see p. 145). Maintaining certain proportions of load in the individual training areas is the real secret of successful competitive training.

	CSE training	BE 2 training	SE 2 training	SE 1 training	SE 1 training	CO training
OBJECTIVE	• Development of competition-specific endurance ability	• Development of basic endurance ability • Increase aerobic/ anaerobic performance capacity	• Development of aerobic/ anaerobic strength endurance ability	• Stabilisation and development of basic endurance ability • Increase aerobic performance capacity	• Development and stabilisation of aerobic strength endurance ability	• Support regeneration • Increase load tolerance for following intensive training
METHOD	• Competition method - • Intensive interval method • Repetition method	• Extensive interval method • Fartlek method • Alternating continuous method	• Intensive interval method • Repetition method • Fartlek method	• Continuous method • Fartlek method	• Continuous method • Alternating continuous method • Extensive interval method	• Short continuous method
INTENSITY	• High to very high • Lactate: above 6.0 mmol/l Heart rate (HR) > 90% of HR max	• Medium – high • Lactate: 3.0-6.0 mmol/l • HR 80-90% of HR max	• High • Lactate: 4.0-7.0 mmol/l • HR 75-95% of HR max	• Low – medium • Lactate: 1.5-2.5 mmol/l • HR 65-80% of HR max	• Medium • Lactate: 2.0-3.0 mmol/l • HR 75-85% of HR max	• Very low • Lactate: under 2.0 mmol/l • HR 60-70% of HR max

(CO: Regeneration and compensatory training
BE: Basic endurance training
CSE: Competition-specific endurance training
SE: Strength endurance training)

Table 1/6.5: Summary of objectives, methods and intensities for training in the training areas of the endurance sports

Intensity of load	Triathlon	Swimming	Cycling	Running	Cross-country skiing
Low	BE 1	BE 1	B 1	BE 1 CRun	SA
Medium	BE 1/BE 2	BE 1/BE 2	BE 2	BE 2 CRun	TA/DA
High	BE 2	BE 2	DFA	BE 2 TR	DFA
Very high	CE	CE	CE	CE	CSE
Very high	SPE	SPE	SPE	TA	BA

SA Stabilising area, BE Basic endurance, B Basic endurance, CRun Continuous run, DA Development area, BE 2 Basic endurance 2, TR Tempo run, CSE Competition-specific endurance, CE Competition endurance, SPE Speed endurance, TA Top area, BA Borderline area

Table 2/6.5: The training fields in selected endurance sports

Sports	SPE	CE	BE 2	BE 1
Swimming	1.8 m/s	1.50 m/s	1.4 m/s	1.25 m/s
Cycling	15 m/s (54 km/h)	12.5 m/s (45 km/h)	11.7 m/s (42 km/h)	8.6 m/s (31 km/h)
Running*	6.6 m/s 110-120%	5.4 m/s 95-105%	5.2 m/s 90-95%	4.3 m/s 70-90%

* derived from 10 km performance

Table 3/6.5: Velocity guidelines for ability development to achieve top-class performances in triathlon or average performances for specialists in the individual sports

Training forms	Sports	Training units (km)	Series (km)	Rate (1/min)	Heart rate (bpm)	Lactate (mmol/l)
Competition-specific endurance (CSE)	Swimming	1 - 2	10 - 20 x 100 m	40 - 46 *	maximum	7 - 12
	Cycling	20 - 40		90 - 140 rpm	maximum	6 - 8
	Running	3 - 10			maximum	6 - 10
	Skiing	1 - 15	10 - 15 x 1		maximum	8 - 12
Basic endurance 2 (BE 2)	Swimming	1.5 - 3	5 - 10 x 300 m	35 - 41	170 - 180	5 - 7
	Cycling	30 - 75	5 - 10 x 6	90 - 120 rpm	160 - 170	3 - 6
	Running	4 - 15	8 - 10 x 1		165 - 175	3 - 6
	Skiing	5 - 20	8 - 10 x 2		160 - 170	3 - 6
Basic endurance 1 (BE 1)	Swimming	3 - 8	4 - 8 x 400 m	30 - 36 *	130 - 140	2 - 4
	Cycling	50 - 200		90 - 100 rpm	120 - 130	2 - 2.5
	Running	10 - 45			130 - 140	2 - 2.5
	Skiing	15 - 50			130 - 150	2 - 3
Compensation	Swimming	1 - 2			< 120	< 2
	Cycling	20 - 50		80 - 90 rpm	< 100	< 1.5
	Running	5 - 10			< 120	< 1.5 - 2
	Skiing	5 - 15			< 130	< 2

Table 4/6.5: Load options in four training areas in selected sports, regulated using sports-methodological and biological measuring indicators.
(Rate of movement in freestyle over 400-1500 m)*

Behind this is the experience gathered on how the use of training stimuli over certain periods affects one individually (Table 4/6.5, see above).

Effective endurance training depends on whether one succeeds in finding the right standard for load (MARTIN et al., 1997). If velocities are not kept to when carrying out training load, under- or overloading of the body is possible, especially when training is too intensive over longer distances. Incorrect adaptation or drops in performance are the result. Keeping to certain proportions in the training areas is dependent on total load. When total load is less, as is usual in fitness or competitive sport, training is usually more intensive (Fig. 1/6.5, see p. 147). In competitive sport, proven proportions of the training areas in the particular sports should be kept to regardless of total load (PFÜTZNER, 1995; FRANZ/PFÜTZNER, 1997). The amount in BE training plays a key role for participation in numerous competitions (Fig. 2/6.5, see p. 148). The number of competitions varies in the endurance sports (Fig. 3/6.5, see p. 149).

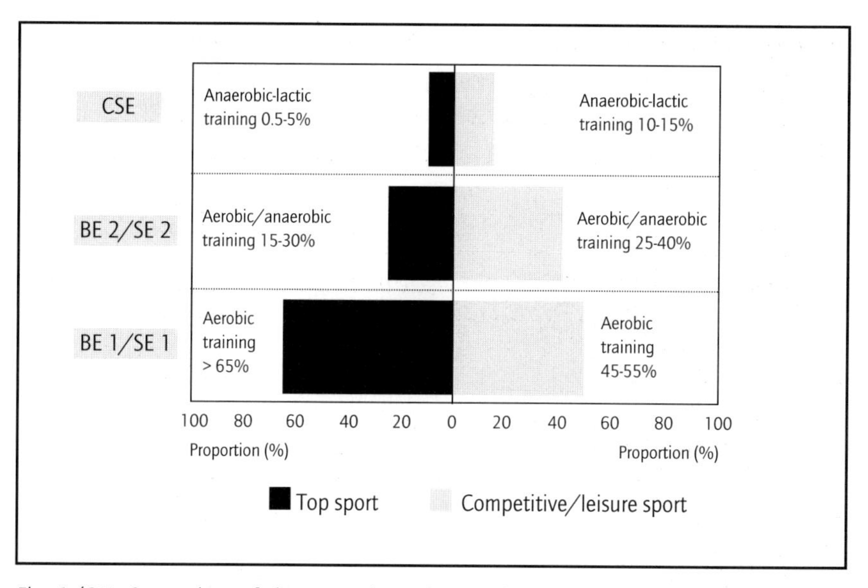

Fig. 1/6.5: Comparison of the proportions of competiton-specific endurance training (CSE), basic endurance (strength endurance) training (BE 2/SE 2) and basic endurance (strength endurance) 1 training (BE 1/SE 1) with top athletes and average competitive or leisure athletes. Because of lower total load, training in competitive or leisure sport is always more intensive.

Summary

The training areas are fixed regulatory areas for the development of functional systems determining performance. The orientation point is individual maximum performance capacity either as an objective or as the current situation. Because load in the training areas occurs in grades of intensity, they are also called intensity areas. The possible range in training sport-specific velocities takes into consideration that training involves residual tiredness and that in its repetition real performance capacity is lower. Intensive training or participation in competitions is always dependent on the absolute amount of basic endurance (BE) training. The higher the amount of BE training, the more competitions are possible. Increasing training intensity or frequent competition participation without carrying out sufficient foundational training (BE training) is always risky.

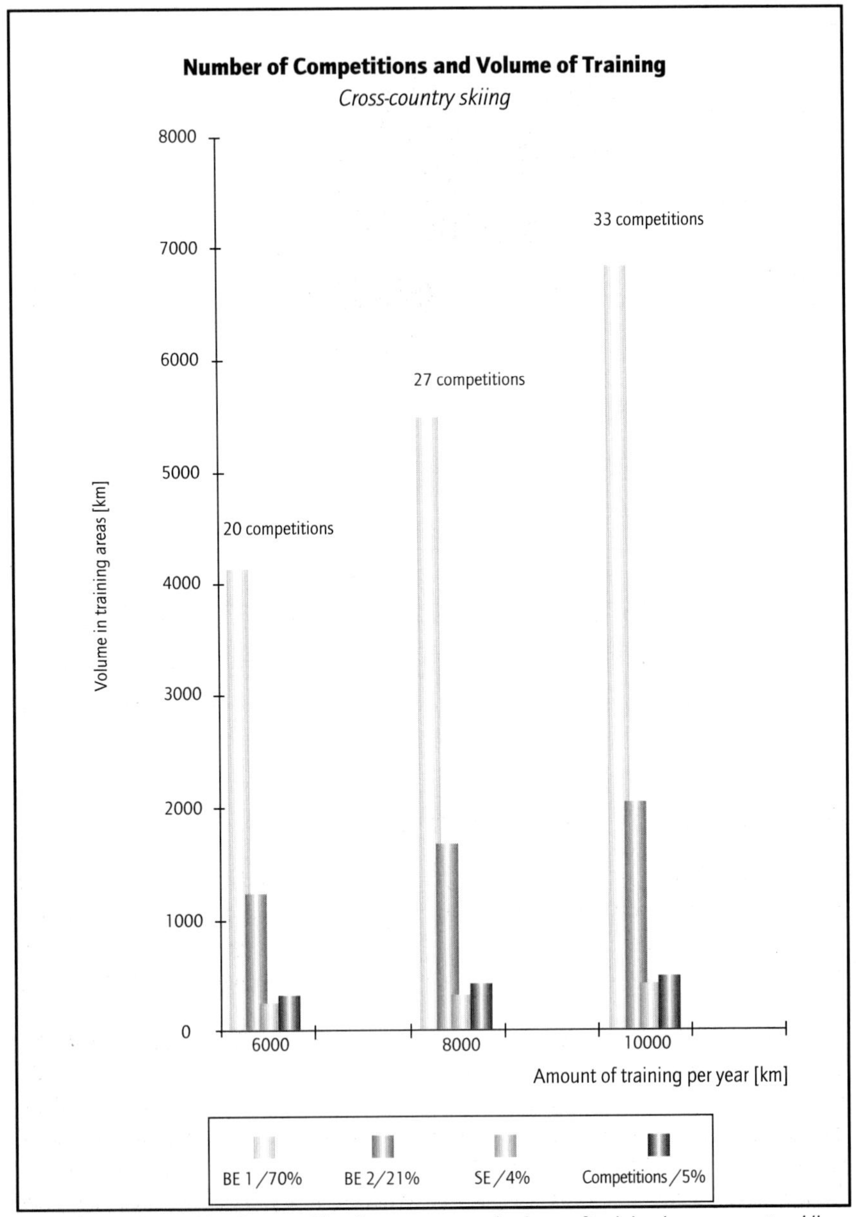

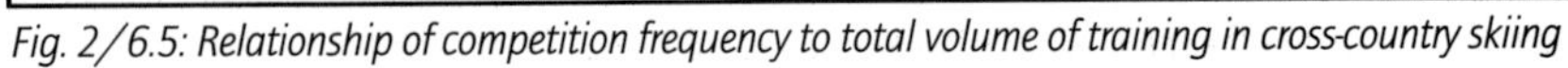

Fig. 2/6.5: Relationship of competition frequency to total volume of training in cross-country skiing

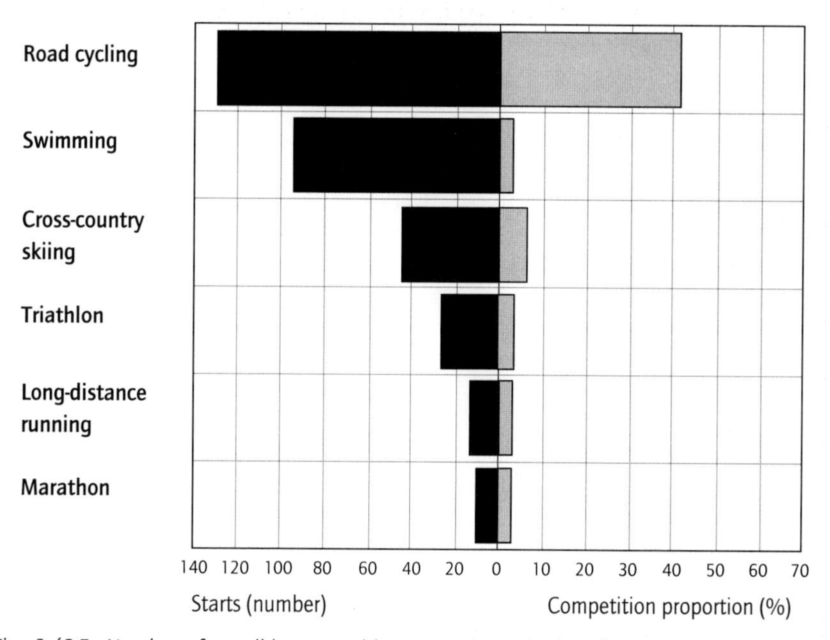

Fig. 3/6.5: Number of possible competition starts in various endurance sports and their proportion of total training volume as a percentage

6.6 Velocity in Endurance Training

Determining targets for the development of competition performance and the main performance factors on the basis of competition analyses creates the foundation for developing abilities (Table 1/6.6, see p. 150). In endurance sports the development of abilities should occur through year-round application of the principles of velocity training (PFÜTZNER/REISS, 1996).

Training sport-specific velocities is a major training principle. The concept assumes that increasing swimming, cycling, running or cross-country skiing velocity over the particular competition distance requires the same increase in velocity over the corresponding training distance. Without higher training velocities, an improvement in competition performance is hardly possible (REISS/PFÜTZNER, 1993; REISS et al., 1996). The required velocities for capacity development are at the same time the basis for structuring the corresponding training standards, they are the main control factors (see Table 1/6.2).

Discipline	SE/S (m/s)	km/h	CE (m/s)	km/h	BE 2 (m/s)	km/h	BE 1 (m/s)	km/h
Swimming	1.8	6.5	1.5	5.4	1.4	5.0	1.25	4.5
Cycling	13.3	48.0	12.5	45.0	11.7	42.0	8.6	31.0
Running	6.6	23.8	5.4	19.4	5.2	18.7	4.2	15.1

Table 1/6.6: Targets for ability development for achieving top performances in Olympic distance triathlon

For this reason the basic requirement in training, especially in BE 2, SE and CE training, is to train over accurately measured distances.

Depending on velocity, endurance training always occurs in two ability groups. The first ability group includes basic endurance and strength endurance and the second group includes competition-specific endurance. Both ability complexes are closely linked and mutually determine each other.

Summary

Endurance training should always occur at predetermined or targeted velocities. This involves exactly measured training distances or performance analysis aids. Documenting competitive training in hours is not sufficient as it allows no assessment of the quality of load. In this way the development of competition-specific endurance can be endangered through velocities that are too low or too high.

6.7 Load Parameters and Training Principles

The key to developing capacities in endurance sports is to create a system of load parameters for the particular sport/event which is the prerequisite for individual training schedules. The schedules serve the development of differentiated abilities. Training the capacities takes place on the basis of sport-specific adapted training principles. The training principles are instructions for the planning and execution of training and claim to be valid for most sports even with differing performance abilities of athletes. Currently there is a confusing number of training principles (SCHNABEL et al., 1995). The following overview lists the training principles which in a narrower sense are related to the "methodological structuring of training" (PFÜTZNER, 1990).

Important training principles for optimal structuring of endurance training are:

1. Principle of orienting sports training to the targeted sporting performance and its structure

Achieving planned sporting performance only succeeds when there is harmony between performance strucutre and training structure. This requires absolute derivation of all sub-goals, contents and structures of training in the individual training stages from the requirements of the performance structure of the sport.

2. Principle of correctly timed and increasing specialisation

In order to achieve high sporting performance in the sport/event, increasingly specialised training on the basis of high motor performance capacity and ability to cope with load must be built up.

3. Principle of periodisation and cyclisation

The development of sporting performance capacity is based on a build-up through the year and over several years. The training sections differ in content as well as methodological structuring of load and are repeated at increasingly higher levels.

4. Principle of consistency and co-ordination in developing performance prerequisites

The targeted development of sporting performance capacity is only possible through a meshing with further sport-specific performance prerequisites which must be trained in a training session or micro-cycle taking into consideration their mutual relationships.

5. Principle of accentuation and continuity

In building-up sporting performance capacity, accentuations must be placed at certain times in structuring capacity development and in the use of training means. It must be ensured, however, that continuous performance development and increase in load is not interrupted for longer periods.

6. Principle of progressive (gradual/rapid/varied) increase in loading

If sporting performance capacity is to be improved long-term, training load must be systematically increased. The necessary adaptations are triggered by increased use of the organ systems relevant to performance and recovery following this.

7. Principle of permanent training control

To ensure an optimal progression of the training process, the effect chain of training planning, performance diagnostics, competition and training analysis must be applied. From this, further derivations for the structuring of training must be made. One-sided evaluation of training and of performance states are of little value in competitive sport.

An important prerequisite for competitive or performance-oriented training is the annual increase in load (see Fig. 2/8, p. 180). The determining of the individual level of total exertion occurs in the form of training time. Here, optimally structured long term performance build-up under consideration of top performance age plays a vital role. In top triathlon, for example, a minimum of 1000 hours of sport-specific training is assumed. These load parameters can be realised as normal or accentuated (Table 1/6.7, see p. 153).

Accentuated training creates a greater load stimulus. In the course of the year the effect of load must be increased through qualitative and quantitative changes in training sessions (greater resistance, increase in average distance) as well as an increase in the proportion of load in the aerobic-anaerobic transitional area (BE 2 training). Here BE 2 training has a key role between aerobic basic training and preparing competition-specific capacity.

Despite increasing specialisation in the build-up over the year as well as accentuation in the stages on the basis of a standardised cyclical structuring, a temporary change of sport should not be omitted (Table 2/6.7, see p. 153). The change of sport has the advantage that afterwards the specific muscular stimulus has a greater effect and there are no training losses in the general cardiovascular and metabolism functions.

The load-recovery ratio has been researched in a number of training courses with the finding that a ratio of 3 : 1 in the micro and meso-cycle is best. Individually suitable proportions can be deduced from training age and are changeable. With increasing intensity the proportion can be changed to 2 : 1. On the other hand, in aerobic build-up training in cycling, ratios of 4 : 1 are possible.

Training content	Swimming		Cycling		Running		Total
	(km)	(h)	(km)	(h)	(km)	(h)	(h)
"Normal"	20 - 25	8 - 10	300 - 350	10 - 12	70 - 80	5 - 6	23 - 28
Swimming accentuation	50 - 60	18 - 21	200 - 250	7 - 9	80 - 100	6 - 7	31 - 37
Cycling accentuation	10 - 15	4 - 6	800 - 1000	27 - 33	50 - 60	4 - 5	35 - 44
Running accentuation	15 - 20	6 - 8	200 - 250	7 - 9	140 - 160	10 - 12	23 - 29

Table 1/6.7: Accentuated ability development and training figures/week in Olympic distance triathlon (men)

Special sport	Triathlon	Cross-country skiing	Duathlon	Cycling	Swimming	Athletics running	Inline skating
Triathlon		XX	XXX	XXX	XXX	XX	XX
Cross-country skiing	XX		XXX	X	XX	XX	XX
Duathlon	XXX	XX		XXX	X	XXX	XX
Cycling	XXX	XX	XXX		X	X	XX
Swimming	XX	XX	X	X		X	X
Athletics running	XX	XX	XXX	X	X		XX

X = low significance
XX = medium significance
XXX = great significance

Table 2/6.7: Possibilities of changing sport for selected special sports

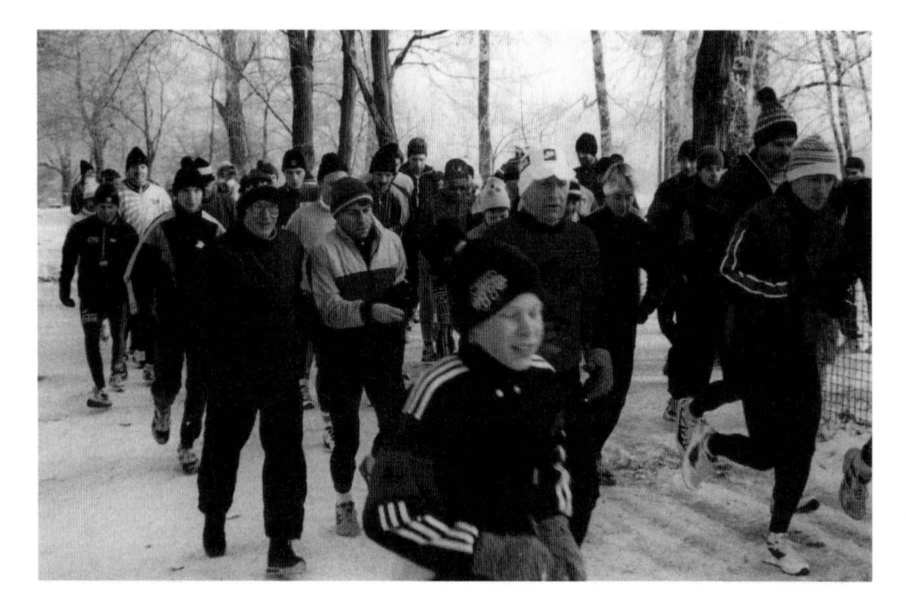

Popular run in winter (-15° C) (Photo: Georg Neumann, Leipzig)

Peak load is best carried out in training camps or in any case where the most favourable training conditions are available, including the training environment. The development of sport-specific basic and strength endurance on the basis of load peaks and using altitude training can take place right up until immediate competition preparation (taper phase).

Year-round training with general and specific training means has an important prerequisite function in making sure of load tolerance. Sport-unspecific training is necessary so that following it, highly specific training load can be processed better. Stable general athletics can also reduce the risk of injury.

In the combination sport triathlon the following methods of increasing load have proved effective:

1. Systematic training change from general to specific means (skiing, swimming, cross-country, mountain bike, running, cycling, coupled training, duathlon, triathlon).

2. Constant increase in the proportion of competition-specific training during the year.

3. Strict application of the cycle method in structuring load, such as bundling of training stimuli (load peak in training camps), strict adherence to load and unloading rhythms etc.

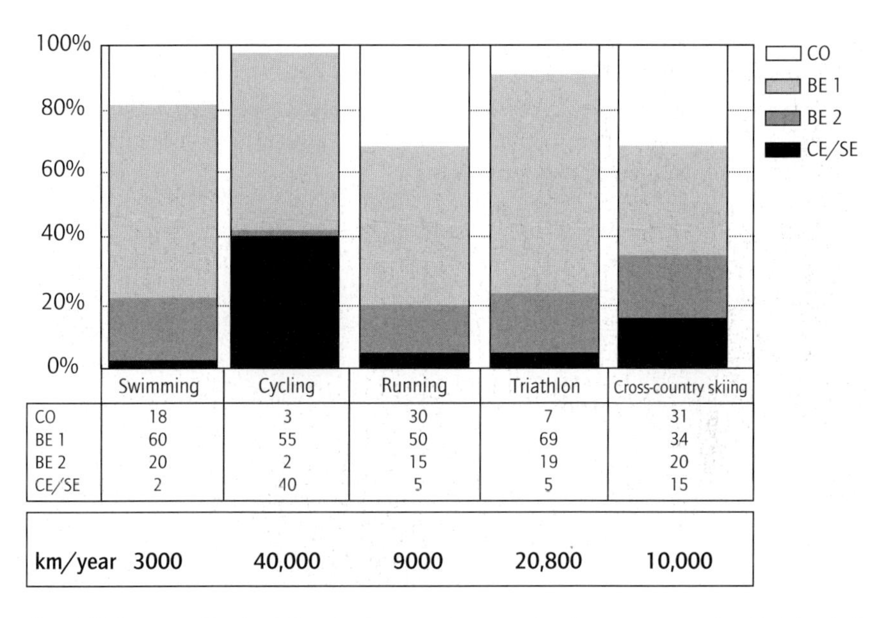

	Swimming	Cycling	Running	Triathlon	Cross-country skiing
CO	18	3	30	7	31
BE 1	60	55	50	69	34
BE 2	20	2	15	19	20
CE/SE	2	40	5	5	15
km/year	**3000**	**40,000**	**9000**	**20,800**	**10,000**

Fig. 1/6.7: Load ratios in ability development in selected endurance sports at a high level of total load

4. Accentuation of the load components, volume, intensity and frequency of training sessions (stimulus density).

5. Gradual increase of intensive proportions in basic endurance training; careful transition from BE 1 to BE 2 training while maintaining proportionality.

6. Selected use of special stimulus factors such as altitude training, training in camps and training on measured out facilities.

7. Constant increase in load resistances over longer duration for the specifically used muscles, giving preference to aerobic strength endurance training.

Training Ratios

Planning the ratios of capacity development in the individual endurance sports is a complicated task of training planning. The ratios are determined by the athlete's performance capacity, the amount of training, the training period, training stages as well as individual prerequisites of the muscle fibre structure. Load ratios vary from sport to sport (Fig. 1/6.7). In order to process the training stimuli, changes in the intensity ratios are necessary in accordance with the requirements of the performance structure.

Whereas runners and cross-country skiiers need high ratios of compensatory training, cyclists and triathletes must compensate less. Through use of the slipstream for example, athletes can organise the necessary compensation themselves.

Summary

The training schedule is a compilation of load parameters and also an expression of the complex organisation of sport-specific body adaptations. Sport-specific performance development is only possible if training structure is in harmony with the requirements of the sport. A number of principles derived from a performance physiology background have established themselves as the basis for the effectivity of competitive training. In summary these are the following:

- Principle of specialisation
- Principle of cyclisation
- Principle of accentuated ability development
- Principle of co-ordination and consistency in capacity development
- Principle of loading and unloading.
- Principle of progressive overload
- Principle of effective training control.

The principles named are complex in character and require a sufficiently high level of exertion for the objectives aimed for. In total, the training concept should be oriented to reaching top performances in the age category of the particular athlete.

7 Performance Structure of Endurance Sports

From a sports methodology point of view, performance structure is seen as the inner structure in the creation of sporting performance. It is influenced by a number of factors and their interrelations. The main factors influencing performance structure include the athlete's personality structure, competition conditions, the influence of the sporting opponent, training structure and the sport-specific performance capacity dependent on the state of adaptation (NEUMANN, 1990, 1991 b; NEUMANN et al., 1995).

In competitions, predetermined distances are covered in the shortest time unless tactical variants cause an athlete to change behaviour. To make sure of performance, certain prerequisites are necessary in training, in the material sector and in organisation. The structure of conditions in training and the interaction of influencing factors in the creation of competition performance are partial factors of performance structure. Training concepts should always be oriented to the requirements of the performance structure of a sport. The criterion for coping with the requirement of the performance structure of a sport or discipline is the competition result (victory, good placing) at the time of the planned performance peak.

In sporting practice it is not insignificant whether e.g. 100 m or 800 m are swum, whether 800 m or 10,000 m are run, whether 4000 m or 120 km are cycled or 5 km or 50 km are skiied. The training-methodological prerequisites and the biological demands are different for the shorter or longer distances in a sport. It is not so much a matter of total load as of the distribution of intensive and extensive training contents. Total load is the central element in training which decides the basic level. In top sport, specialists in the individual distances have clearly developed on the basis of a high volume of total training. The boundaries for the various performance structural requirements in training are often very close together, as for example for 200 m or 400 m swimming or for 800 m or 1500 m running. Athletes in excellent shape can also be successful in neighbouring performance structures, i.e. over shorter and longer distances. In preparation for performance at the annual peak, athletes compete under- and overdistances for training-methodological reasons.

Performance structure is subject to constant methodological and technological influences. If these are insufficiently or not regarded, performance fall-backs are the consequence (Table 1/7, see p. 158).

Sports	Element
Swimming	Dolphin movement - backstroke
Cycling	Aerodynamically favourable seat position
Running	High quality of intermediate and finishing sprints
Walking	Fast walking while keeping to rule 192
Triathlon	Repeal of slipstream rule
Canoeing/rowing	Individual adaptation of paddle and paddle surfaces
Cross-country skiing	Modified freestyle techniques
Biathlon	Two second shooting rhythm
Speed skating	Use of folding skates

Table 1/7: New elements in the performance structure of endurance sports

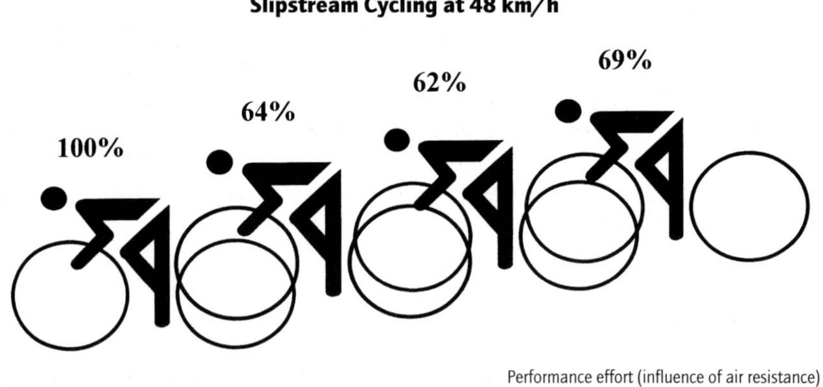

Fig. 1/7: Changed performance effort in slipstream cycling

The underdistance is chosen to develop sport-specific speed and the overdistance to stabilise the endurance foundations for the special distance. In track cycling, strenuous cycle tours are carried out in preparation for the special distance. In order to set the world record of 4:11 min in the 4000 m individual pursuit on the track, Englishman Boardman prepared by participating in the Tour de France 1996. As a result of this unusual tour load of nearly 4000 km he developed a very high aerobic basic performance capacity which was exploited for the following intensification of velocity. The previous load thus took place in another performance structure, whereby through slipstream cycling a great deal of energy can be saved (Fig. 1/7).

The performance structure of sport is described differently from the point of view of single events. Performance structure must not only be recorded with regard to its sports-methodological content but also to its biological (performance physiological) basis. Complex performance diagnostics supplies objective data for this purpose (see chapter 10.4).

The main contents of training are derived from the requirements of the performance structure (NEUMANN/PFÜTZNER, 1992). The endurance sports are a very inhomogeneous group of sports with regard to their requirements and are therefore divided into short, medium and long duration endurance sports. Short duration endurance (SDE) includes race endurance from 35 s to 2 min duration. Medium duration endurance (MDE) represents sports with a race time of over 2 min up to a 10 min duration. The requirements of long duration endurance (LDE) are very differentiated. All race performances over 10 min represent long duration endurance. The dominance of aerobic performance prerequisites is typical for LDE. Within LDE the ratios vary greatly. With increasing duration of load the use of carbohydrates decreases while fat conversion increases (see chapter 4.5). The change of energy supplier during longer load leads to a gradual decrease in competition velocity. The highest velocities are achieved in endurance sports through aerobic and anaerobic glucose breakdown. At the points where there is a clear change of energy supplier to ensure performance, LDE is further subdivided. Corresponding to the performance-physiological peculiarities of competition performances a difference is made between LDE I, II, III and IV (NEUMANN, 1990 and 1991). Below the physiological basis of performance structure in selected sports is shown.

7.1 Running

In athletics running, competitions are carried out in a great time range. Competitions run in the areas of SDE and MDE exert the cardiopulmonary functional system at the top end of the scale (Table 1/7.1, see p. 161). The 400 m running distance already is 50 % covered by aerobic foundations. With the 400 m run we have a performance structure borderline situation because from a training-methodological point of view it can be prepared for either from the sprint side (200 m) or from the fast endurance side (800 m). For the choice of the sport-methodological method, the deciding factor is the athlete's hereditary muscular speed or endurance tendency.

The other extreme are runs over very long distances. For a long time now the marathon has no longer been the crowning training goal. While top athletes are satisfied with three marathon starts per year with excellent times (under 2 h 10 min for men and 2 h 30 min for women), a German doctor managed to take part in 111 marathon runs in one year by using unusual logistics. For him the running time played a secondary role.

Amongst the "slower" runners the longer running distances are becoming increasingly popular and are an expression of great training application and stable motivation in the way they live their lives. For some runners the training motive is the collection of participation certificates in ultra runs (marathon and longer). Of course the key prerequisite for this is that the support apparatus and locomotor system can cope with the frequent sport-specific load and that there is sufficient time for recovery between the long duration competitions. At any rate the world's best "collector" of ultra runs (H.P. from Hamburg) could point to 830 starts by 1999. At the moment there are no limits to load tolerance in endurance sports in sight. Running is a component of combination sports such as triathlon, duathlon, winter orientation runs or modern pentathlon.

Although in running comparable velocities are reached through the combination sports, a performance structural analysis shows clear differences (Table 2/7.1, see p. 162).

Fast running is one of the most strenuous forward movements in endurance sport. In total load, at 6000 to 8000 km/year or 150 to 250 km/week, runners rank below cyclists, triathletes or swimmers. At a speed of 13 km/h it would be possible to do 260 km with a net training time of 20 h/week. This is possibly the reason many runners who have a full-time job train alone and thus neglect the necessary professional peripheral conditions to ensure load tolerance and adaptation (physiotherapy, nutrition, group training, altitude training, change of sport etc). The consequences of insufficient management are often muscle injuries which disrupt the build-up of training. The "catching up" training after training interruptions is then too intensive and without enough breaks. This leads to accelerated performance development with high instability and a lack of top performances.

Running speed is dependent on the volumes of training annually in the particular sport and the average training velocity. If runners train 8000 km per year and triathletes run 0.5 m/s slower with only 3000-4000 km/year, this training difference leads to changes in the performance structure of running.

Performance Structure Running (Competition)						
Measurement Factors:	**SDE** **35 s – 2min** 400 m, 800 m	**MDE** **> 2 min– 10 min** 1000 m, 1500 m, 3000 m, 3000 mH	**LDE I** **> 10 min – 30 min** 5000 m, 10,000 m	**LDE II** **> 30 min – 90 min** 12 km- 25 km	**LDE III** **> 90 min – 360 min** 42.2 km- 80 km	**LDE IV** **> 360 min** 100 km, 160 km, 24 h, 48 h
Heart rate (bpm)	190-205	190-205	180-195	175-190	120-180	100-150
Oxygen uptake (% VO_2 max.)	95-100	97-100	88-96	85-93	60-85	50-65
Energy generation % aerobic % anaerobic	47-60 53-40	70-80 20-30	75-80 20-25	85-90 10-15	97-99 1-3	99 (1)
Energy consumption kcal/min. kcal/total	59 50-100	45 100-350	34-38 400-800	24-27 850-2200	18-23 3,100- 6,480	14-17 6800-12,000 (24 h)
Lactate (mmol/l)	18-25	16-22	8-14	8-12	1-3	1-2
Free fatty acids (mmol/l)	0.400 **	0.400 **	0.800	0.900	1.2-2.5	1.8-3.0
Serum urea (mmol/l)	5-6	5-6	6-7	6-8	8-10	9-16
Cortisole (nmol/l)	200-400 **	200-400**	200-500	400-800	500-1000	800-1200

* Dependent on velocity and body weight
** Stress lipolysis (adrenaline stress)

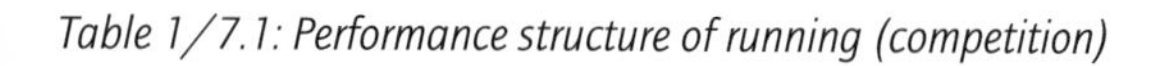

Table 1/7.1: Performance structure of running (competition)

Motion Analysis of Long-Distance Runners and Triathletes at Top Level (n = 26)										
Running velocity (m/s)		Vertical velocity (m/s)		Flight time (ms)		Stride length (m)		Stride frequency (1/s)	
		Runner	Triathlete	Runner	Triathlete	Runner	Triathlete	Runner	Triathlete
4.5	x	0.67	0.49	105	77	1.52	1.48	2.97	3.03
	±s	0.22	0.15	30	19	0.09	0.09	0.21	0.19
5.0	x	0.64	0.47	112	88	1.65	1.61	3.05	3.11
	±s	0.23	0.18	28	15	0.10	0.08	0.18	0.17
5.5	x	0.63	0.45	117	96	1.76	1.72	3.14	3.21
	±s	0.23	0.13	26	14	0.10	0.08	0.19	0.16

Table 2/7.1: Comparison of motion analysis of runners and triathletes (GOHLITZ, 1994)

Comparisons showed that the running velocity of triathletes at 2 mmol/l lactate was 0.9 km/h (0.25 m/s) slower. To keep up with a runner at 19 km/h the triathlete has to constantly produce 1 mmol/l more lactate, take in 2-4 ml/kg.min more oxygen and regulate the HR 7-10 bpm faster than the runner. At 4.5 to 5.5 m/s the stride length of top runners is 4 cm longer than that of top triathletes (GOHLITZ, 1994). Triathletes' running requires much more biological effort than that of long-distance runners. On the other hand, the high total load of triathletes leads to identical metabolism regulation (fat and carbohydrate metabolism) and a greater heart volume (see chapter 4.4). This example shows clearly that independent of the sport, performance structure is linked to highly specific training.

7.2 Cycling

As in running, the range of possible load in cycling (racing bike for road and track, mountain bike) is great. Cycling load is a major element in combination sports (duathlon, triathlon).

With race load of up to 90 min duration, energy generation results mainly from the breakdown of glucose (Table 1/7.2, see p. 164). When the glycogen stores have been exhausted, fat metabolism becomes the main energy supplier (see chapters 4.5.2 and 4.5.3). It is typical of cycling that over short distances (track cycling) there is a high use of anaerobic metabolism.

In road cycling there is a trend similar to that in running of increasingly covering long and overlong distances. The classical long tours (Tour de France, Giro d'Italia etc.) are a proving element for pros and attract increasingly large audiences. In addition to the tours an extreme endurance sport is developing. Already well-known are the crossing of the USA on a bike or running (4700 km), swimming the English Channel (40-50 km at water temperatures of 15-16°C) or circumnavigating the earth (about 20,000 km cycling distance in 80 days, first done in 1997 by Hubert Schwarz). A feature of these extremes is a low average velocity coupled with long travelling times (about 500 km/day). Individual cycling races are carried out over 560 km (Trondheim-Oslo) at an average of over 35 km/h (over 16 hours).

The particular problem with cycling is placing training in intensity areas. Because of the group effect (slipstream), the second and third cyclist need 30 % less energy or strength endurance (see Fig. 1/7). In a large field of cyclists the demands are even less. This is of significance for the classification of cycling training according to load areas. In its biological effects, only about 1/3 of a cycling race is a real individual competition. The other two thirds are forms of qualitatively valuable BE 1 and BE 2 training. Professionals and competitive athletes therefore deliberately use tours to raise the quality of their training load. In doing so they have variable loading options in group or individual training.

Cycling training is a form of load which is easy on the support aparatus and locomotor system and allows load of over 40 h/week or over 1000 km/week. This results in possible annual load of 40,000 to 55,000 km.

7.3 Swimming

In swimming there is a trend towards adding both shorter and longer distances to the programmes of top swimmers. This points to the use of many possibilities of metabolism use (Table 1/7.3, see p. 165). This applies to swimming over the short distance (50 m) and over longer distances (5 and 25 km), which is recognised by the awarding of international titles (European and world championships). Independent of this, extreme swimming is increasing. This includes the spectacular Channel crossings, river swimming (up to 80 km) or 24 hour swimming. Swimming is the basis of combination sports such as triathlon, flipper swimming and diving. The mastery of swimming technique is of decisive significance for swimming performance. If "clean" swimming technique is not learned at the optimal motor learning age (6 to 10 years), with increasing age there is only a small chance of learning effective swimming technique. Those swimmers in the combination sports who are not from the swimmer field are considered "bad" swimmers.

Performance Structure Cycling (Competition)						
Measurement factors:	SDE 35 s - 2min	MDE > 2 min - 10 min	LDE I > 10 min - 30 min	LDE II > 30 min - 90 min	LDE III > 90 min - 360 min	LDE IV > 360 min
	1000 m Track, cycling sprint	3000 m women, 4000 m men (individual team), Keirin, MB downhill	Hill-timed competitions point competitions	30-60 km, timed competitions 40 km triathlon, 30-50 km MB	60-80 km timed competitions 80-250 km road, 180 km long triathlon, 55-70 km MB	>250 km road, multi-triathlon, extreme competitions <500 km
Heart rate (bpm)	185-205	190-210	180-195	175-190	140-180	100-150
Oxygen uptake (% VO_2 max.)	95-100	97-100	90-95	80-95	60-85	40-55
Energy transformation % aerobic % anaerobic	50 50	80 20	85 15	95 5	98 2	99 (1)
Energy consumption kcal/min kcal/total	55-60 60-70	40-45 150-230	22-28 280-660	20-25 750-1800	12-20 1800-9900	8-12 8600-12,000 24 h and more
Lactate (mmol/l)	14-18	16-22	12-14	8-12	1.5-4	1.0-2.0
Free fatty acids (mmol/l)	0.5*	0.5*	0.8	0.9-1.0	1.2-2.0	1.5-3.0
Serum urea (mmol/l)	6	6	7	7-9	8-10	9-15
Cortisole (nmol/l)	200-400 **	200-400**	200-450	400-800	500-900	600-1200

* Stress lipolysis (adrenaline stress)
** Dependent on velocity and body weight

Table 1/7.2: Performance structure of running (race)

Performance Structure Swimming (Competitions)						
Measurement factors	SDE 35 s - 2min	MDE > 2 min - 10 min	LDE I > 10 min - 30 min	LDE II > 30 min - 90 min	LDE III > 90 min - 360 min	LDE IV > 360 min
Swimming distances	50 m, 100 m (200 m)	200 m, 400 m	800 m, 1500 m	5 km	25 km	> 30 km
Heart rate (bpm)	180-200	180-195	170-185	150-160	120-140	100-130
Lactate (mmol/l)	13-16	10-13	8-10	4-8	2-4	1-2
Energy transformation % aerobic % anaerobic (alactic)	20 80 (20)	40 60 (10)	80 20	90 10	95 5	98 2
Energy consumption kcal/min kcal/total	60-80 50-160	45 90-450	30 450-870	25 870-2250	20-25 2250-6120	15-20 > 6120
Free fatty acids (mmol/l)	0.4-0.5*	0.4 - 0.5	0.6 - 0.9	0.6 - 1.4	0.7 - 1.9	0.8 - 2.0
Serum urea (mmol/l)	4-6	4-6	4-6	5-8	6-9	7-11
Cortisole (nmol/l)	150-250	150-250	400-700	400-800	400-900	500-800

* Stress lipolysis (adrenaline stress)
** Dependent on velocity and body weight

Table 1/7.3: Performance structure of swimming (competitions)

Performance Structure Triathlon (Competition)						
Measurement factors	LDE II > 30 min - 90 min Sprint triathlon (750 m S, 29 km C, 5 km R)	LDE III > 90 min - 360 min (105 - 180 min) Short triathlon (1.5 km , 40 km C, 10 km R)	(LDE III) (240 - 300 min) Middle triathlon (2 km S, 80 km C, 20 km R)	LDE IV > 360 min (8-15 h) Long triathlon (3.8 km S, 180 km C, 42.2 km R)	(LDE IV) (22-30 h) Double long triathlon (7.6 km S, 360 C, 84.4 km R)	(LDE IV) (33-57h)** Triple long triathlon (11.4 km S, 540 km C, 126.6 km R)
Heart rate (bpm)	180-195	160-190	140-160	120-150	110-140	100-130
Oxygen uptake (% VO_2 max.)	85-95	80-90	70-80	60-70	55-65	40-60
Energy transformation % aerobic % anaerobic	 90 10	 95 5	 98 2	 99 1	 99 (1)	 99 (1)
Energy consumption kcal/min kcal/total	 25 1500	 20 2400-3600	 15-18 4320-6480	 11-15 7200-9900	 10-12 12,000-16,000	 8-10 19,800-25,000
Lactate (mmol/l)	8-12	5-9	2-4	1-2	1-2	1-2
Free fatty acids (mmol/l)	0.800	1000-1400	1300-1900	2.0-2.5	2.0-2.7	2.0-3.0
Serum urea (mmol/l)	5-7	7-9	8-10	9-12	9-14	9-16
Creatin/cinase (µmol/s.l)	10	10-25	10-30	10-60	20-70	20-70
Cortisole (nmol/l)	400	300-600	400-600	600-1000	800-1000	800-1200

* Dependent on velocity and body weight
** Interruption through sleep

Table 1/7.4: Performance structure of triathlon (competition)

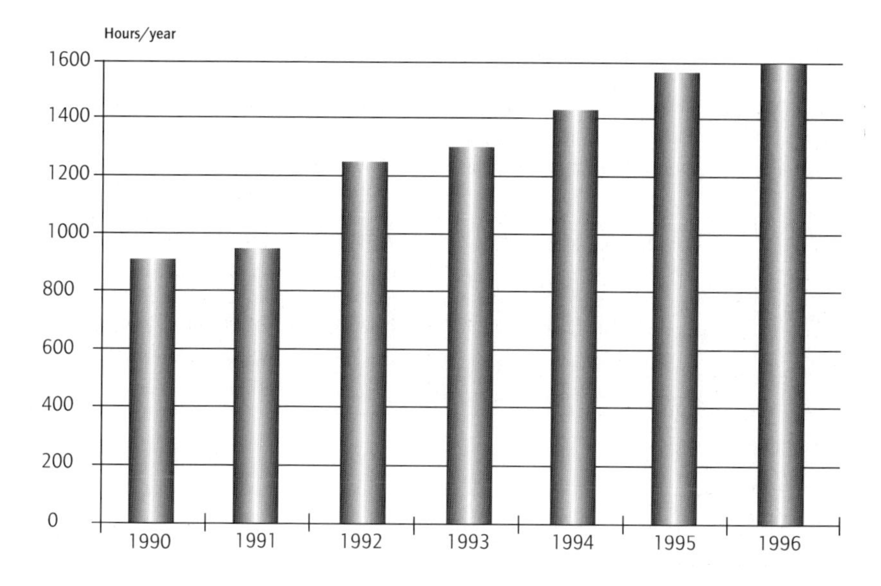

Fig. 1/7.4: Increase in total training load over seven years of a top athlete in triathlon

The sparing of the support apparatus and locomotor system of the body through swimming makes it possible to swim up to 20 km daily or over 120 km per week. Through volume swimming, however, specific speed decreases. For this reason, series training over short distances and short breaks is the typical training principle in competitive swimming.

7.4 Triathlon

The sport triathlon is a typical long duration endurance sport with greatly varying use of the functional systems (Table 1/7.4., see p. 166).

Triathlon combines popular endurance sports. In the twenty years it has existed this sport has spread worldwide. Because of the necessity of training in three sports, an unusually high load tolerance level of athletes both in fitness sport and in competitive sport has been achieved. In triathlon the principle of sport-specific load and unloading of muscle groups is practised in an almost ideal way. The specificness of muscular load is especially apparent in the change from cycling to running (PFÜTZNER et al., 1994). When for example in the ultra triathlon after the 180 km cycling an athlete is still capable of running a marathon, this phenomenon can only be explained by the emptying of the glycogen depots in the cycling-specifically loaded muscles. Cycling training uses different leg muscle groups than running.

The diversity of muscular load and also the potential load tolerance called for have been realised in an exemplary fashion in triathlon. As a result of the change of sport in random sequence (swimming, running, cycling) the limits of load tolerance in training are high. Together with road cyclists, at about 1600 training hours per year top triathletes are the leaders in load amongst endurance athletes (Fig. 1/7.4, see p. 167).

Performance Structure Cross-country Skiing (Competition)				
Measurement factors	LDE I > 10 min -30 min 5 km F 10 km F, C	LDE II > 30 min - 90 min 15 km F, C 30 km F	LDE III > 90 min -360 min 50 km F, C to 100 km	LDE IV > 360 min > 100 km
Heart rate (bpm)	180-200	170-195	140-175	110-140
Oxygen uptake (% VO_2 max)	90-95	80-90	50-85	40-60
Energy transformation % aerobic % anaerobic	 80-90 10-20	 90-95 5-10	 90-98 2-10	 95-99 1-5
Energy consumption kcal/min kcal/total	 25-30 500-800	 20-25 800-1800	 16-20 1800-5760	 14-16 5760-12,000 (24 Stunden)
Glycogen depletion (leg muscles %)	40-50	50-60	70-80	85-95
Lactate (mmol/l)	12-16	10-14	2-8	1-2
Free fatty acids (mmol/l)	0.4-0.6	0.6-0.8	0.8-1.0	1.2-2.0
Serum urea (mmol/l)	5-7	7-8	7-10	8-13
Cortisole (nmol/l)	400-500	600-700	600-900	700-1200

* Dependent on velocity and body weight

Table 1/7.5: Performance structure of cross-country skiing (competition)

Training in three sports, which is well-tolerated muscularly, makes it possible to carry out the ultra triathlon in the multiple version. While the triple ultra triathlon is already an official competition, extreme athletes have already managed the deca version in Mexico (38 km swimming, 1800 km cycling and 422 km running). This load would not be possible if muscular load tolerance and energetic supply through constant food intake did not permit it.

7.5 Cross-country Skiing

In cross-country skiing too there is a trend whereby the distances of 5 to 50 km so far usual in international competition are being extended. As a result, the times of previous competition load of 15 to 100 min for women and 25 to 135 min for men over single distances have been clearly moved into the area of several hours. The increase in participant numbers in long distance races (e.g. Vasa cross-country) confirms the trend (see Fig. 4/1). The mass cross-country ski races are so popular because they can be managed without great preparation. Also, cross-country skiing is one of the milder forms of forward movement with a high level of total body load. Improvements in ski materials and wax mean increasingly higher average velocities over all distances and at all performance levels. Cross-country skiing velocity is dependent on the gliding conditions of the snow and is thus an unreliable measure of the level reached. For the assessment of the state of development of biomotor abilities in cross-country skiing, the biological monitoring options of load regulation are particularly important (see chapters 10.4 and 10.5). It is a characteristic of the performance structure of cross-country skiing that the aerobic performance foundations are the dominating element (Table 1/7.5, see p. 168). This also corresponds to the selection criteria for cross-country skiing, in which the successful skiiers have a proportion of 60 to 80 % of slow twitch muscle fibres (STF). In cross-country skiing, multiple starts in close sequence are possible. In international competition weeks, individual women cover a total of 65 km and individual men 115 km. The double and multiple starts are undertaken by athletes with stable basic endurance ability and high motor variability and who easily manage the change from freestyle technique to the classical skiing technique. The exploitation of personal strengths (freestyle or classical skiing) leads to the development of specialists over certain distances.

Performance capacity on the skiing treadmill in summer and autumn only roughly corresponds to the performance that follows on snow. Whereas on the skiing treadmill a high level of basic endurance with limited technique suffices, skiing on snow requires a higher level of forward moving technique. The brief finding of the push-off point makes classical cross-country skiing more demanding than the longer lasting push-off in freestyle.

Performance comparisons of cross-country skiers with biathletes are interesting. The latter have a clearly different performance structure to cross-country skiing, characterised by the constant interruptions to skiing for shooting. Covering distances without breaks at high velocity is difficult for biathletes, they could not maintain the pace of cross-country specialists. This highlights the differentiated requirements of the performance structure which are prepared for with training. Nobody would consider letting a race walker compete against a runner.

Summary

The framework of conditions in training and the interaction of influencing factors in the development of competition performance are described as performance structure. The training concepts of sports must always be oriented towards the performance structure of a sport. The criterion for dealing with the requirements of the performance structure of a sport or event is always the competition result at the time of the preplanned performance peak. The performance structure of a sport is subject to constant change which is derived from changed competition regulations, shortened or lengthened competition distances, increases in difficulty and other technological influencing factors. Projected performance development in a sport is the prognosis performance structure.

8 Long-term Development of Performance

The long-term development of performance involves a training process over several years which begins in childhood. Each sport has a different starting age for competition-oriented training in childhood. In endurance sports, training is systematised and involves four stages. These are basic training, build-up training, follow-up training and high performance (top-class) training (Table 1/8, see p. 172). Beforehand the child participates in general training in the sport. During this time training is diverse and is independent of particular sports; training of movement is emphasised (MARTIN/ROST, 1996).

Talents for endurance sport can be recognised both in basic and in follow-up training (Table 2/8, see p. 172). The time range for entering a sport is great. In swimming it begins earliest, in rowing latest.

In the long-term development of performance, two courses are possible. The first involves training the young person in the sport right from the beginning, i.e. from childhood to top performance age. The second course is possible through a deliberate change of sport (HOTTENROTT/BETZ, 1995).

These are the lateral entrants to a sport. This way is taken especially in combination sports like duathlon, triathlon, biathlon etc.

In analysing top performance age it is noticeable that there is neither a tendency to lower or to higher age. From the age of 20 onwards, top performances are possible in the endurance sports (Fig. 1/8, see p. 177). All later winners have trained constantly for eight to twelve years, on average ten years. It is still uncertain how long these athletes can stay at the top. There are many influences here. It is amazing that the individual performance limit can be stretched to the middle of the 30th year (Table 3/8, see p. 177). In the long duration endurance sports the top performance age of both sexes is between 28 and 32 years.

In the long-term development of performance the use of training contents, i.e. training means and methods must be very subtly differentiated.

Basic Training

Basic training begins after general and diverse basic motor training. In basic training the objective pursued is to teach children sporting technique and to develop the co-ordinative abilities initially necessary for the sport. Biomotor abilities are developed broadly and not primarily sport-specifically. The child must learn motivation for training and for the time being decide on a sport.

Sport/age level*	Swimming (years)		Cycling (years)	Running (years)	Triathlon (years)	Cross-country skiing (years)	Endurance sports in total (years)
	male	female					
Basic training	9 - 11	8 - 10	10 - 14	11 - 13	11 - 14	12 - 14	8 - 14
Build-up training	12 - 14	11 - 13	15 - 16	14 - 15	15 - 16	15 - 17	12 - 17
Follow-up training	15 - 19	14 - 17	17 - 18	16 - 18	16 - 18	18 - 20	14 - 20
High performance (top) training	> 20	> 18	> 19	> 19	> 19	> 20	18 - 30

* *Depending on development (biological age), sex differences and sport-specific requirements, variations of one to three years are possible.*

Table1/8: Long-term development of performance in selected endurance sports

Indicators for the Recognition of Endurance Talents

Basic Training (Time of Diverse Basic Training in Sports)	Build-up Training (Time of Development of Sport-specific Performance Capacity)
• **Talented for endurance sports** (Enjoys running, cycling, swimming, cross-country skiing)	• **Noticeably good performance capacity in the sport** (Stable endurance performance up to 60 min)
• **Drive for longer performances** (Diverse flexibility, staying power up to 30 min)	• **Above average performances in speed motor activity for the sport** (Liveliness, pace variability)
• **Aptitudes for speed motor activity** (Sprinting speed, motor switching ability, reaction speed)	• **Excellent test results on checking endurance capacity**
• **Co-ordinative capacities for sporting technique** (Running, swimming, cycling)	• **High load tolerance of the support apparatus and locomotor system** (Stable health, few consequences of incorrect exertion)
• **Basic prerequisites for changing a sport** (Running, rowing, skiing)	• **Competition motivation** (Ability to improve offensive use of performance capacities, competition character)

Table 2/8: Indicators for the recognition of endurance talents. Modified from REISS et al. 1993.

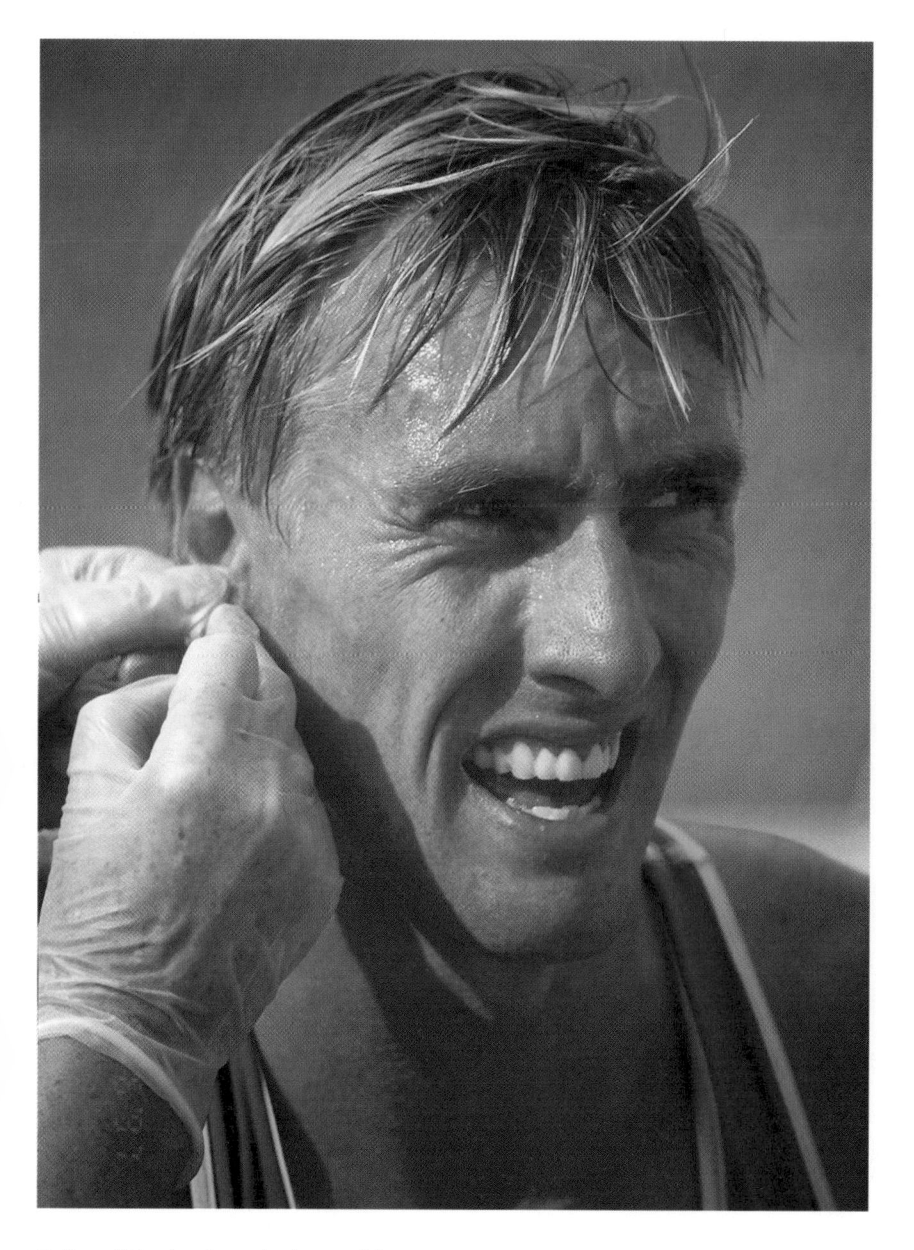

Taking of blood to determine lactate (Photo: Georg Neumann, Leipzig)

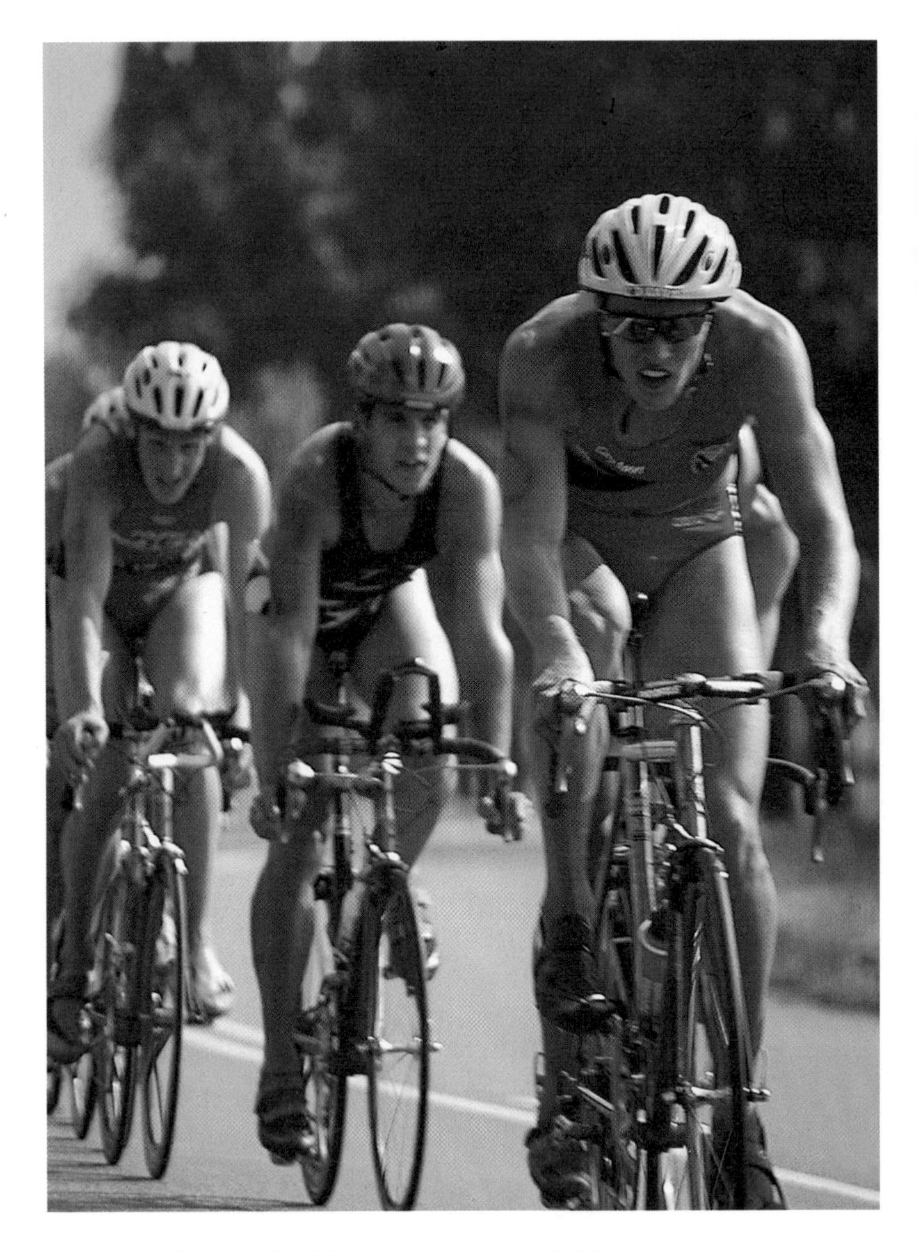

Slipstream cycling in triathlon (Photo: Georg Neumann, Leipzig)

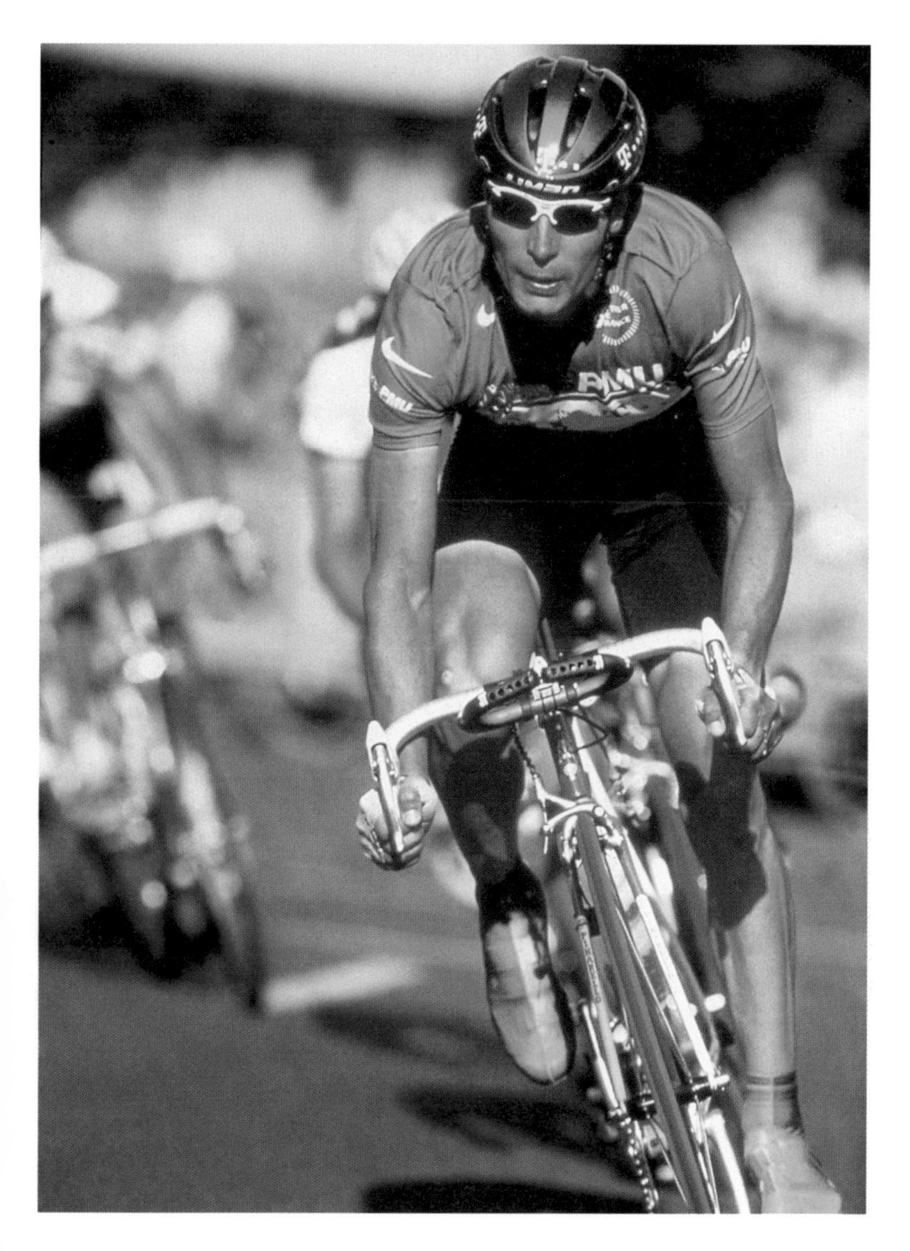

(Photo: Polar)

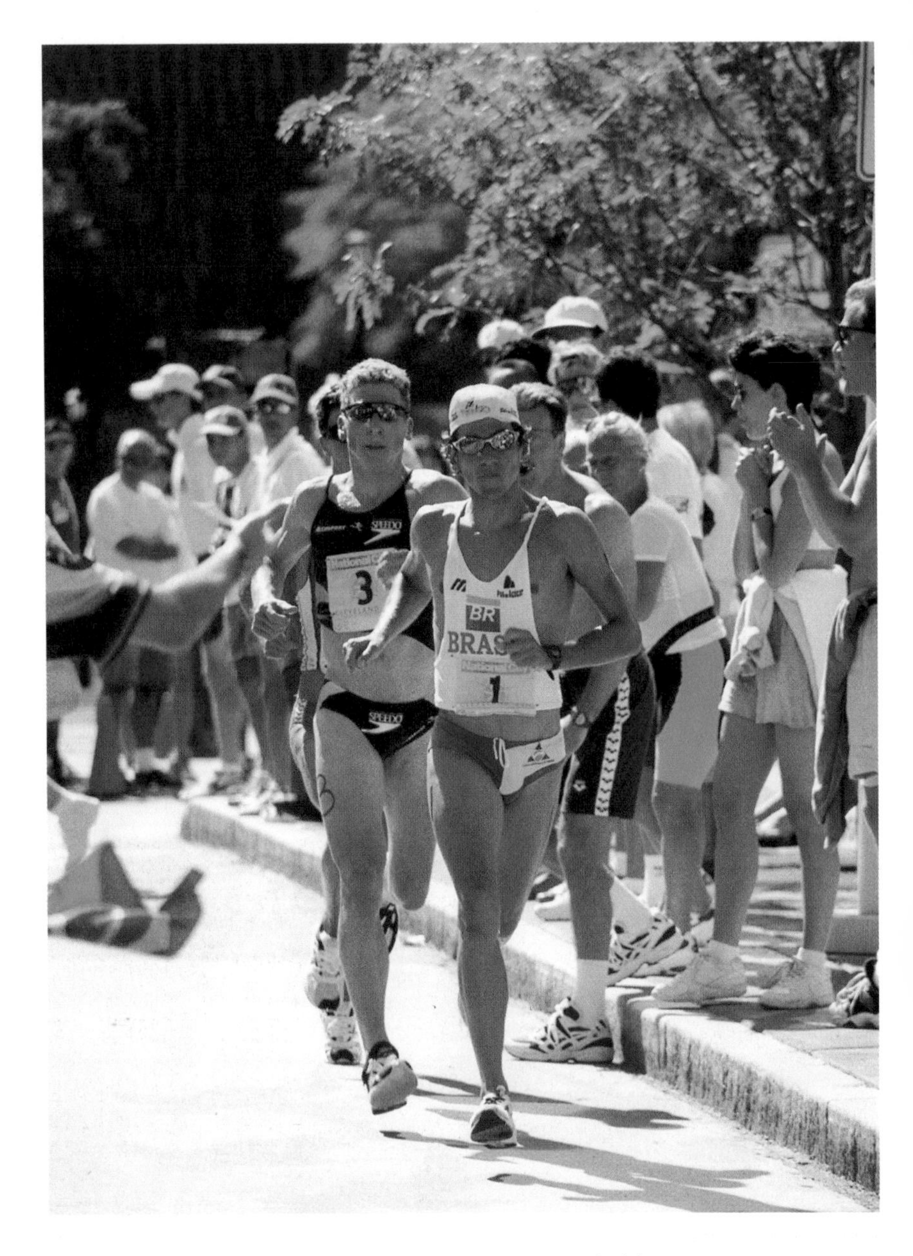

Triathlon competition on a hot day (Photo: Georg Neumann, Leipzig)

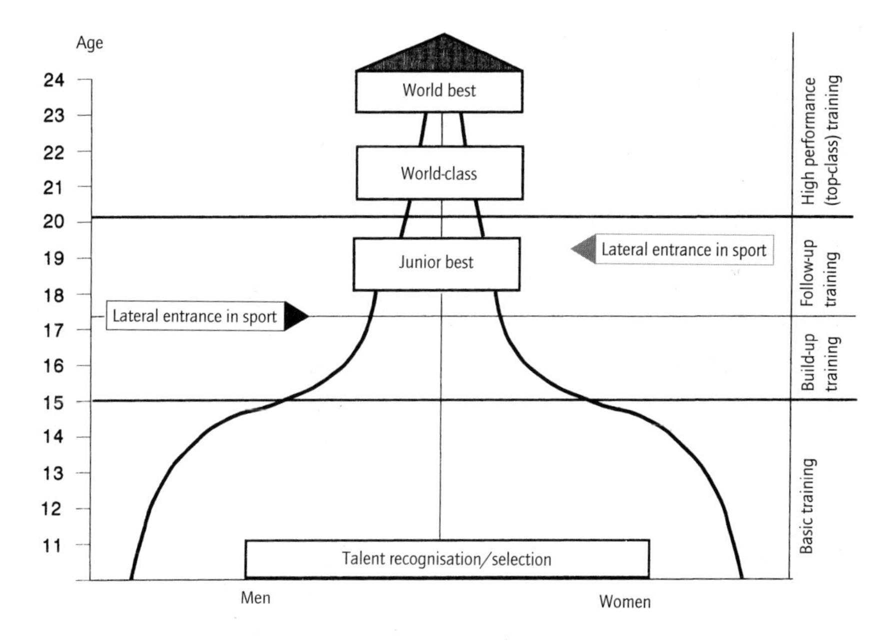

Fig. 1/8: Pyramid system in long-term development of performance and characterisation of the possibility for lateral entrance in the endurance sports

	World Championships		European Championships	
Placing	Men	Women	Men	Women
1-3	31 ± 3	28 ± 3	24 ± 3	25 ± 4
4-10	27 ± 6	26 ± 4	25 ± 4	28 ± 3
11-20	26 ± 3	27 ± 5	26 ± 3	26 ± 4
1-20	28 ± 4	28 ± 4	25 ± 4	27 ± 3

Table 3/8: High performance age in triathlon/Olympic Distance (figures in years). Averages from competition results in the period 1990-1996.

Build-up Training

Build-up training is the continuation of basic training in a sport and is characterised by a diverse development of sporting performance. The volume of load is increased in the physical fitness area and there is initial, resistance-emphasised training. It is important that the weights or resistances are not greater than the young person's own body mass. Sport-specific and general speed must be trained further. Sporting technique is further developed in conjunction with fine co-ordination and motor variability. Endurance training "in advance" is not a good idea and would also make the athlete "slow" (NEUMANN et al., 1990; NEUMANN, 1991 c). Endurance capacity cannot be stored. Increases in the volume of training should only be introduced at the end of the junior age period.

Follow-up Training

Follow-up training is the last phase before entering high performance or top training. The transition lasts 2-4 years even for successful juniors. Men's performance in the individual sports is so high that this time must be planned for. Only after 2-3 years at the earliest can one reckon with first follow-up level performances in the men's class. The emphasis in follow-up training is on a definite increase in the volume of training altogether. The first training goal is to cope with a large volume of training. On this base, 1-2 years of qualitative elements of endurance training can be built up. Aerobic basic training that has not been carried out is difficult to catch up on in this period. The main feature of additional training is to achieve a high level of ability to deal with load. With increasing age (age classes), norms for performance development are laid down in the individual sports (Table 4/8, see p. 179).

High-performance (Top-class) Training

In the high-performance training period top performances are aimed for. Training conditions become increasingly more professional. The available time framework should not disrupt training. It becomes necessary to decide whether to carry on one's occupation or not. Giving both equal priority leads to conflict situations. High-performance training has three stages which are dependent on age and success.

1st Stage of High-performance Training

Successful male and female juniors begin high performance training at the age of 20 to 21. They have about three years in which to reach the world best in the sport. In this time the biomotor abilities must be developed to a personal highest degree so that the desired increase in forward propulsion performance occurs (Table 5/8, see p. 179). The development of the aerobic energy flow rates (VO_2 max) needs at least three years to reach the individual maximum.

	Swimming 400 m		Cycling 20 km		Running 5 km	
Age	Men	Women	Men	Women	Men	Women
18 years	4:35	5:00	28:00	30:00	16:00	18:00
19 years	4:25	4:50	27:00	29:30	15:30	17:30
20 years	4:20	4:45	26:30	29:00	15:00	17:00
	Swimming 1500 m		**Cycling 40 km**		**Running 10 km**	
Age	**Men**	**Women**	**Men**	**Women**	**Men**	**Women**
18 years	18:15	19:15	57:00	62:00	34:00	37:00
19 years	17:45	18:45	55:30	60:00	33:00	36:00
20 years	17:30	18:30	54:00	59:00	32:00	35:00
21 years	17:15	18:15	52:30	57:30	31:00	34:00
22 years	16:45	17:45	51:30	56:30	30:30	33:30
23 years	16:30	17:30	50:30	55:00	30:00	33:00

Table 4/8: Age-linked performance prognosis (min, s) in triathlon (swimming: 50 m length; cycling: individual timed cycling, flat, no wind; running: 400 m track)

Running Structure

In running training over several years the movement patterns change

- Performance improvement over several years of training is always coupled with an increase in stride length.
- In training the increase in stride length and the decrease in stride frequency is always dependent on a definite improvement in of the biomotor abilities.
- Increased stride frequency and decreased stride length are signs of a definite decrease of the biomotor abilities.
- When climbing, stride length decreases and stride frequency increases.
- 40 measured running cycles are representative for changes, i.e. about 80% of the covered distance over 100 m.

Table 5/8: Running structure

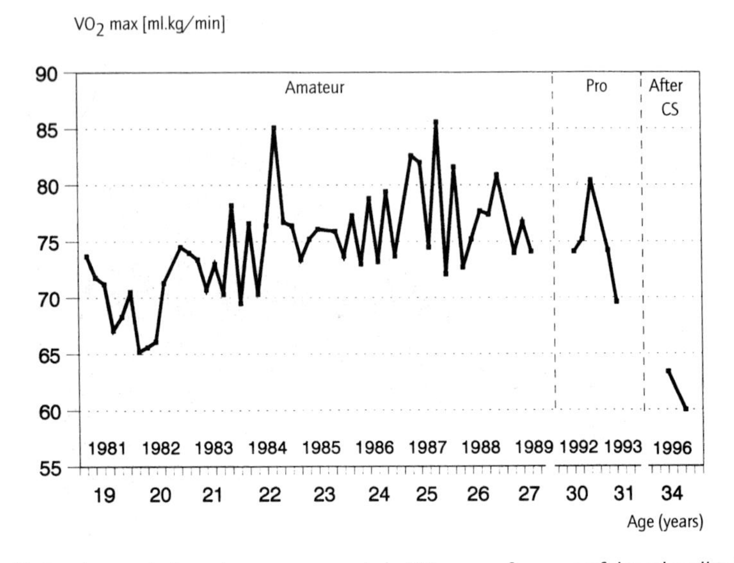

Fig. 2/8: Development of maximum oxygen uptake VO_2 max of a successful road cyclist (world champion). VO_2 max is subject to training related fluctuations in the course of the year. CS = competitive sport

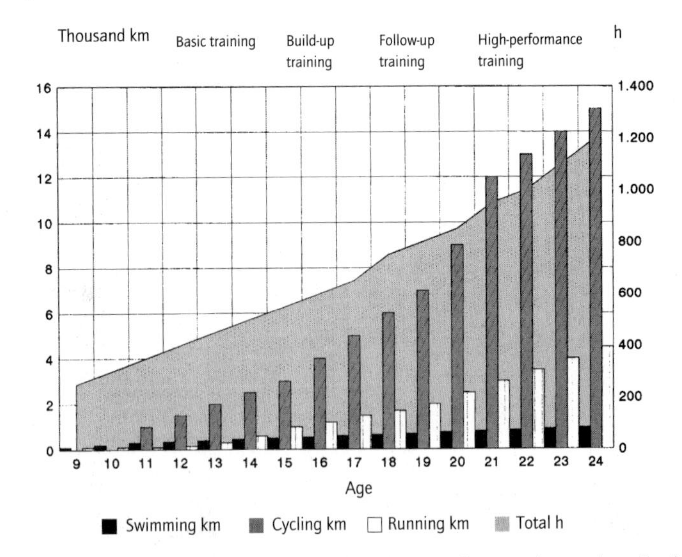

Fig. 3/8: Training load requirements in swimming, cycling and running in long-term performance development for triathlon

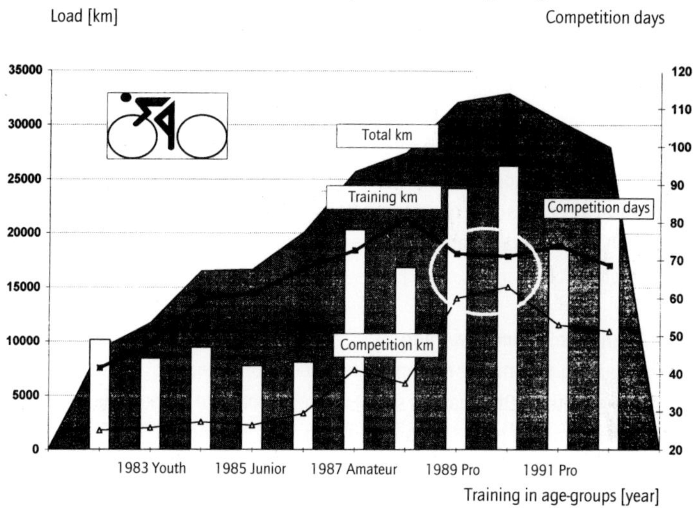

Fig. 4/8: Load data of a talented cyclist who went professional. When the number of competitions dominated and endurance training decreased, performance stagnated and the career soon ended

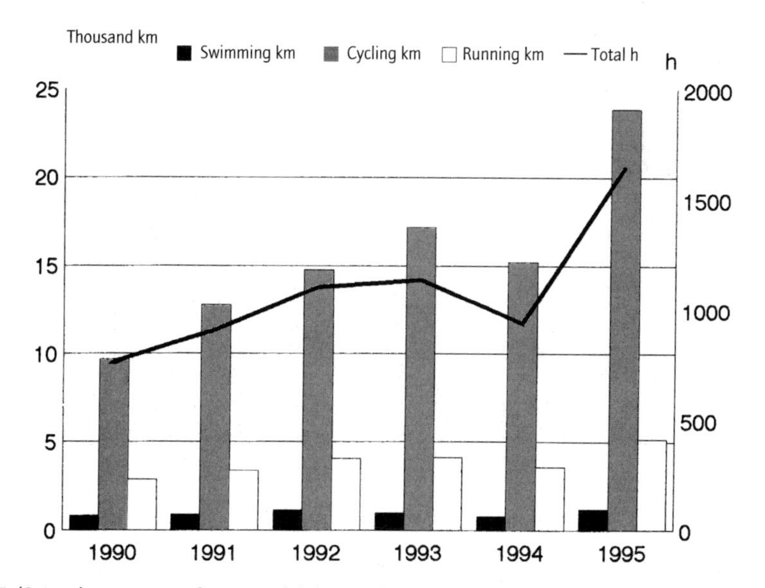

Fig. 5/8: Load parameters of a successful short and long-distance triathlete from junior age onwards

2nd Stage of High-performance Training

In this training phase, at the age of about 24 years world best performance must be achieved or further developed. When the top has been reached, the trend to constant performance improvement in the training years must be followed. This means that training must be structured increasingly effectively. Every year new stimuli must be applied in training. Increasingly physiological performance reserves are used in training, such as medium altitude, climate training or competition series etc. Once a certain level of aerobic performance has been reached it is not always possible to maintain or reproduce it over several years (Fig. 2/8, see p. 180). Talented athletes manage to remain among the world best for about five years and in some cases longer.

3rd Stage of High-performance Training

After years of training the top is no longer reached, front placings no longer occur. At the beginning of the athlete's 30th year his social interests begin to reorientate. Sports-specifically he begins to slow down and moves to longer distances in his sport. 10,000 m runners become marathon runners, short triathletes become ultra triathletes or cross-country skiers become participants in mass events.

Every sport has its own load parameters and performance norms for long-term performance development. These serve as framework co-ordinates for training (Fig. 3/8, see p. 180). In performance development over several years there is a basic relationship between the increase in load and performance, unless major faults have been made.

As long as the basic relationship between training and competition frequency is correct, performance will develop positively. If these elementary rules of performance development are broken, then stagnation and a decrease in performance occur. This is especially so when as a result of too many competition basic aerobic training is neglected (Fig. 4/8, see p. 181). Commercial temptations in pro sport do not invalidate the physiological laws of individual ability to handle load. If the load-unloading rhythms are not right, the greatest sporting talent is of no use at all. Talents also need regular planned unloading in training. In performance training of junior or young athletes the increase in load need not be linear, intermediate years of temporarily reduced load do not hinder further growth in performance (Fig. 5/8, see p. 181).

Summary

Competitive sport lives from sporting talent discovered early and supported over longer periods. Early talent seeking and supporting is a decisive factor in long-term performance development. The prominent stages of development in long-term performance development are basic training, build-up training, follow-up training and high-performance training. The ages during these training stages can differ greatly from one endurance sport to the other. As a rule, ten years of training are necessary to achieve top performances. In endurance sports the age of top performance is between 25 and 30. In long-term performance development the world best in a sport should always be used as the basic yardstick for training. Successful high-performance training is only possible under professional conditions.

9 Cyclical Structuring of Training

The development of sport-specific performance capacity occurs in shorter and longer phases of training also known as cycles. The content of the cycles is a sequence of load-stress regulations interrupted by regenerative periods. Only the planned alternation between load and recovery allows one to make full use of one's adaptive potential.

In endurance sports the post-competition period clearly influences the cyclisation of training load. In order to make training comprehensible, the training year is divided up sports-methodically into sections of varying duration (cycles) and contents.

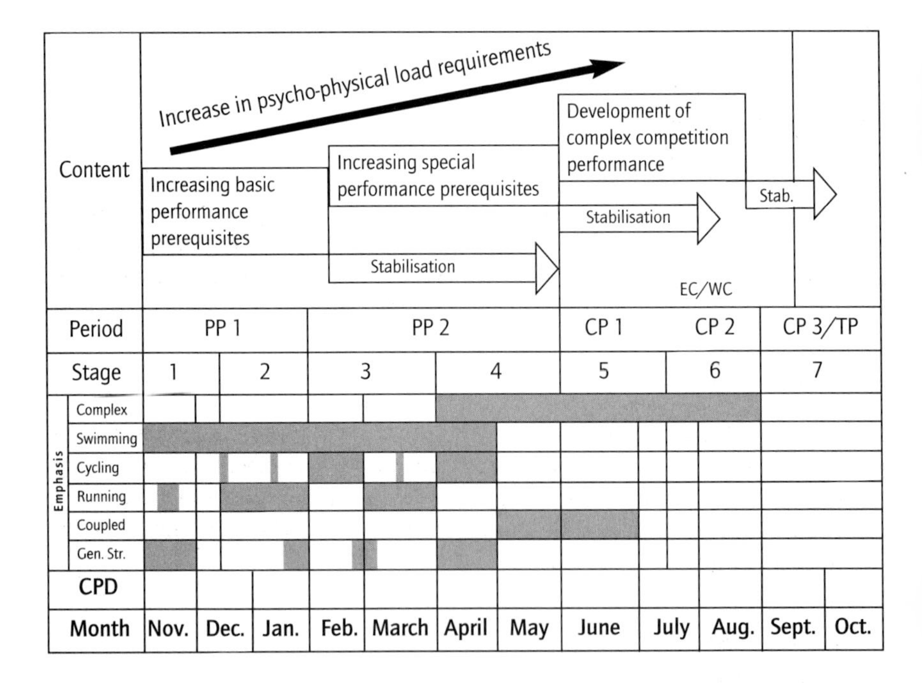

Fig. 1/9.1: Structuring of training in periods. Performance development occurs in the preparatory periods (PP 1 and PP 2) and competition periods (CP). The transitional period (TP) finishes training. Complex performance diagnostics (CPD).

9.1 Annual Cycle

The annual structure of training is called the annual cycle, which is structured differently over several years. To achieve top performances, independent of performance categories and age, a training process must be planned and structured.

Training should always be oriented to the yearly performance peak.

For systematic performance development over the year, training is structured in periods which can extend beyond the calendar year (Fig. 1/9.1, see p. 184).

Summer and winter sports have a different time periodisation. In summer sports the preparation period (PP) begins in October and lasts until May of the following year. In winter sports the PP lasts from April until November. This is followed by the competition periods, i.e. from June to September for summer sports and from December to March for winter sports.

Periodisation can be single or multiple. In seasonal sports single periodisation is more common, in indoor sports double or multiple periodisation occurs more. The training cycle usually consists of:

- **three preparatory periods**
- **one competition period**
- **one transitional period.**

For more detailed planning these periods are divided further into stages (Table 1/9.1, see p. 186). The training-methodological contents for the 52 weeks in the year are different in the individual periods. In particular there are variations in intensity proportions and the use of training means (Fig. 2/9.1, see p. 187).

Preparatory Period 1 (PP 1)

In PP 1, training of basic (general) abilities for the sport takes place. Basic performance prerequisites are: general endurance, general strength and general motor activity. Additionally there are exercises for flexibility, stretching and relaxing capacity of the muscles. Training is mainly sport-unspecific, with preference given to general and semi-specific training means. Competitions in other sports are also possible.

Preparatory Period 2 (PP 2)

The objective of PP 2 is the development of special performance prerequisites in close connection with the development of sporting technique and under training conditions as specific to the event as possible. The proportion of semi-specific training means increases, coupled with increased load.

Period	Stage	Weeks	CE/SPE (%)	BE 2 (%)	SE (%)	BE 1 (%)	CO (%)
PP 1	1	4	3	14	11	67	5
PP 1	2	9	3	14	5	73	5
PP 2	3	9	3	15	2	70	10
PP 3	4	8	5	19	2	62	12
CP 1	5	6	10	17	2	51	20
CP 2	6	7	4	19	2	66	9
TP	7	9	3	10	3	80	4

Training data swimming (week)

Period	Stage	Weeks	CE/SPE (%)	BE 2 (%)	SE (%)	BE 1 (%)	CO (%)
PP 1	1	4	2	5	4	85	4
PP 1	2	9	3	8	18	68	3
PP 2	3	9	3	7	14	73	3
PP 3	4	8	1	6	22	66	5
CP 1	5	6	9	4	7	69	11
CP 2	6	7	4	5	10	74	7
TP	7	9	1	2	9	81	9

Training data cycling (week)

Period	Stage	Weeks	CE/SPE (%)	BE 2 (%)	SE (%)	BE 1 (%)	CO (%)
PP 1	1	4	3	4	7	72	14
PP 1	2	9	4	17	13	55	11
PP 2	3	9	4	19	11	52	14
PP 3	4	8	8	16	5	54	17
CP 1	5	6	13	4	3	57	23
CP 2	6	7	11	16	4	50	19
TP	7	9	2	8	5	73	12

Table 1/9.1: Training data swimming, cycling, running/week

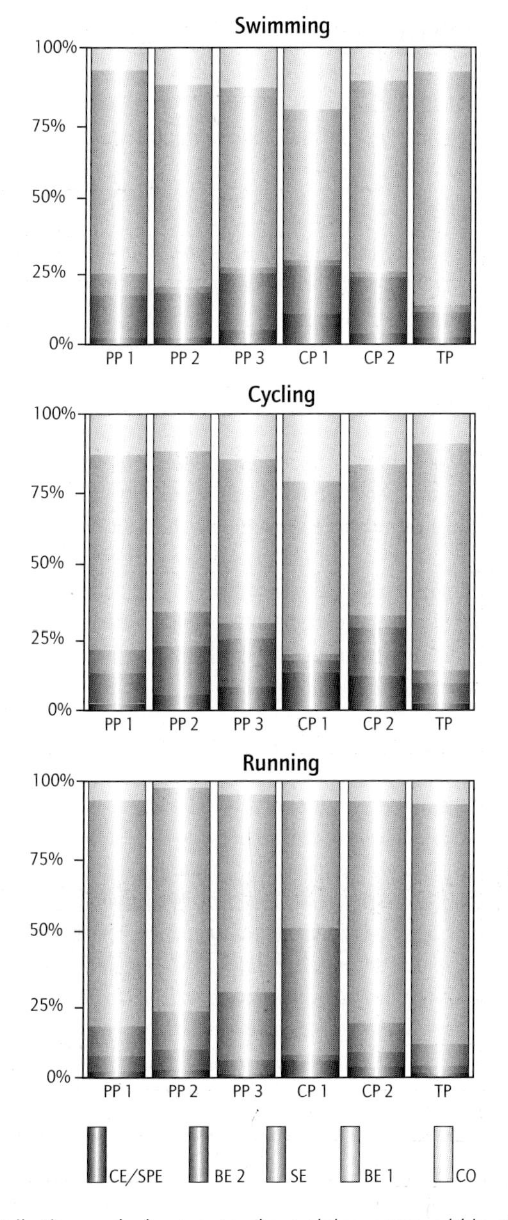

Fig. 2/9.1: Distribution and changes to the training areas within the preparatory and competition periods in three sports in triathlon

Preparatory Period 3 (PP 3)

In PP 3, competition-specific performance prerequisites are developed. Competition specific training forms and build-up competitions are used. Semi-specific training means are increasingly replaced by specific ones. The total volume of training reaches an annual peak.

Preparatory Period 4 (PP 4)

PP 4 is a special form and is used for double periodisation. Both climate and altitude training camps can be combined with PP 4, which serve the direct preparation for the following second competition series.

Competition Period 1 (CP 1)

The competition period is usually seasonally limited. Several competitions develop competition performance capacity. The aim here is to achieve personal top performance at the peak. Competition performance is dependent on the beginning level from PP 3 that was started with. The stability of basic aerobic performance capacity, which to a certain extent was trained in advance in PP 3, decides to a large extent the successes in the competitions that follow. If the beginning level was too low, after the 3rd competition already the ability to improve may be missing. In the competition period the amount of training must decrease, as a rule by 10-15 % in comparison to PP 3. Between competitions compensation training takes place and BE training to maintain form. This is usually neglected.

Competition Period 2;3 (CP 2;3)

In this period competition-specific performance capacity is stabilised. This is done through selected competitions. In order to reach top performance, performance at the peak time is especially carefully prepared through direct competition preparation (DCP). In the classical sense the duration of DCP or tapering time is 4-6 weeks, but increasingly this is broken up by contractual competition participation. Planned individual top performance results thus become uncertain. In normal DCP the basic elements of annual performance development are trained in abbreviated form. The decisive prerequisite for DCP or tapering time is that the total amount of training is reduced by 20 to 30 %. The reduction in load is necessary for performance-physiological reasons so there is not too much residual tiredness and so that a kind of overcompensation in the release of performance capacity occurs.

Post Competition Period, Beginning of the Transition Period

In this period the competitions at the end of the season take place without any particular pressure to perform. Sport-specific performance capacity is spread more thinly and gradually decreases. In endurance sports races over shorter distances are common.

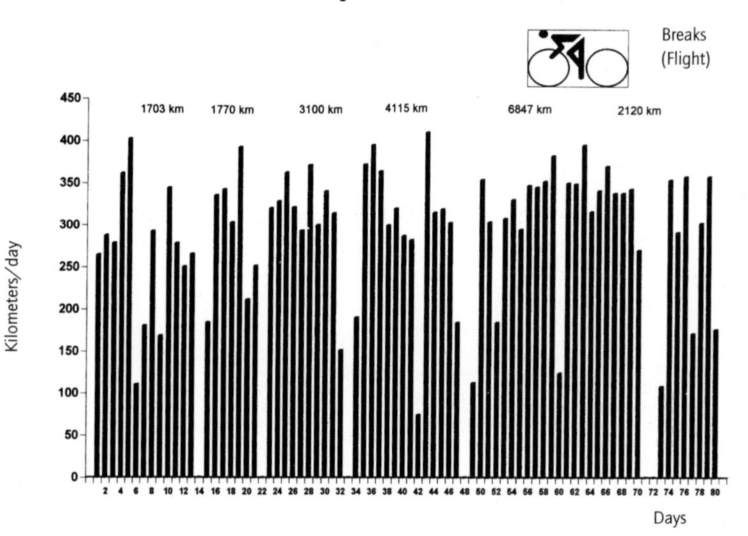

Fig. 3/9.1: Extreme macro-cycle of about 19,700 km cycling trip in 80 days around the world (Hubert Schwarz 1997)

Transition Period (TP)

The TP begins fluidly after the last race. It can also begin as a vacation. Initially it serves psychological recovery and the introduction of rehabilitation measures. Load begins with general training means, often training is in a different sport.

The principle of periodisation is not enough for the exact structuring of the relationship between load and unloading (regeneration). Therefore another cyclically structured sports methodological principle of order was introduced. The cycles in the annual training structure are called macro-cycle, meso-cycle and micro-cycle. The **macro-cycle** is the largest training cycle and covers a training year or 2-3 larger periods of time within a year. An extreme macro-cycle was practised by Hubert Schwarz in 1997 during his cycling trip around the world in 80 days (Fig. 3/9.1).

9.2 Meso-cycle

The meso-cycle (MEC) covers a period of several weeks (2-4 weeks). In it, vital adaptations to training load take place. In content it is further divided into micro-cycles which cover a period of a week. During the MEC phases of load and recovery take place and there is thus enough time to develop sport-specific abilities in a complex. Sports-methodically it has proved useful to standardise the sequence of meso- and micro-cycles because they represent the smaller and still comprehensible series of training sessions. The following capacity complexes are trained in the meso-cycle:

- MEC for development of a general performance base,
- MEC for emphasised development of BE and SE capacities,
- MEC for complex performance development and development of CSE (Fig. 1/9.2).

Meso-cycle for Development of a General Performance Base

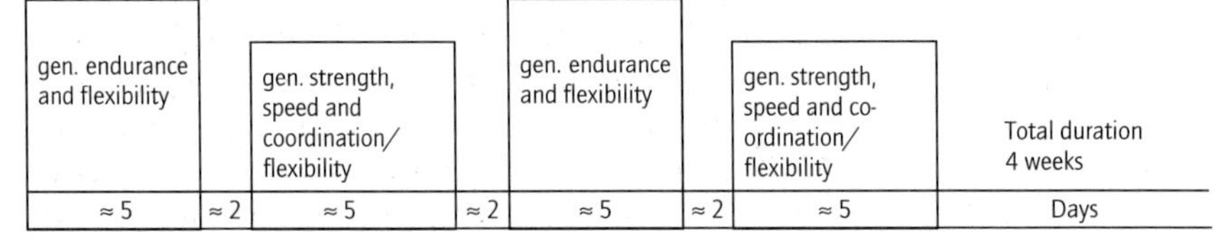

Meso-cycle for Emphasised BE/SE Development

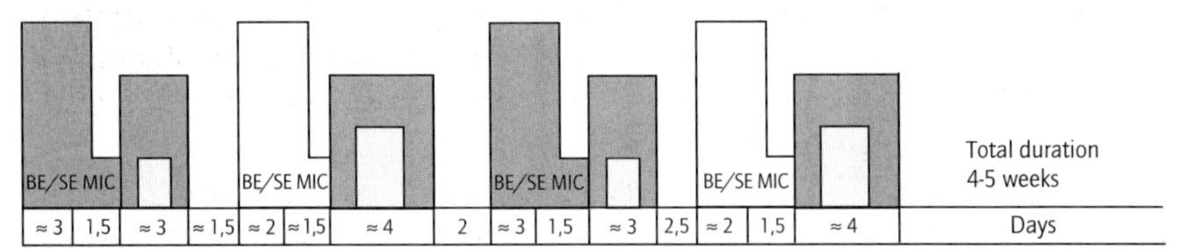

Meso-cycle for Emphasised CSE Development and Development of Competition Performance

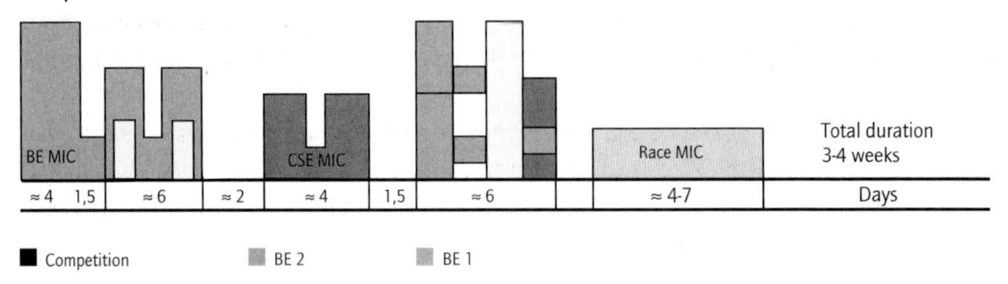

Fig. 1/9.2: Various examples of meso-cycles (MEC) structured with different contents. Above, MEC for development of a general performance base. Centre, MEC for training of basic endurance (BE) and strength endurance (SE). Below, MEC to develop competition-specific endurance (CSE). A number of training days with the same content are grouped together as a micro-cycle (MIC).

The MECs for the development of basic and strength endurance consist of the following content sequence of training sessions:

- **1st week: BE 1 and SE 1 training**
- **2nd week: BE 2 and SE 2 training**
- **3rd week: Complex motor activity training (BE 1, CE and SE).**
- **4th week: Reduction in load for regeneration and compensation.**

9.3 Micro-cycle

The micro-cycle (MIC) is the smallest training cycle. It consists of several training sessions (TS) and is usually planned as a weekly cycle. The emphasised use of a training means is the focus of weekly training. In the MIC, series of great load and following fatigue come close together and must be accommodated sports-methodologically. The current state of performance capacity decides the sequence in which load and unloading are alternated (Fig. 1/9.3, see p. 192). The preferred load rhythm is 3 : 1. In the case of intensive load the 2 : 1 rhythm can also be used.

As already mentioned, the micro-cycles are components of the MEC and usually represent the training within a week. The MICs are thus differentiated for the development of endurance (BE 1 and BE 2), strength endurance (SE) and competition-specific endurance (CSE) (Fig. 2/9.3, see p. 193). Combinations are possible.

In the micro-cycle there is individual borderline area load which adds up. Unloading periods, which should be previously planned in certain rhythms, are especially necessary for processing stimuli. Athletes often underestimate the necessity of unloading, also at times when they feel good physically. Often the subjective judgement of the need for unloading is deceptive. When a reduction in load has been omitted there usually follows a sudden performance collapse which then requires longer breaks to overcome it. This reduces total load, performance development is interrupted.

The MICs which are meant to help prepare a higher performance state are called transformation micro-cycles. Through them energetic overcompensation is prepared through the use of major unloading. There is a reduction of load of 30 to 50 % of usual total volume. Load intensity is not affected by this.

9.4 Direct Competition Preparation or Tapering (DCP)

Direct competition preparation, DCP for short, is a methodological category that developed historically. It served to create the best organisational conditions for training so that, freed from pressure, individual top performance could be prepared for training methodologically.

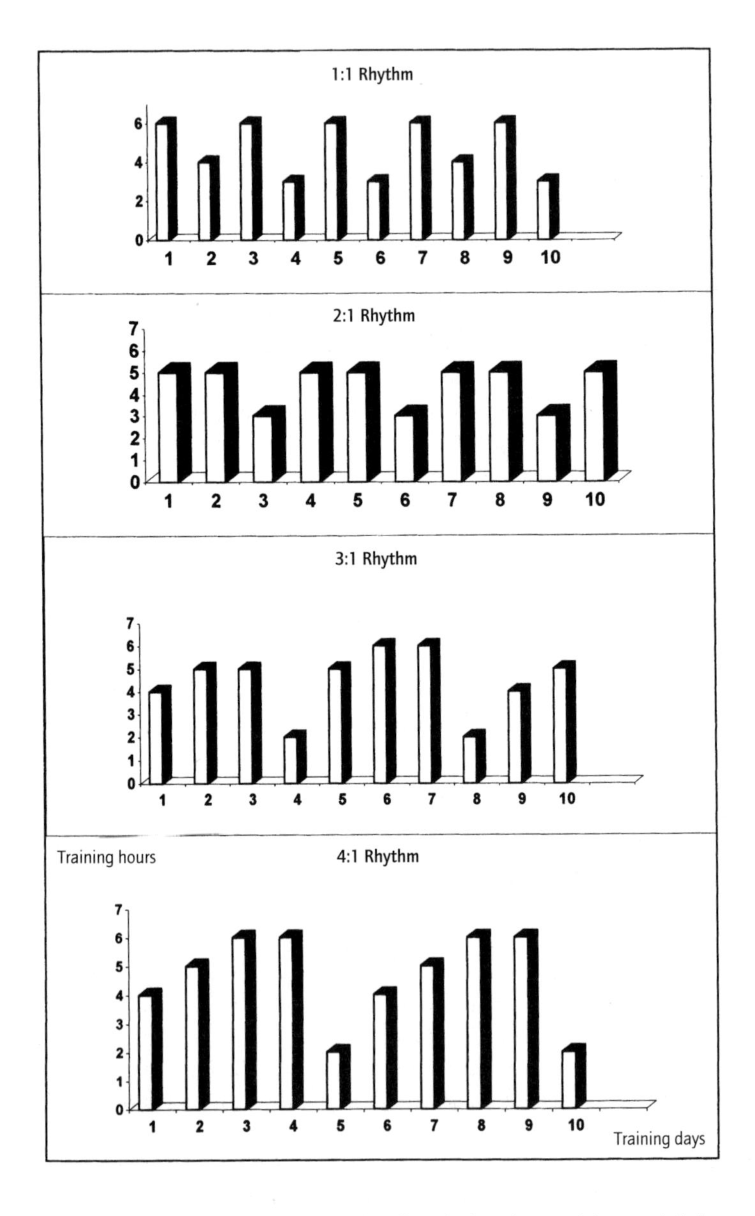

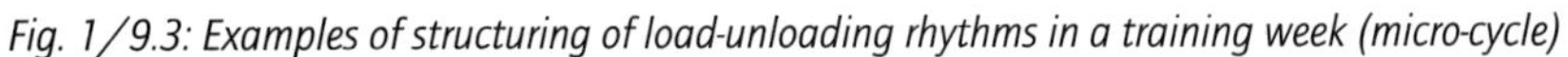
Fig. 1/9.3: Examples of structuring of load-unloading rhythms in a training week (micro-cycle)

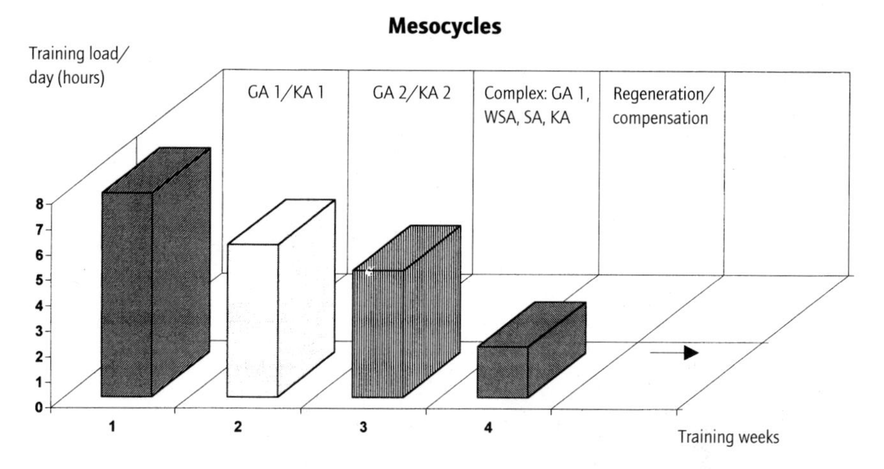

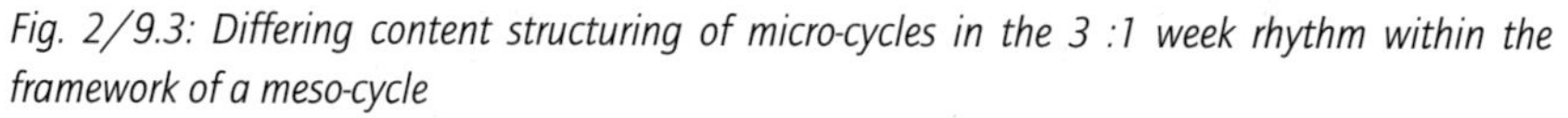

Fig. 2/9.3: Differing content structuring of micro-cycles in the 3 :1 week rhythm within the framework of a meso-cycle

The basic idea behind DCP has been kept alive. The structural contents had to be adapted to new sport-specific conditions.
Valid principles of DCP or Tapering are:

1. Reach the greatest total load by about three weeks before the performance peak.
2. DCP starts with high beginning performance.
3. Increase in load in the intensive CSE area.
4. Keep to the preparatory period of 4-6 weeks.
5. Use of altitude training in the first half of DRP.
6. The time sequence of the MEC for complex ability development must be worked out backwards from the first competition date.

When the greatest adaptive loading stimulus of the year is applied in the DCP, this must end about three weeks before the first competition. The remaining training time is necessary for the processing of the loading peak and for development of complex performance capacity for the competition. The training stimulus is transformed, which is the reason for the term transformation cycle. The first competition after a load peak or after an altitude training camp should take place ten days later at the earliest. In the intermediate period performance instability is too high, it can affect up to 70 % of athletes. This means the majority of athletes do not reproduce their personal best performance. In DCP, training load should be greatly dynamised and in competitive training it should be accompanied by biological measurements (Fig. 1/9.4, see p. 194).

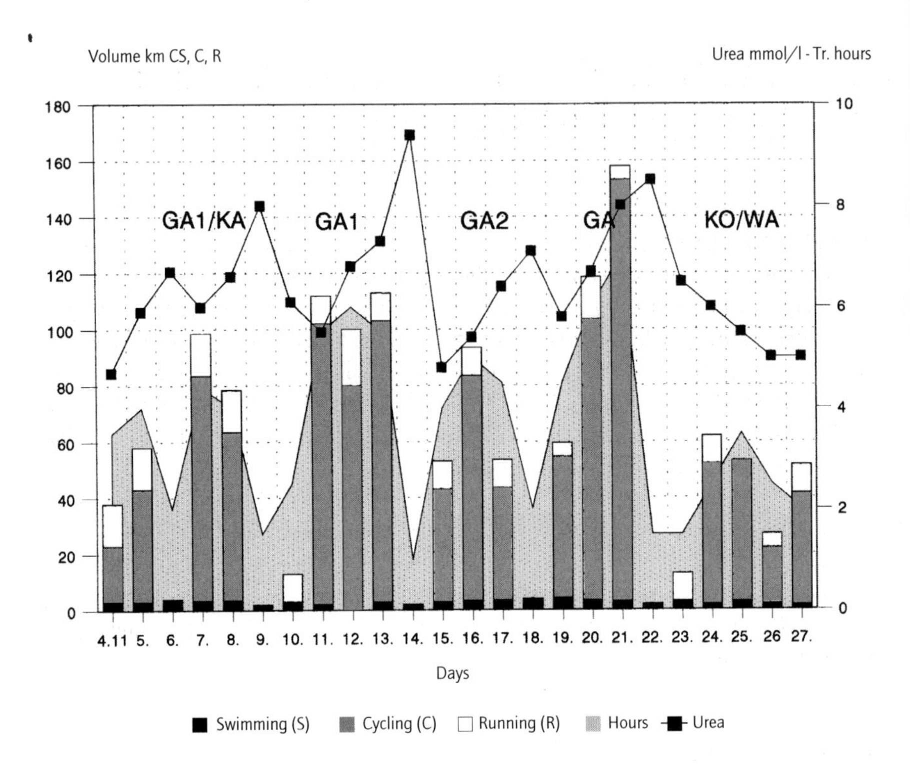

Fig. 1/9.4: Support for the regulation of load in direct competition preparation (DCP) with the aid of determination of serum urea concentration (urea) in the morning. The urea always reacts to the training stimulus a day later. Average urea readings of six squad triathletes in an altitude camp.

Summary

The annual structure of training is divided into cycles. A difference is made between macro-, meso- and micro-cycles. In addition, load during the training year is prescribed in periods, such as preparatory period, competition period and transition period. The periods can be broken down further still into individual training stages. If there is one performance peak per year, there is single periodisation in the training structure. Multiple periodizations are possible depending on main competitions.

10 Control of the Training Load in Endurance Training

Training is characterised by the sequencing of training sessions according to sports-methodological guidelines or empirical ideas. Criteria here are duration, speed, intensity areas as well as load-unloading rhythms. The sports-methodological loading guidelines are not always accurate, especially when the structuring of load intensity is uncertain owing to the weather, course profile, frictional resistance and other factors. With the use of biological measurement factors the intensity of load and its stimulating effects can be assessed with more certainty. Both an increase in performance capacity and the continuing effects of residual tiredness can have varying effects on training load. The use of biological regulating factors is useful for registering these states.

The use of biological measurement factors does not replace training planning and training analysis. A weakness of current competitive training is the neglect of exact training recording and evaluation. In addition to training analysis, competition analysis is of great significance because it allows conclusions about the effects of training (Fig. 1/10, see p. 196).

10.1 Training Planning

The starting point for all considerations with regard to performance development is training planning. In addition to registering and classifying the performance capacity of an athlete, performance goals must be set for him and the necessary programme for training and competitions laid down.

The following working steps should be observed when planning training:

1. Characterisation of the starting situation
2. Formulation of the performance goal and of sub-goals
3. Determination of structuring of training and competition
4. Working out of a training plan on the basis of training data and
5. measures for the organisation of training.

The starting point for planning is the actual level of performance and training age as well as the time objectively available for training. Performance development in clear-cut regulation areas, known sports-methodologically as training areas, is aimed for.

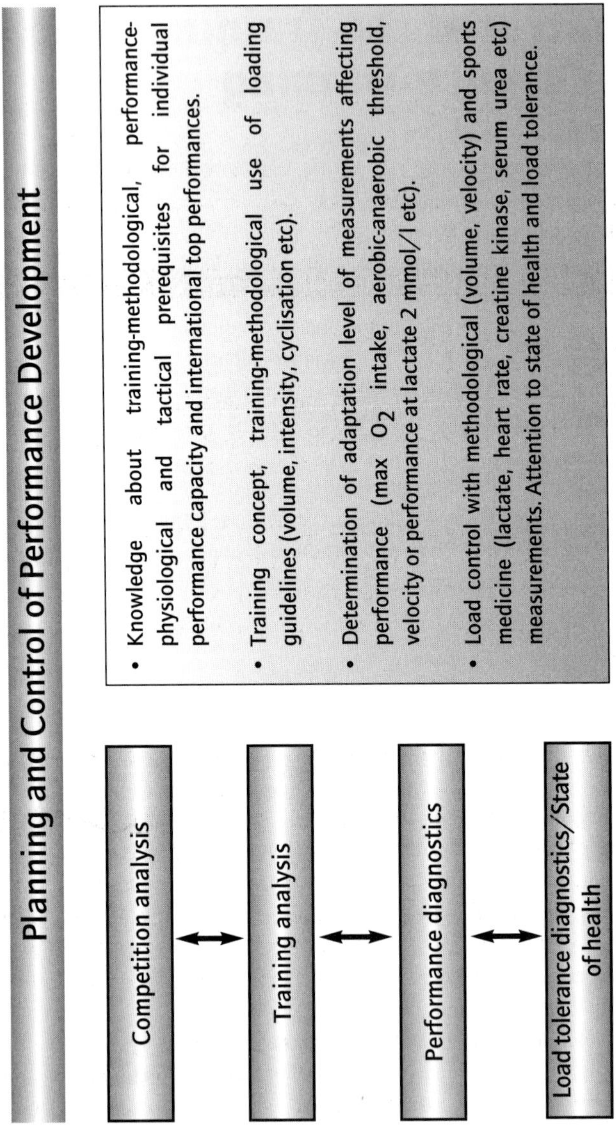

Planning and Control of Performance Development

Competition analysis ↔ Training analysis ↔ Performance diagnostics ↔ Load tolerance diagnostics/State of health

- Knowledge about training-methodological, performance-physiological and tactical prerequisites for individual performance capacity and international top performances.
- Training concept, training-methodological use of loading guidelines (volume, intensity, cyclisation etc).
- Determination of adaptation level of measurements affecting performance (max O_2 intake, aerobic-anaerobic threshold, velocity or performance at lactate 2 mmol/l etc).
- Load control with methodological (volume, velocity) and sports medicine (lactate, heart rate, creatine kinase, serum urea etc) measurements. Attention to state of health and load tolerance.

Fig. 1/10: Planning and regulation of performance development in competitive training. The requirements are competition analysis, training analysis, performance diagnostics and health check.

Summary

The training plan is an instrument for the preparation of increasing performance in predetermined periods. The contents of the training plan are based on load parameters in the sports which are available as training data. Load is applied in training areas and the quality of execution can be checked with methodological and biological indicators.

10.2 Training Analysis

Uncovering the reasons for the development of sporting performances calls for knowledge of the contents of training carried out. A prerequisite for this is the documentation of training, i.e. the reflection of training carried out in the form of training data.

Training which has been standardised and made comprehensible sports-methodologically makes analysis easier. In training planning already the development of the individual biomotor abilities should be thought out and indicated with appropriate data. To make training analysis easier and use it as a regulatory instrument, training should be structured according to fixed content rhythms.
The sequence is:

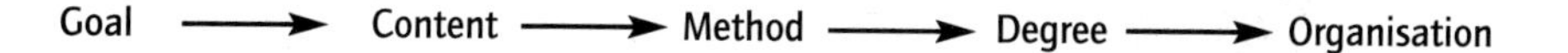

Training recording should be structured in accordance with these contents (Fig. 1/10.2, see p. 198). The top of the record contains general data about the person. When recording data in the training sessions, begin with the year, the week, the day of the week and the particular training session in the course of a day. After that the training goal is given. For example, for basic endurance training in the aerobic area write BE 1. Further training goals in ability development are entered as competition endurance (CE), strength endurance (SE) etc.

Then come the training means. For the fulfilment of the training goal individual external conditions can be laid down. As training means both the individual sports such as swimming (S), cycling (C), running (R) and complex training forms such as duathlon and triathlon etc. should be entered.

The training methods are laid down according to usual training terminology and include e.g. the continuous method, the interval method, the repetition method as well as the competition

Year	Week	Day	TS	TMeans	Conditions	Method	Intensity (%)	Volume (km)	Hours	Velocity (m/s; km/h)	HR, Lactate	Total Time (h, min)	Comment
98	3	Mo	2	Cycling	flat	BE 1	70	110	4	28	131/ ...	4	Frost
98	3	Tu	1	Running	cross-c.	BE 1	75	15	1	4.2	145/2.5	90 min	Rain

Fig. 1/10.2: Example of a training protokol

and control method (MARTIN, 1991; HARRE, 1986; SCHNABEL et al. 1995; ZINTL, 1990). More details are in chapter 6. After this follows a comment on training intensity, the basis of which is current competition velocity, and details of the volume of training in kilometres.

The frequency of repetitions and the training time (without preparation and follow-up) are important parameters for assessing the training session. Details on training velocity for major training contents should not be left out, they characterise the quality of training. The training record can be individually extended. Possibilities are notes about biological regulatory factors such as heart rate and lactate. At the end of the record comes the total training time. Details on one's psychophysical feeling complete the training record. Training follow-up can be complemented by a training journal. Subjective processing of load, the emotional state and other details of importance to the athlete can be recorded here.

After daily recording of training contents, there should be a training analysis after about 4-6 weeks, especially at times when performance diagnostics are carried out.

The objective of training analysis is the evaluation of training content covered in the form of a comparison of target and result. In this way the reasons for the current performance state and performance reserves become recognisable. With the evaluation of training on the basis of tables and graphs, better overview of load is possible.

The training analysis should concentrate on the following points:

1. Presentation of training contents and structures which determine performance in the dynamics of their progression.
2. Structuring of intensity in the main training areas.
3. Cyclical structuring of training load.
4. Dynamics of load and recovery in the micro- and meso-cycles.

Summary

The objective of training analysis is the set and actual comparison of training content and the intention of recognising the current state of performance and uncovering reserves. The training analysis is an important prerequisite for further structuring of loading, assessment of the effectiveness of training and also for complex performance diagnostics. The assessment of adaptations is only partially or in fact hardly possible without detailed knowledge of training.

10.3 Competition Analysis

Competition performance is the result of training carried out beforehand. Here it is proved whether training effort was effective with regard to performance.

A systematic analysis supports penetration into the structure of competition performance and allows the uncovering of individual performance reserves. The more exactly competition structure can be analysed, the more accurate are the conclusions for training. The findings from competition analysis are the basis for planning of prognosis performance and in particular influence further competition-specific training (Fig. 1/10.3).

The competition analysis has a performance diagnostic character.

The evaluation of the competition can be done on the basis of the analysis of the time progression, the velocities in certain sections, behaviour at the start, the main velocity, behaviour in the finish, incline structuring, mastery of descents, movement rate and cycle distance (Table 1/10.3, see p. 201).

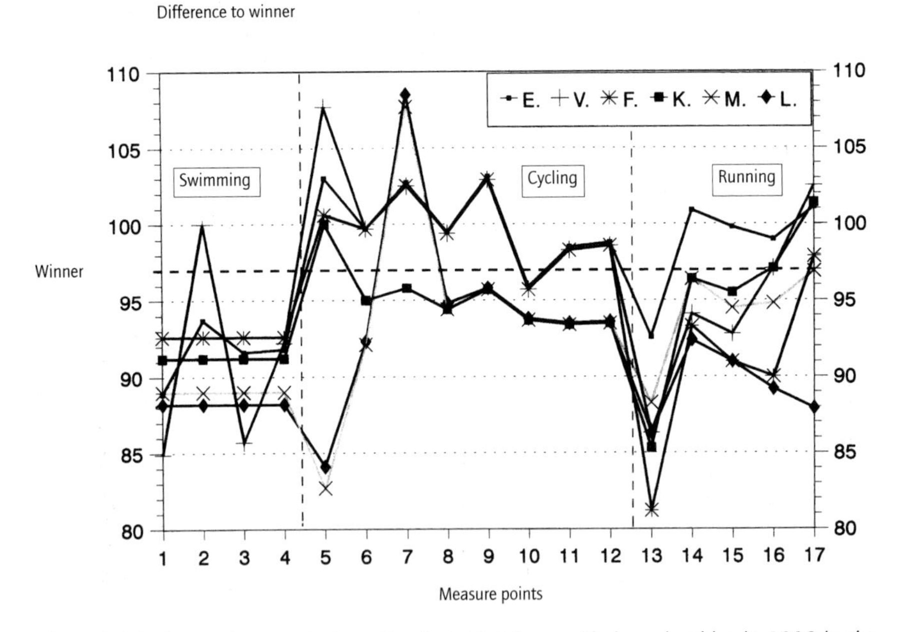

Fig. 1/10.3: Competition analysis at the short triathlon world championships in 1996 in the USA. The illustration shows the time variations (in per cent) of the German participants in comparison to the winner in all three sections.

Emphases in Competition Analysis		
	Triathlon	Cross-country skiing
Race performances: World Cup (WC), European Championships (ECh), World Championships (WCh)	WC, ECh, WCh,	WC, ECh, AC
Performance comparison with world best	**% Amount behind**	**% Amount behind**
Performance over shorter and longer distances	Sprint triathlon (0.8; 20;5 km) Short triathlon (1.5;40;10 km)	5; 10; 15 km 30; 50 km
Performances in sub-events	Swimming, cycling, running	Freestyle, classical
Velocity in course of race	Start, changeover, course, finish	Start, course, finish
Specific performances	Neoprene, changeover, slipstream cycling	Incline, flat
Sporting technique	Movement structure	Stride structure
Tactics	Speed burst and finishing sprint	Inclines, finishing sprint
Biological measurements	Heart rate (HR), lactate	HR, lactate

Table 1/10.3: Emphases of competition analysis

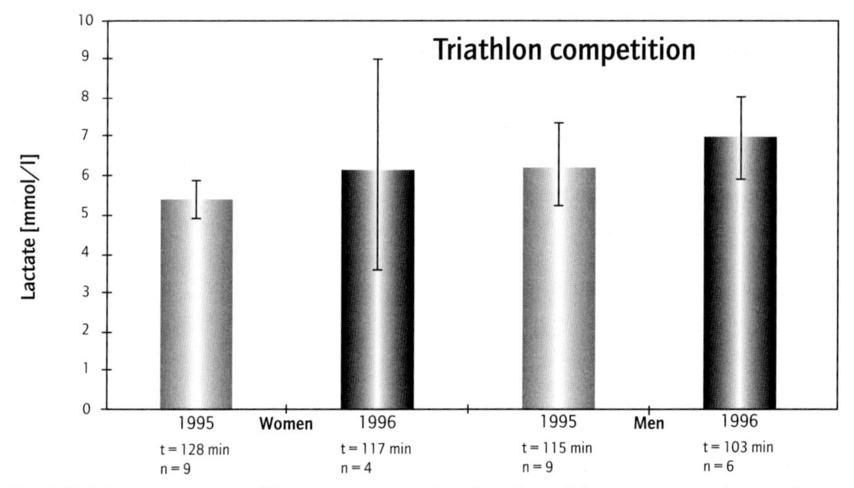

Fig. 2/10.3: Measurement of lactate concentration of male and female squad athletes after a qualifying competition in short triathlon

In particular competition technique should also be checked. The data from the competition analysis can be evaluated with the aid of video technology and also manually. The results of the competition analyses give athletes and coaches important hints for structuring of races. Orientation values for training can be extrapolated from aspects of competition performance.

In addition the use of selected performance-physiological measurements in competitions completes findings on competition structure. In endurance sports, heart rate and lactate measurements are preferred because they allow objective indications of the level of exertion and effort (Fig. 2/10.3, see p. 201).

Summary

The analysis of competition performance by means of the measuring of sector times, determination of movement rate, cycle distance, start and final sprint behaviour, etc. is a realistic measurement for training control. Through it the level of development of complex competition specific endurance performance capacity can be assessed. This analysis can be meaningfully complemented by measurement of heart rate, lactate and other factors. Competition structuring and final performance are useful orientation points for the evaluation of performance diagnostic findings.

10.4 Control of Loading by Sports-methodological and Sports-medical Indicators

If diagnostics are carried out under conditions of real training it is a load control measure. Training control, on the other hand, is a more comprehensive form of taking influence and requires data from daily load testing with various measurement units. The diagnostic prognosis is limited in load tests but it has the advantage of specificness and the registration of states that change in daily training (REISS/GOHLITZ, 1994).

The control of load with sport methodology and sports medicine measurement units occurs in a short-term (daily) and medium-term form:

- **Short-term load or training control** includes measures which help to assess the effectiveness of stimuli in every single training session. Sport-methodological regulatory measures are supported with the aid of suitable biological measurements. Both procedures help prepare sport-specific adaptation.

- **Medium-term training control** involves test loads in the laboratory or the carrying out of field tests. The purpose of these tests is to complexly register and assess over longer periods the state of adaptation or performance reached. Methods favoured are functional and performance diagnostics tests in the laboratory as well as test competitions.

The decisive method for controlling load is still the assessment of the duration and the velocity of training loading. Only registering loading time is uncertain as a regulatory measure because in this case the qualitative factor of training, velocity, is neglected. Increasingly athletes' behaviour is recorded on video at certain points of the training or competition. In this way e.g. length of stride in running, cycle rate in swimming, pedalling rate in cycling and other factors characterising movement structure can be recorded. Changes in forward movement technique when tiredness sets in can also be recorded.

The secret of performance development in sport is based on increasing sport-specific velocity coupled with a total volume necessary to achieve this. The ratios of intensity and duration of load can be changed as a result of the findings of daily loading control. The decisive adaptations in the muscle take place via the average training velocity achieved over a sport-specific distance. To ensure a speed that is an effective stimulus in the particular training areas it is advantageous to use biological measurements. The biological measurements used in daily loading control are not very numerous. Measurements that have proved useful for years are:

- Heart rate (HR)
- Blood lactate
- Blood serum urea
- Blood creatine kinase.

The control of load using biological measurements cannot make good sports-methodological shortcomings in the structuring of load. As the processing of load and the reaction of the body to this are of a complex nature and also vary individually, the experience of coaches or experts in the sport cannot be done without. We emphasise this because the number of athletes who control load themselves and do not call on qualified assistance is increasing. At the latest when failure in competitive training occurs, use should be made of advice and a complex training analysis.

In order to make the procedure for daily loading control comprehensible, the following **complex state assessments**, which can be registered with a number of measurements, are possible:

- **Loading intensity**
- **Level of exertion**
- **Loading summation**
- **Load tolerance**
- **Regeneration state**
- **Performance stability**

Using these categories of state, reality can be better recorded than by limiting loading control to one or two measurement factors.

10.4.1 Assessment of Loading Intensity

The main criterion for the assessment of loading intensity is the combination of duration and velocity of a performance in the sport. These influence HR and lactate in typical ways.

Heart Rate Measurement

The HR only needs a short time to adjust itself to the prescribed level of load. The better the training state, the more quickly a steady state of HR regulation is reached. Well-trained athletes need one to two minutes and untrained persons need four to six minutes for the HR to regulate itself to a steady state. In the regulation field of 120 to 175 bpm the HR is suitable for differentiating demands on the body in an aerobic metabolism situation. The metabolism situation is aerobic when the lactate concentration is under 2 mmol/l.

With increasing muscular tiredness the HR rises gradually or sometimes rapidly. Despite the feeling of effort applied, with tiredness velocity decreases. The HR gives direct feedback information on the biological effort to achieve performance. The greater the biological effort, the higher the HR.

Experienced athletes regulate their endurance performance capacity in competitions by keeping to a certain HR regulation field. They know that when they overload themselves they go above a certain upper HR level. In long duration competitions the number of athletes is increasing who regulate their performance capacity with the aid of HR measurement and who are constantly aware of their load tolerance. Going above an HR borderline area during long duration load, which for young athletes is between 180 to 190 bpm and for older athletes between 160 and 170 bpm, signals a loading borderline situation and is usually linked with the addition of anaerobic metabolism. An increase in HR during long duration load indicates that the chosen velocity is too high.

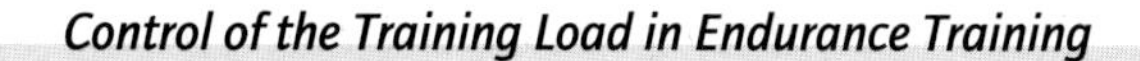

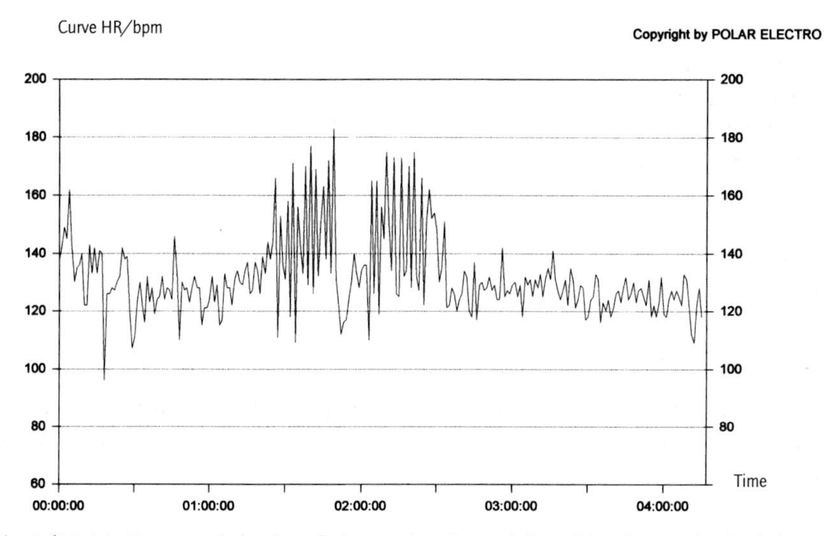

Fig. 1/10.4.1: Heart rate behaviour during road cycling training of four hours. The rise in heart rate between the 90th and 150th minute is due to incline training on hills.

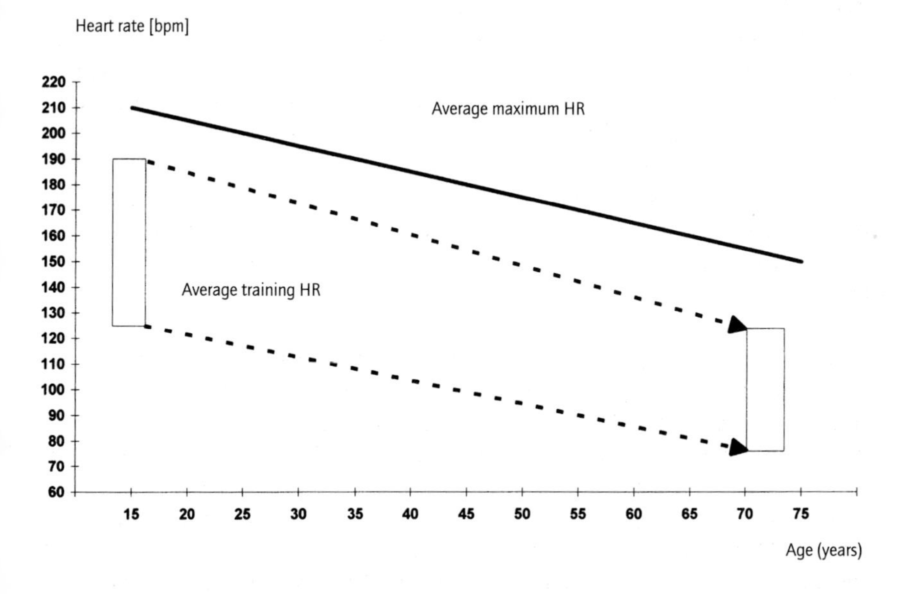

Fig. 2/10.4.1: Maximum heart rate (HR) with increasing age and area of loading HR

The advantage of HR measurement lies in the constant ability to differentiate intensity and duration of load both in training and in competitions (Fig. 1/10.4.1, see p. 205).

For training control the measurement of maximum HR is of less significance. Maximum HR is subject to too many influences, such as mobilisation capacity, age, sex, etc. (see chapter 4.1). Women generally have higher maximum HR values in younger years than men. With increasing age the maximum HR goes down (Fig. 2/10.4.1, see p. 205). The main influence on the lowering of maximum HR comes from the decrease in sport-specific speed motor activity due to lack of training. Older athletes no longer achieve such high velocities in training and competitions.

The HR level allows conclusions on possible lactate development and the use of energy.

In the region of maximum HR lactate always develops. If the HR reaches about 90% of the individual maximum value, it is no longer possible to deduce the level of lactate development from this. If e.g. a HR of 190 bpm is reached, then the athlete is in the upper regulation level of the cardiovascular system. In metabolism there can be a lactate concentration of 5 or of 13 mmol/l. This means that when the cardiovascular system is at the upper end of the scale, lactate development can increase further.

Often the training HR is derived from the maximum HR. The existence of a number of formulae documents the uncertainty about the estimation of the right individual training HR (Table 1/10.4.1, see p. 207). The formulae are general guidelines and were developed at a time when ongoing HR measurement was not yet possible. Individual and ongoing measurement of the HR makes it possible to better classify load training methodologically.

In the individual sports, training state and sporting technique clearly influence the HR regulation level. With increasing performance capacity the HR goes down at comparable velocities, the same applies to improved sporting technique (see Fig. 1/4.1).

In the individual sports, HR measurement is accompanied by a number of typical peculiarities.

Heart Rate in Running Training

When running on flat ground, over a longer period, HR regulation is very stable. Nevertheless, minor changes in velocity or in energy use (incline) immediately lead to a rise in the HR of 3 to 7 bpm. This observation makes it possible for athletes to approach inclines more slowly and not go above a certain level of effort.

Untrained people or those with little training react to increases in velocity in running with a much more pronounced HR increase than trained athletes. With improved training state a change in running velocity has less effect on the cardiovascular system.

Loading Control with the Heart Rate (HR)	
Maximum HR and Age	
Recommended estimates	**Examples**
• 200 - 1/2 age	50 years = 175/min
• 220 - age	50 years = 170 / min
• 210 - 0.8 age	50 years = 170 / min
Deviations of ± 10 bpm are considered as normal	
Load HR Running Training	
Intensity (velocity)	
low (slow)	125 - 140 / min
moderate (medium)	145 - 155 / min
high (fast)	160 - 170 / min
competition (maximum)	165 - 200 /min

Table 1/10.4.1: Loading control with heart rate (HR)

In comparison to other endurance sports, with running load the HR regulation level is always somewhat higher because one's own body weight is also accelerated. Because basic motor activity for running is well-developed in a wide circle of athletes, the highest individual maximum HR values are found in running.

Heart Rate in Cycling Training

Velocity in cycling is influenced by a number of disruptive factors. These include wind, road surface, inclines, descents, cycling position and bicycle material etc. They make themselves noticeable in a high fluctuation of the HR. To keep cycling velocity constant, the muscular strength endurance effort must be constantly changed and that leads to greater HR fluctuation (Fig. 3/10.4.1, see p. 208).

The course profile has the greatest influence on the HR. After the hill climb with full cardiovascular load follows the descent and this allows a partial recovery in the cardiovascular system.

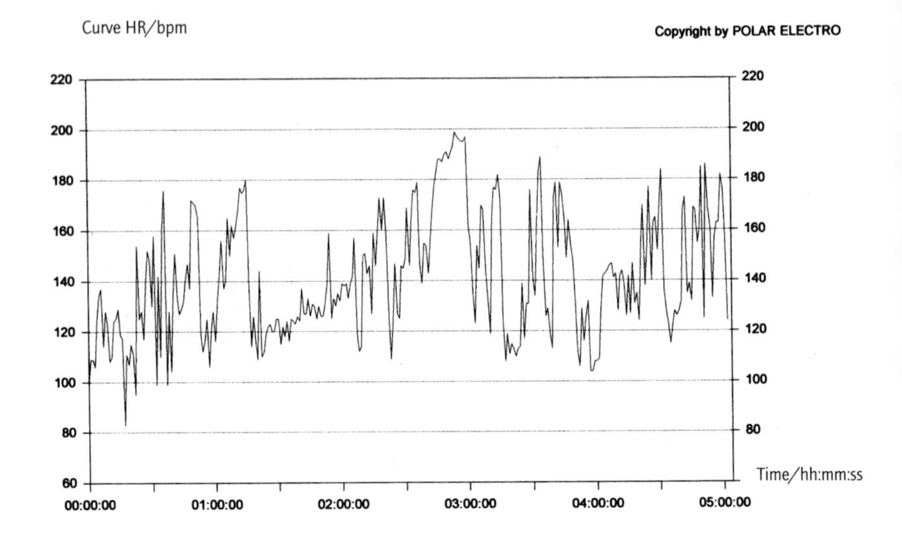

Fig. 3/10.4.1: Heart rate during a road race over 160 km

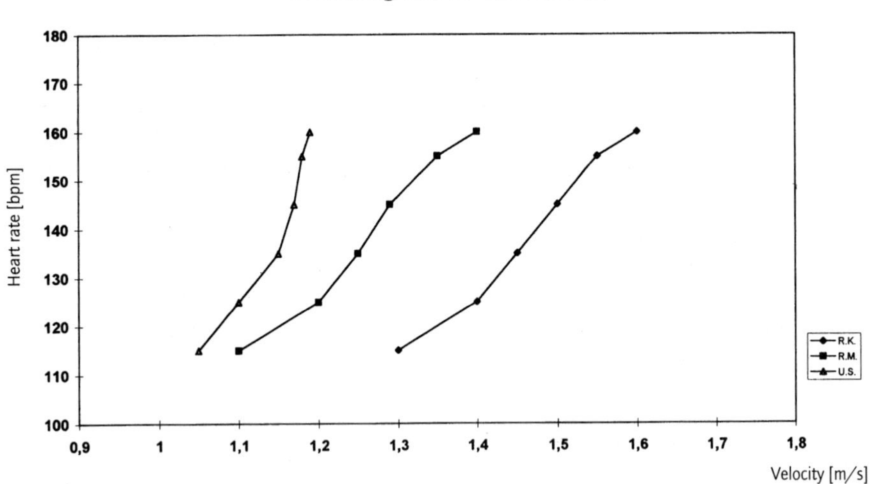

Fig. 4/10.4.1: Increase in heart rate of triathletes with varying performance capacity in swimming. Swimmer S. with the lowest performance and inadequate swimming technique showed the steepest HR rise.

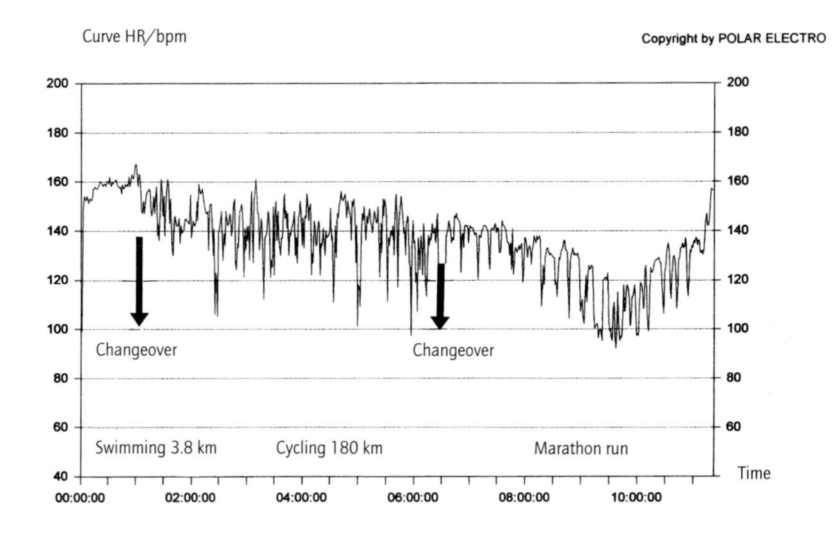

Fig. 5/10.4.1: Heart rate during an ultra triathlon successfully completed by an athlete with diabetes type II in Hawaii.

Heart Rate in Swimming

In swimming HR regulation is greatly influenced by the technique of forward movement. Differentiating ability for movement processes and swimming velocity ("feeling for water") characterises mastery of swimming velocities. Athletes with inadequate swimming technique (e.g. triathletes) reach their maximum HR earlier and also at lower swimming speeds (Fig. 4/10.4.1, see p. 208). Swimmers with poorer technique have a lower maximum load HR in the water than those with better technique. Before the cardiovascular system reaches the top of the regulation scale, poor swimmers are already muscularly exhausted.

If the load intensity in swimming is given as a percentage of best performance, the result is that at comparable intensity the HR in the submaximal load region is 10-15 bpm lower than in running. In swimming, competitive athletes do not usually reach their maximum HR, with the exception of special swimmers.

Heart Rate in Cross-country Skiing

Monitoring of loading intensity using biological measurements is especially necessary in cross-country skiing because changing friction conditions on snow and the course profile make assessment of load more difficult. Cross-country skiing velocity can change suddenly through changing gliding conditions alone even when biological effort is constant. "Faster" snow supports movement motor activity and thus causes a greater rise in HR than "dull" snow. Similarly, freestyle technique leads to a greater rise in HR than does the classical skiing technique.

As a result of the course profile the cross-country skier quickly changes his HR regulation level. After full load on a climb where he reaches his maximum HR he can recover on the descent, or else actively maintain his pace with stick work. On longer descents the HR decreases to below 100 bpm. With increasing tiredness HR goes down less on descents, i.e. the athlete's recovery gets less and less. Recovery is disrupted if the HR does not fall more than 30 beats within a minute. Similarly to cycling, cross-country skiing has a broad HR regulation level. During skiing in aerobic metabolism the HR fluctuates from 100 to 170 bpm. This statement is analogous for ski treadmill load.

Heart Rate in Triathlon

Both in short and in ultra triathlons the HR is dependent on the sport being practised. In triathlon competitions there is a gradual increase in HR from the swimming through the cycling to the running. The HR level is between 150 bpm and up to 185 bpm in competitions. During sport changeovers the HR only decreases briefly by 15 to 20 bpm so that altogether there are high demands on the cardiovascular system the whole time (Fig. 5/10.4.1, see p. 209).

Assessment of Loading Intensity through Lactate

The determination of the lactate concentration in the blood is of central importance in training control and for the assessment of loading intensity.

In training practice, lactate measurement is done using various methods, most only require 10 to 20 μ/l of blood.

Lactate measurement can now be carried out by athletes themselves. Paper strip measuring technology (Accusport®) is available at an affordable price. With this measuring process, with or without someone else helping, lactate concentration can be determined from a drop of blood from the pad of the finger in only a minute.

Within the framework of loading control lactate determination allows the following information:

- **Assessment of the direction of the metabolic effects of training load**
  Here a conclusion is drawn from the level of lactate concentration whether metabolism load was aerobic, aerobic-anaerobic or mainly anaerobic.

- **Mobilisation capacity of motor activity**
  The lactate concentration arrived at is dependent on the involvement of the fast twitch muscle fibres (FTF) in the sport-specific movement programme and thus decisively dependent on velocity. The lactate is mainly developed by the FT fibres included in the movement programme.

- **State of development of submaximal aerobic performance capacity**
  Using increases in stages of performance or velocity the submaximal sport-specific performance capacity at a fixed lactate value (2, 3 or 4 mmol/l) can be ascertained. The determining of the lactate performance curve or the anaerobic threshold can be carried out with laboratory or field tests (see chapters 10.3 and 10.4) .

- **Classification of loading intensity (velocity) in the intensity areas of the sport**
  Training occurs in a certain spectrum of metabolism regulation.
  The level of lactate concentration is dependent on the particular training velocity. Training velocities are classified into the intensity or training areas of the sport.

- **Effect of training means**
  The training means, such as cycling, running, ski treadmill, swimming etc. change in their use in the sport or are a fixed element of training.
  Depending on technical and motor mastery of them, their effect on metabolism varies. The effect of the training means on anaerobic metabolism and thus on lactate development is of methodological interest.

- **Application of training methods**
  The training methods, such as the continuous method, interval or tempo changing methods, have varying effects on metabolism. With the aid of lactate measurement their effect on metabolism (aerobic or anaerobic) can be determined (HOTTENROTT/ZÜLCH, 1995).

With lactate measurement the energetic components of training load are registered. Increasing lactate concentration means crossing of the upper limits of aerobic performance capacity and compensation through anaerobic energy metabolism. The prerequisite for this statement is that velocity is checked over a measured or comparable test distance. If the lactate concentration decreases at the same or at higher velocity, then an increase in aerobic performance capacity is likely. An exception would be great muscle tiredness. In the reverse case the same velocity and a higher lactate concentration means a decrease in aerobic performance capacity and an increase in anaerobic capacity (Fig. 6/10.4.1, see p. 212).

If training in a fitness or competitive sport is begun at a low level, usually the lactate concentration is higher than generally recommended in order to ensure a certain velocity. At the beginning of training, lactate can temporarily rise to 4 or 6 mmol/l during load. This reaction is physiologically normal.

Improvement in performance capacity can be recognised in a decrease in lactate concentration. The HR reacts even more sensitively to performance improvement, it signals a functional adjustment already after eight days of training (see Fig. 3/3).

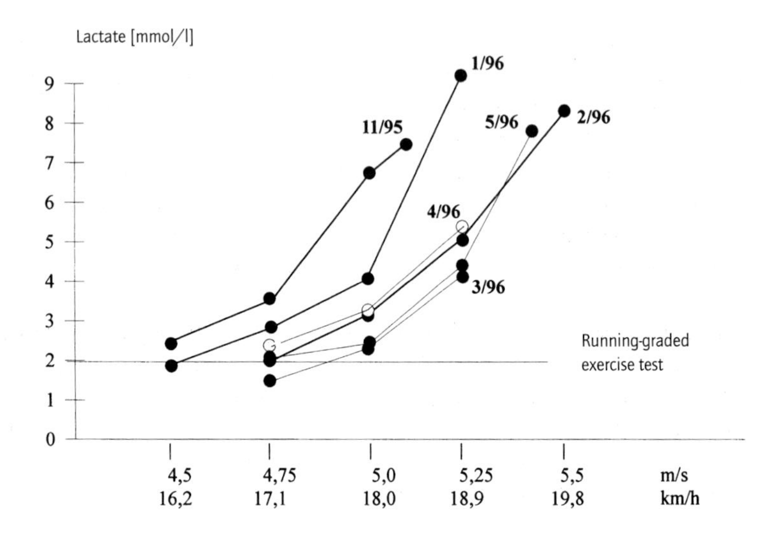

Fig. 6/10.4.1: Monthly performance diagnostics on the treadmill in the 4 x 4 km graded exercise test of a top triathlete. Although a move to the right of the lactate performance curve can be made out, current after-effects of training also lead to a temporary "move to the left" of the lactate performance curve (e.g. 4/96 as opposed to 3/96)

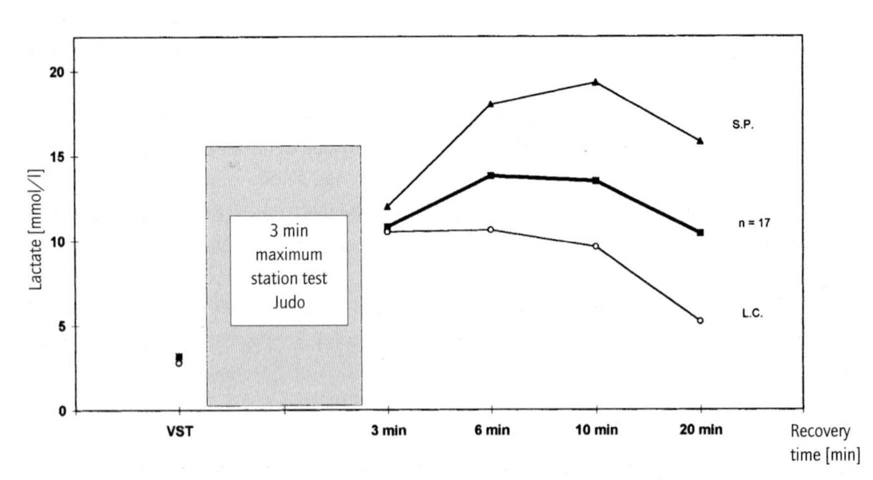

Fig. 7/10.4.1: Different examples of lingering lactate concentration after intensive specific graded exercise test load in judo

In performance-oriented training, velocity is always the leading factor and not automatically metabolism regulation. Training with higher anaerobic ratios leads to faster performance development, but it is unstable. Brief intensity increases incorporated in training are useful for motor activity. The lactate increase that then occurs is quickly broken down again during load and does not hinder the development of aerobic performance capacity. If the record breaking African runners had made their high velocities in training dependent on the level of lactate concentration, then their performance development would probably not have occurred to the extent it did or it would have been slowed down for biological reasons.

Maximum lactate development is also dependent on load duration. The highest lactate values are reached during intensive cyclical load between 60 s and 120 s (see Fig. 4/5.2). Lactate development is linked to the muscle glycogen store and stops when it is exhausted. This state is reached after competitions of over two hours duration. In sporting practice it is repeatedly seen that a top marathon run is finished in 130 min with a lactate of under 3 mmol/l. Slower marathon runners only reach lactate concentrations up to 2 mmol/l.

The level of lactate concentration after long duration load documents the metabolic steady state. The balance between lactate development and lactate breakdown can be raised considerably. Sport-specifically, lactate concentrations of about 8 mmol/l can be maintained in competitions for one or two hours. The amount of the constant lactate level is always dependent on the aerobic performance level. The aerobic performance level determines to a large degree the velocity level with lactate development that can be kept up. A high lactate level as a result of speed bursts disturbs aerobic energy metabolism considerably. Experienced endurance athletes avoid unnecessary speed bursts or have deliberately practised them out of competition-tactical necessity. A constant high lactate concentration in competitions characterises the stability of endurance performance capacity. Endurance stability is a separate diagnostic category which can be registered through longer sport-specific test load.

Factors which negatively influence lactate development include lack of glycogen and the state of fatigue of motor activity, whether acute or chronic (overtraining).

The timing of lactate measurement depends on the type of load. The shorter intensive load lasts, the later lactate should be measured. Lactate needs a certain amount of time for distribution in the body.

If high load lactate development is expected, then blood should only be taken after three minutes or more (Fig. 7/10.4.1, see p. 212). The lactate developed in the blood after brief load reaches the blood with a delay. If it is measured too early, lactate mobilisation ability is underestimated.

Lactate determination is especially informative after competition. Through comparisons of velocity (performance) and the level of lactate concentration, conclusions can be drawn about the state of development of aerobic and anaerobic sport-specific performance capacity or race specific endurance (CSE). In competitions the lactate values only rise when velocity increases. In order to decide for sure whether the increase in performance is based on aerobic or anaerobic foundations, complex sport-specific performance diagnostic laboratory tests are necessary (see chapter 10.5).

10.4.2 Assessment of Level of Exertion

Intensive short and long duration loads lead to stress regulation in the body. The increase in hormones of the suprarenal gland (adrenaline and noradrenaline) makes it possible to register stress regulation. During intensive short duration stress the adrenaline in particular rises. Adrenaline is the typical stress hormone which winds up the cardiovascular system and metabolism. Adrenaline raises the HR, blood pressure and glycogen breakdown in the liver. In emergency situations the blood sugar level is raised. Under load the use of energy is increased with the aid of adrenaline.

Under stress the adrenaline concentration rises from 0.3 mmol/l at rest to 8 mmol/l. Adrenaline only begins to rise when load is higher than 75 % of maximum oxygen intake. This corresponds to the beginning of subjectively felt exertion. When load ends, adrenaline normalises within 30 minutes, so it is not so suitable for intensity control.

In the case of long duration stress a rise in adrenaline is not so typical, but rather in noradrenaline and the suprarenal gland hormone cortisole. After intensive endurance load the cortisole concentration rises from a resting value of 150 nmol/l to as much as 1300 nmol/l (see Fig. 2/12).

Because cortisole increases the breakdown of the substrates during load, it ensures the supply of energy from carbohydrate, protein and fat metabolism for extreme load. Because determining hormones as a whole is complicated, they are not routinely used in training control. An increased cortisole concentration as a result of load has an inhibiting effect on the immune system. High concentrations of cortisole have an immune depressive effect.

Exertion under load can be indirectly derived from the HR. The HR usually reaches its individually highest level under stress loads.

10.4.3 Assessment of Load Tolerance

Coping with training demands is a characteristic of load tolerance and reflects a certain level of adaptation. The target organ representative for load tolerance in sport is the muscle. The muscle is not only an organ that develops strength, but is also a highly sensitive sense organ which reacts to stretching stimuli. Stretching stimuli regulate the degree of muscle movements. If muscular load tolerance is exceeded through unaccustomed short or long duration load, the cell constant enzyme creatine kinase (CK) enters the bloodstream. Measuring CK activity in the blood is a suitable measurement factor for assessing muscular load tolerance. Under normal conditions CK can only be found in very small concentrations. In case of energetic bottlenecks and/or mechanical muscle disruptions the CK activity in the blood increases. In accustomed training the CK level is about 2 to 5 μmol/s.l. In training where stimuli take effect it rises to as much as 15 μmol/s.l. After extreme endurance load rises in CK of over 60 μmol/s.l. occur (see Fig. 1/4.5.4). These high readings are sure signs of muscular overloading and structural destruction as a result of exceeding muscular load tolerance limits and also strain the kidney function. The raised CK level can be found several days after great load with a decreasing tendency. A clear drop in the CK increase indicates that muscles are loadable again. Clinical norm values of CK are not applicable in competitive sport because they are regularly exceeded by the muscle load. Apart from extreme increases they have no practical consequences for training.

Great increases in CK activity in the blood, not explainable through load, can also be a sign of major muscle dissolution (rhabdomyolysis) and calls for urgent consultation of a doctor.

10.4.4 Assessment of Summation of Load

Several training sessions a day in close sequence are a characteristic of competitive training. The new training stimulus meets with muscles that have not yet recovered. The lack of glycogen during load leads to greater protein breakdown in the muscles. As a result, urea in the blood rises. This is used for training control. From the level of serum urea, conclusions about the degree of protein use and protein breakdown can be drawn. In normal competitive training the serum urea concentration rises to 5 to 7 mmol/l in men and 4.5 to 6 mmol/l in women. The advantage of determining serum urea is that the increase in urea remains for several days after load (see Fig. 3/4.5.3)

For best results urea is measured daily and well before training begins. Direct post-load concentration and recovery capacity over night are included in this reading. The trend in the change in the serum urea provides information on the summational effect of training and at the same time allows conclusions regarding recovery capacity. If serum urea exceeds 9 mmol/l early on several days in a row, then load is too high. It must be reduced considerably or a break must be taken. A break of one day lowers morning serum urea by 1 to 3 mmol/l on the following day. If training continues despite high serum urea, then the ground is prepared for overtraining. The athlete enters a catabolic metabolism situation which blocks adaptation in the muscle.

With increasing load duration, serum urea concentration rises. After eight hours of training a day, similarly high urea values are reached as after a 100 km run. Extreme urea values are measurable after ultra triathlons (Ironman), 100 km runs or multiple ultra triathlons. Directly after load they are between 12 and 17 mmol/l and remain high for a week with decreasing tendency. This shows clearly that from a metabolism point of view, muscular tiring continues for at least a week.

Reductions in training load also have an effect on the decrease in serum urea concentration; the day after, a relief in urea decrease of 0.5 to 2 mmol/l can be registered.

10.4.5 Assessment of Regeneration

For the assessment of regeneration after sporting load, measurement factors which have a long lasting effect are useful. As HR and lactate return to their original levels within a few minutes or 30 minutes at the most, they can only be used for direct assessment of recovery. An exception here is the resting HR (resting pulse). The resting HR is a fine indicator for disturbed regeneration or overloading caused by training. A rise in resting HR of 6-8 bpm already indicates incomplete regeneration or the beginning of overtraining. The resting HR also rises early when illnesses begin, usually more than 10 bpm.

A new supportive piece of information for training regulation is the measuring of the variability of the resting HR. In a recovered state, the variability of the HR is greater than in a regeneratively disturbed state. Tiredness restricts variability (see chapter 4.1).

Greatly disrupted regeneration also leads to a higher HR during training or test load; under accustomed load it can be 10 bpm higher (Fig. 1/10.4.5, see p. 217). If this occurs, an analysis of loading and unloading should be made.

An increased HR at rest or under load can contain three pieces of information: disturbed regeneration, beginning overtraining or a developing illness. In this case a break is the safest decision. For further information see chapter 12. CK and serum urea are indirect measurement factors for assessing regeneration. Increased values point to incomplete regeneration.

10.4.6 Assessment of Performance Stability

Performance stability is a new category in the assessment of loading ability and in training control. For experienced coaches it is a matter of course to think of the stability of performance development according to the requirements of performance structure. The simplest sign of performance instability is a clear drop in velocity in the last third of the training or competition distance which goes beyond the physiological measure.

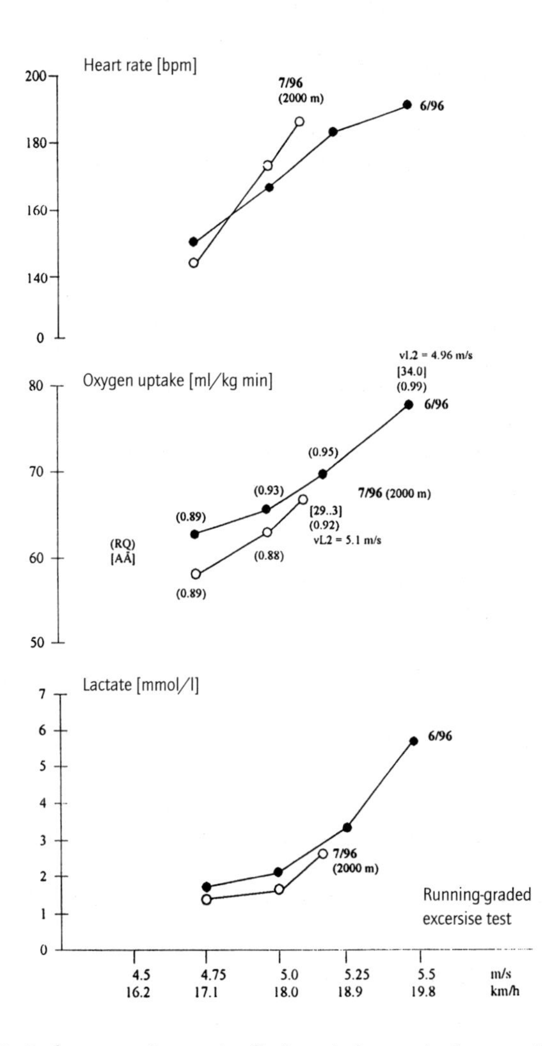

Fig. 1/10.4.5: Performance diagnostics findings before and after an ultra triathlon. A top athlete made himself available eight days after an ultra triathlon for the diagnostics. Tiredness is measurable in the steep rise in HR, the decrease in oxygen uptake and lactate concentration. A classic example of disturbed regeneration.

Performance instability can be clearly recognised when there are multiple competitions on one day (qualifications) or on several days in a row. The main cause is often too low a level of aerobic performance capacity or training for a shorter competition distance. Experience in competitive sport has shown that the best individual 10 km running time is no guarantee for the stable running of the marathon distance. The course averages for marathon training are considerably longer (and thus take more time) than for a 10 km training. Performance stability and thus the state of adaptation for a particular performance structure can be objectively checked through sport-specific performance diagnostics.

10.5 Sport-specific Functional and Performance Diagnostics

Medium-term training regulation is based mainly on laboratory performance test procedures and on test competitions. Laboratory tests help to register and complexly assess the state of adaptation in the functional systems determining performance. Competitions are the simplest diagnostic measure for documenting performance development. Competition results only allow limited corrections to training because the subcomponents of the coming about of performance are not known. Uncovering the foundations of aerobic and anaerobic performance is only possible through laboratory tests.

The common test procedure for this is *spiroergometry*. The main principle of spiroergometrical testing is increasing load on the treadmill or cycle ergometer. At the allocated testing points HR, lactate and oxygen intake are measured. The diagnostic conclusion is based on two factors. One is the assessment of the change in measured values at a prescribed load. Here the structure of the prescribed load (test record) and the sport-specificness of load are of secondary importance. The diagnostic conclusion is oriented to the description of changes to the measuring factors at prescribed and comparable load (Fig. 1/10.5, see p. 219). Relationships to specific performance capacity are usually not possible or intended. Naturally the borders between functional diagnostics and performance diagnostics conclusions are often thin or they are not differentiated.

The other performance diagnostics test strategy is oriented towards measuring performance or velocity during sport-specific ergometry. The physiological measurement factors are put into relationship with concrete performance or velocity. The diagnostic judgement is based on changes in individual performance or velocity in a longitudinal section and on physiological measurement factors (see Fig. 2/8).

Further details can be found in special literature on sports medicine functional and performance diagnostics (HECK, 1990; NEUMANN/SCHÜLER, 1994; CLASING et al. 1994; ENGELHARDT/NEUMANN, 1994 etc).

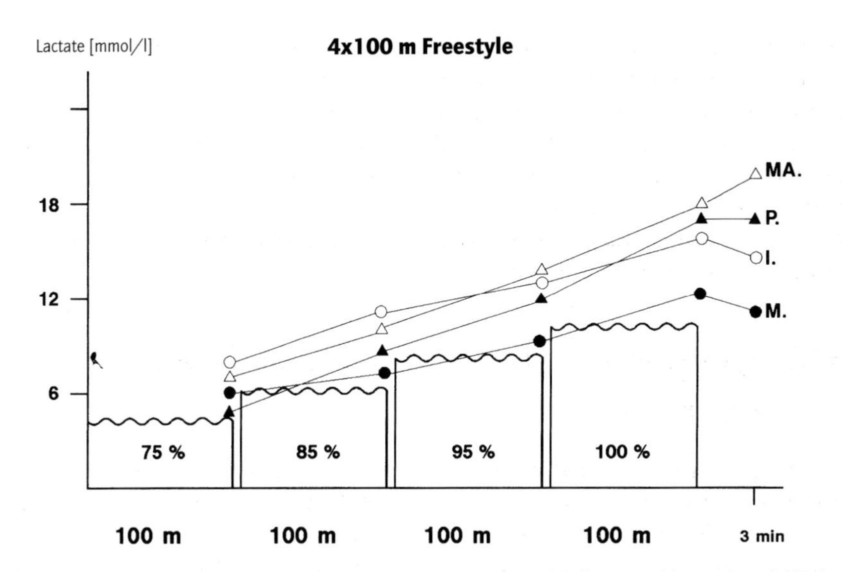

Fig. 1/10.5: Swimming graded exercise test over 4 x 100 m with fitness athletes. They fulfil the requirements with high anerobic energy use (lactate).

10.5.1 Sports-medical Functional Diagnostics

Sports-medical functional diagnostics is based on standardised ergometer load where the changes to physiological measurement factors like HR, lactate or oxygen intake are registered. Of the multitude of tests, those which are objective, reliable and valid for conclusions in sport have established themselves.

The combination of ergometer load with breathing functional diagnostics (breathing gas analysis) is called *ergospirometry* or *spiroergometry*. Spiroergometry has been a long established method in functional diagnostics (HOLLMANN/HETTINGER, 1990). The favoured load devices are the cycle ergometer and the treadmill.

Cycle Ergometry

On the ergometer load is increased in stages. In relationship to performance capacity the level of the starting stage, cycling duration at the stages and increases between the stages are selected. With athletes one generally begins with a load of between 50 and 100 Watt (W) and three minutes at each stage. Jumps in load are between 25 and 50 W, whereby for well-trained athletes it is usually 50 W. The test objective is the subjective loading limit. During load the HR, oxygen intake (VO_2) and lactate are measured. Under these test conditions HF and VO_2 rise linearly and lactate non-linearly (exponentially).

The criteria for the evaluation of spiroergometric tests when loading limits are reached are maximum oxygen intake (VO_2 max), maximum HR and maximum lactate concentration. From the dynamics of lactate increase the lactate performance curve or the anaerobic metabolism threshold are calculated. For the determining of the lactate performance curve the ergometer performance is related to a fixed lactate value. Lactate 2 or 3 mmol/l is favoured as an orientation point. Because lactate increase has individual characteristics it was originally calculated with various mathematical formulae. In most cases the exponential increase in lactate applies.

The point of change in the steep lactate increase can be registered with certainty using a mathematical compensatory calculation of the individual values measured. By determining the bending point of the lactate increase as a lactate performance curve and the breakdown of lactate in the first minutes of recovery, the so-called individual anaerobic threshold is calculated (STEGMANN et al., 1981). Lactate development and lactate breakdown are included in the calculation of the individual anaerobic threshold. The individual anaerobic threshold of long duration endurance athletes can be at 2.5 mmol/l and by less well endurance trained persons at over 4 mmol/l lactate. Another variant of individual threshold determining is the addition of 1.5 mmol/l after reaching the minimal increase in lactate concentration above the resting value during load.

The apparent contradictions in determining the "true" threshold are academic in nature and practically have no influence on training in the individual intensity areas. Metabolism regulation during load can only be influenced in certain control areas and not selectively.

With the fixed threshold the point of change in the lactate curve is determined at a fixed lactate concentration. This can vary slightly from the individual threshold depending on the athlete's fibre distribution and his training regime. With the fixed threshold performance is determined at 2 mmol/l lactate as PL2 and velocity as vL2. For competitive sport practice the differences between fixed and individual lactate thresholds are not of significance. When determining the fixed threshold, four measuring points are sufficient, for the individual threshold more measuring points are needed.

In competitive sport the change in the lactate performance curve in relationship to performance capacity and the degree of training load are assessed (Fig. 1/10.5.1, see p. 221). Lactate concentration of 2 mmol/l and below is considered a characteristic of aerobic metabolism. Between the lactate concentrations of 2 and 4 mmol/l is the aerobic-anaerobic metabolism transition area.

Treadmill Ergometry

On the treadmill the athlete runs against the belt running velocity. Performance on the treadmill is given as velocity, in metres per second (m/s) or kilometres per hour (km/h). The starting velocity depends on the running level. Untrained persons begin at 9 km/h (2.5 m/s), trained athletes at about 12 km/h (4.0 m/s).

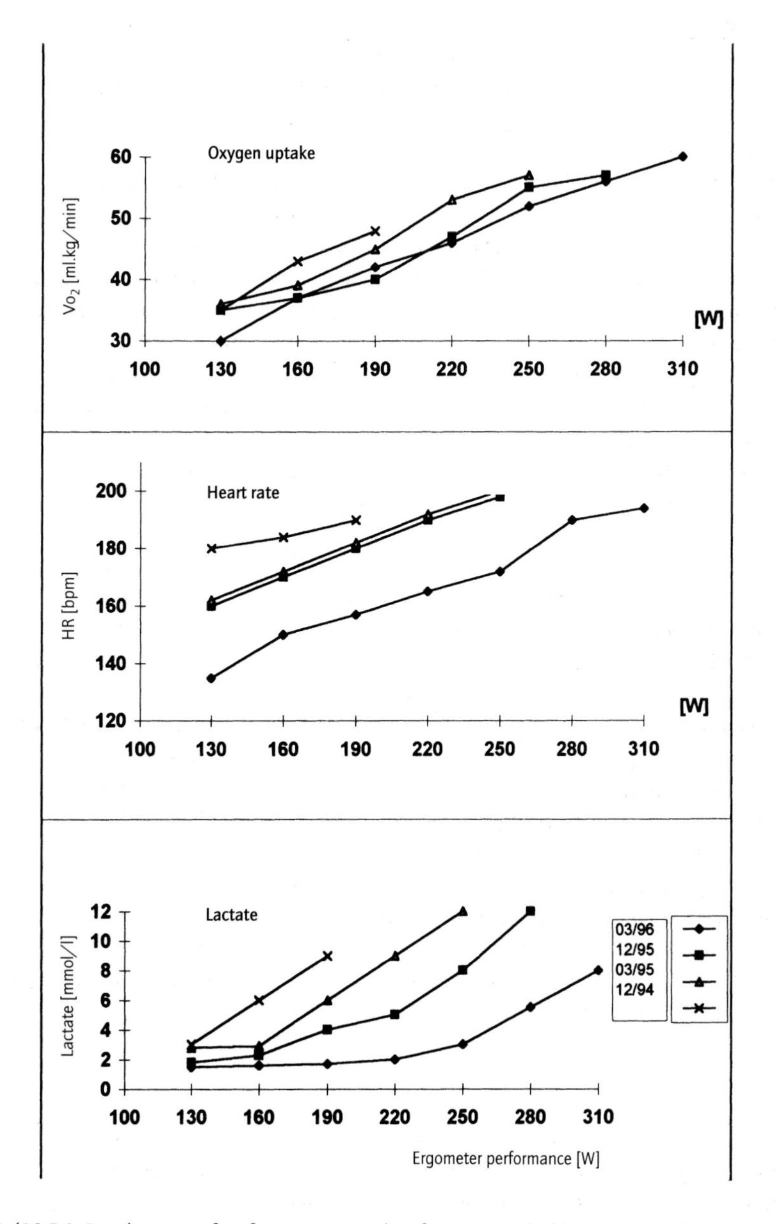

Fig. 1/10.5.1: Development of performance capacity of a woman triathlete on the cycle ergometer

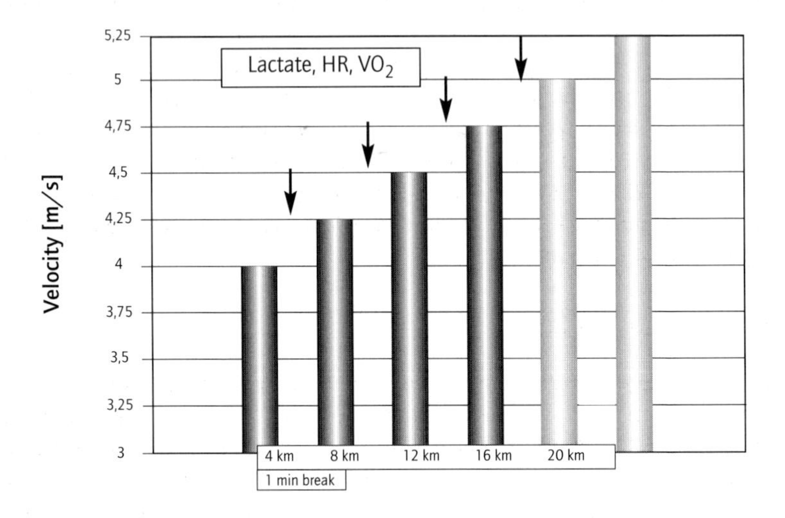

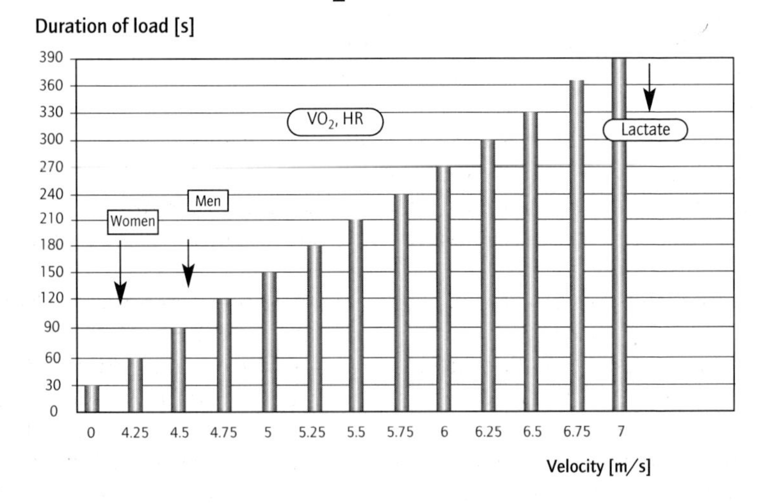

Fig. 2/10.5.1: Scheme of test structure of a distance related 4 x 4 km graded exercise test and maximum test in running. The treadmill remains level.

The duration of each stage on the slightly tilted belts is between 3 and 6 min. 2 km/h or 0.25 m/s is chosen as the increase in velocity. Between stages there is a one minute break in which blood is taken for lactate determination. As in cycle ergometry, HR, oxygen intake and lactate are measured. To better meet the requirements of sporting practice for training regulation, load is not only applied over fixed times but also fixed distances. The distances are selected according to the performance state. Those with the poorest performance run the shortest distances. For top athletes three and four km at one stage are preferred (Fig. 2/10.5.1, see p. 222). In this way endurance stability can be tested at the same time. Experience shows that there is a great difference in load whether altogether only four km (4 x 1 km) or 16 km (4 x 4) must be run.

10.5.2 Sport-specific Performance Diagnostics

Sport-specific performance diagnostics is oriented to sport-specific performance capacity through the application of sport-specific special ergometers and the relationship of the test results. To a certain extent test structuring is done in such a way that it can be repeated and also allows comparisons of treadmill tests with field tests. The application of distance-related graded exercise tests makes a direct comparison of laboratory and field tests possible (Fig. 1/10.5.2, see p. 224). In the sport-specific performance diagnostics the graded exercise test principal is also predominant (Fig. 2/10.5.2, see p. 225).

For the individual sports **special ergometers** have been developed:

Swimmers	:	**Current channel, rope pulling ergometer**
Rowers	:	**Rowing ergometer**
Canoeists	:	**Canoe ergometer**
Cyclists	:	**High performance cycling ergometer**
Runners/Walkers	:	**Large treadmill**
Cross-country Skiers	:	**Tippable treadmill, rope pulling ergometer**
Triathlon	:	**Cycle ergometer, treadmill, rope pulling ergometer** etc.

In sport-specific ergometry, sport-specific performance or velocity is measured, to which the relevant biological measurement factors are allocated (PFÜTZNER/NEUMANN, 1992; NEUMANN/MÜLLER, 1994). The emphasis in the assessment is on the changed effort in managing performance. The sports medicine criteria for assessing aerobic and anaerobic performance capacity are also valid in sport-specific ergometry (see chapter 4.4). The emphasis in sport-specific ergometry is on creating a relationship between training load, the direction of the effects of training and the direction of adaptation (Fig. 3/10.5.2, see p. 225). In this way sports-methodological and reliable recommendations for training are possible (Table 1/10.5.2, see p. 226).

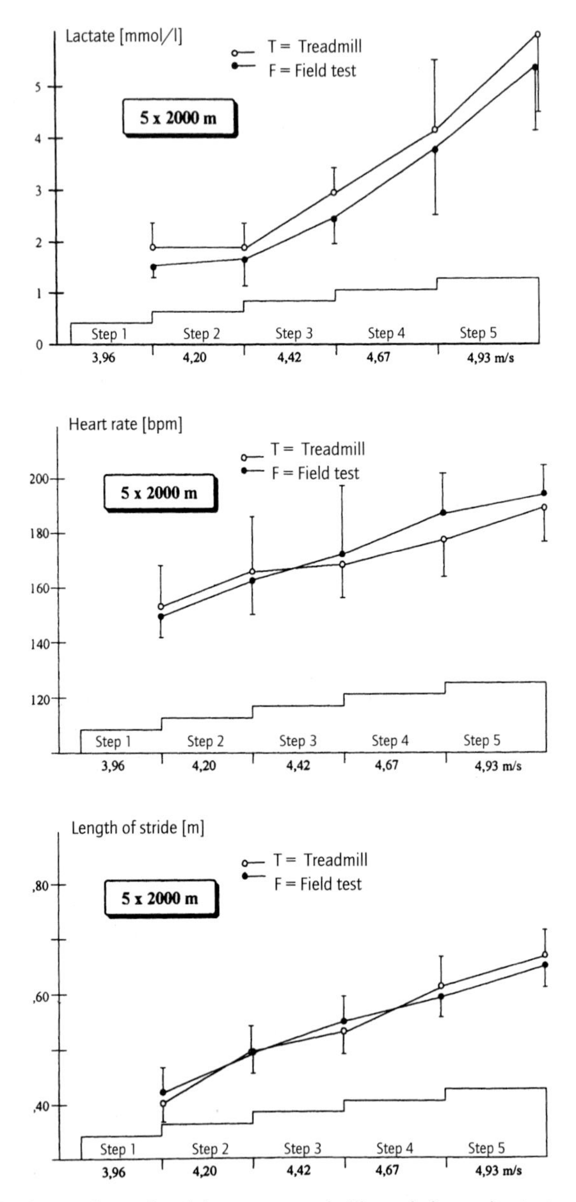

Fig. 1/10.5.2: Comparison of a laboratory treadmill graded exercise test with a field test. Average values of five athletes. The parameter differences were coincidental.

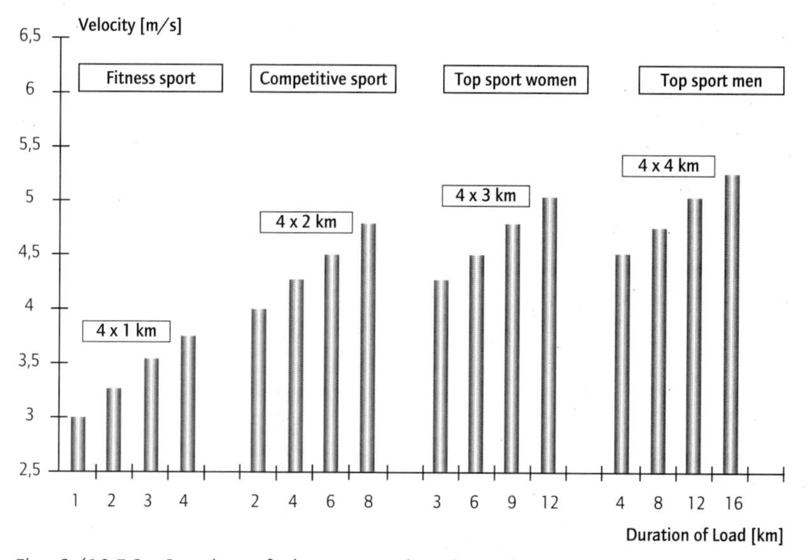

Fig. 2/10.5.2: Overview of the structural variants in the incrememtal exercise test in relationship to the performance capacity of the athletes

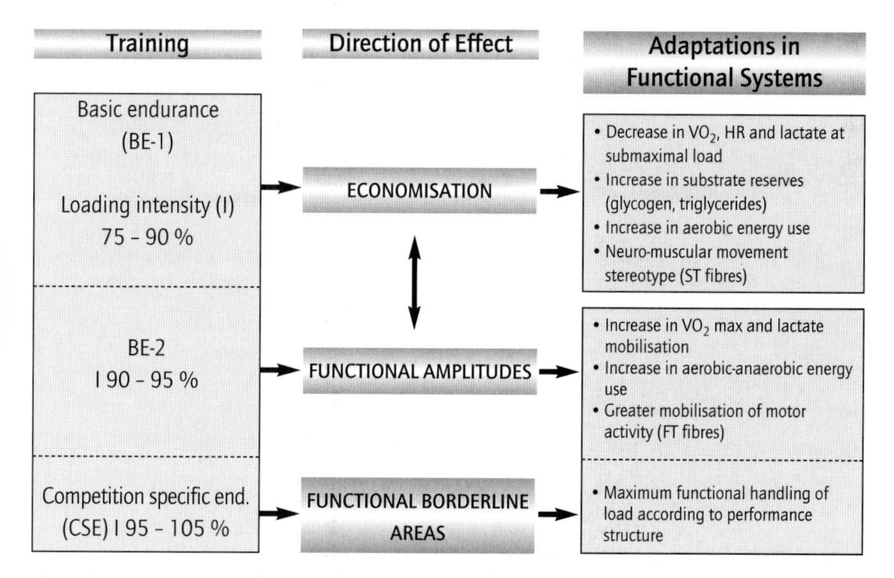

Fig. 3/10.5.2: Overview of training, direction of effect of training and possible adaptations

Velocity Guideline for Running Training According to Results from Submaximal 4 x 4 km Incremental Exercise Test (Level Positioning). vL2,3 = Velocity at 2 or 3 mmol/l Lactate in the Graded Exercise Test

Training Fields	Velocity	Adaptation goal
Speed endurance (SPE)	> 115 % competition tempo10 km (target time)	Motor activity training, speed reserve, final acceleration
Competition specific endurance (CSE)	> 95 % competition tempo 10 km, under distance training/competition tempo runs (15-20 x 400 m and/or 6-8 x 1000 m)	Development of competition-specific endurance capacity, tempo toughness
Basic endurance 2	90-95 % competition tempo 10 km, tempo runs over 6-8 km x 1000 m and/or 10-15 x 400 m	Development of aerobic-anaerobic performance base for CSE
Basic endurance 2	> 95 % of vL2 or > 90 % of vL3 over 10-15 km (jog)	Development of aerobic-anaerobic oxygen uptake and stability of aerobic endurance capacity for higher velocity areas
Basic endurance 1	80-90 % of vL2 or 75-85 % of vL3 over 10-18 km or 20-25 km	Development of basic aerobic performance, increase velocity at vL2,3

Tab. 1/10.5.2: Velocity for running training

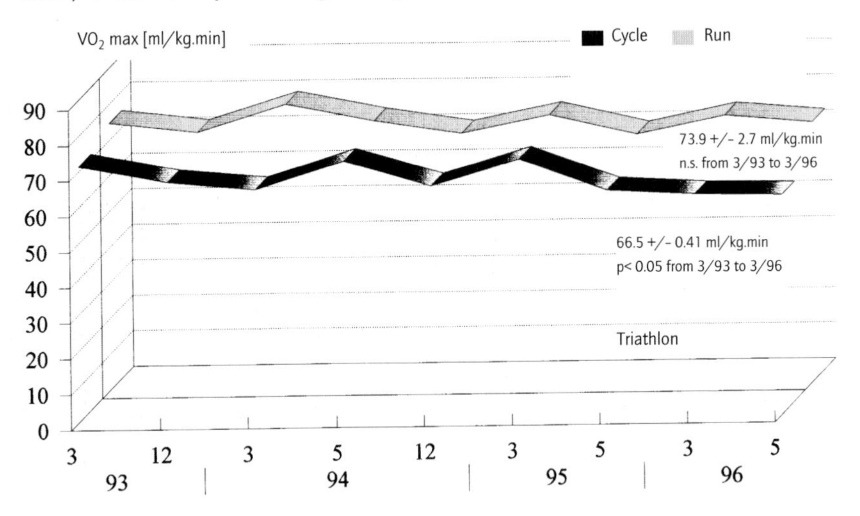

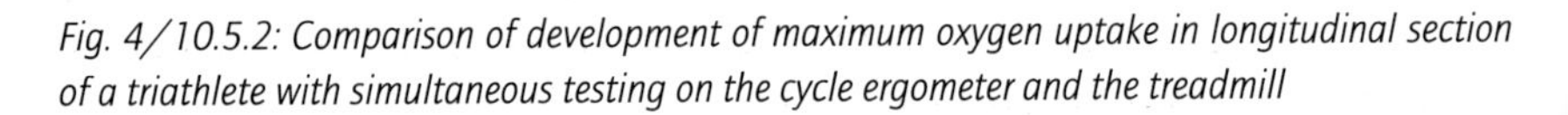

Fig. 4/10.5.2: Comparison of development of maximum oxygen uptake in longitudinal section of a triathlete with simultaneous testing on the cycle ergometer and the treadmill

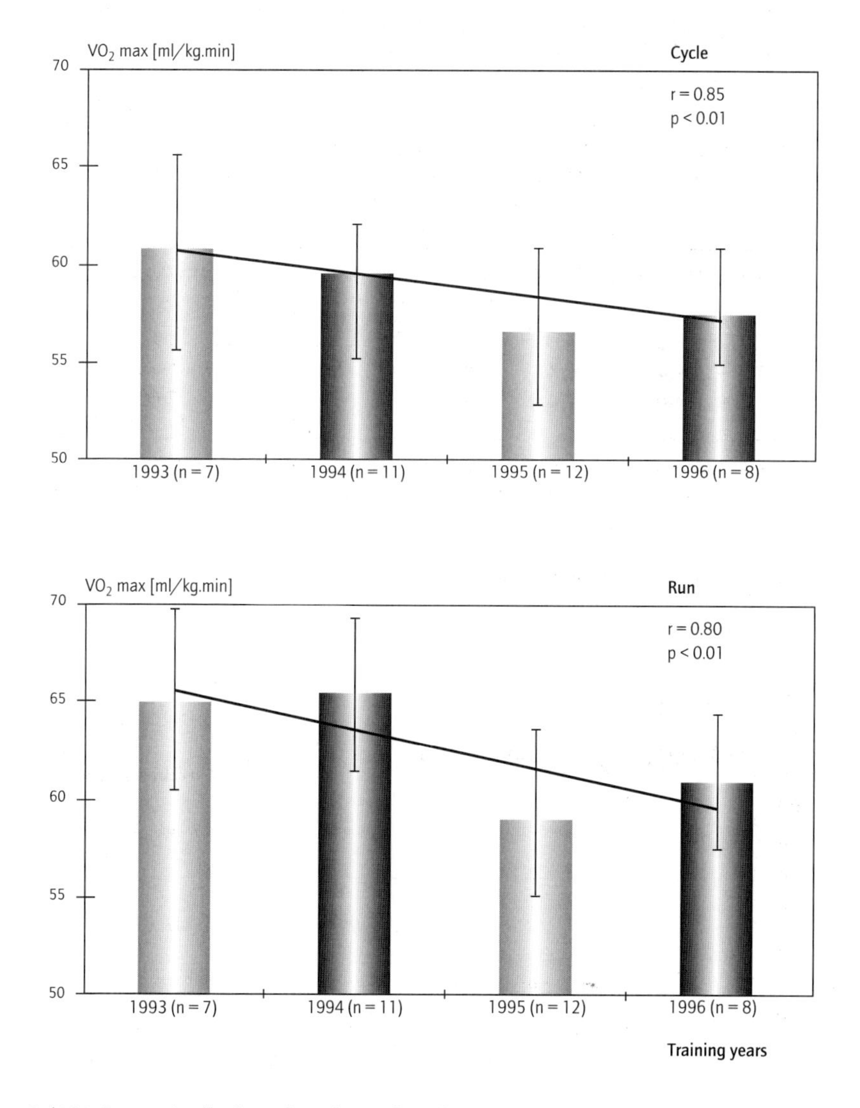

Fig. 5/10.5.2: Longitudinal section data of performance diagnostics tests on the cycle ergometer and treadmill of female athletes. Maximum oxygen uptake went down on both ergometers as a result of changed training content.

Field Tests in the Endurance Sports	
Sport	**Incremental Exercise Test****
SWIMMING	
Short duration swimming	8 x 100 (200) m
Medium duration swimming	8 x 200 m
Long duration swimming	5 x 400 m
Short triathlon	4 x 400 m
RUNNING	
Middle-distance running	6 x 2000 m
Long-distance running	Men 4 x 4000 m Women 4 x 3000 m
Short triathlon, duathlon	Men 4 x 4000 m Women 4 x 3000 m
CYCLING	
Road	4 x 6-8 km
Track	4 x 5 km
Short triathlon, duathlon	4 x 6 km
CROSS-COUNTRY SKIING	4 x 5 km 4 x 5 km
CANOEING, ROWING	
Canoeing	4 x 1000 m
Rowing	3 x 1000 m

** *Favoured monitoring factors are velocity, heart rate and lactate. Velocity is increased according to sport-specific standpoints and performance capacity of the athlete in submaximal intensity areas. The last stage usually involves a current load limit (over 95 % of performance capacity). Two graded exercise tests are unreliable.*

Tab. 1/10.6: Field tests in endurance sports

To get a good idea of sport-linked adaptation, triathletes are a good example. Through the application of cycle and treadmill ergometry, differences in the training effort for cycling and running in triathlon are recognisable. They are expressed in a difference in maximum oxygen intake (Fig. 4/10.5.2, Figure 5/10.5.2, see pp. 226 and 227).

For repetition of tests in sport-specific ergometry, a time span of six weeks is recommended. An adaptation to a higher performance level needs this time (see chapter 3). As the development of performance capacity and the biological effort required for it are in the field of vision of diagnostics, it is advisable to only carry out the tests at times in which sport-specific performance capacity is normal and not overlapped by too much residual tiredness (see Fig. 1/10.4.5). This means that after competitions or directly after training courses, diagnostics are falsified by continuing tiredness. A typical example is glycogen exhaustion and the low lactate development during load that is linked with it. In determining the lactate speed curve in running or the lactate performance curve in cycling, glycogen exhaustion gives the impression of an improvement in submaximal performance capacity. The curves of lactate increase move to the right, i.e. in the direction of higher performance (see Fig. 1/10.4.5). In order to exclude the false impression of greater performance capacity or to safely confirm performance improvement, in addition to lactate measurement the determining of HR and oxygen intake are also necessary. Deriving training recommendations from lactate regulation only is very one-sided and risky too.

10.6 Field Tests

Field tests are carried out at training or race locations. They are done according to the principle of graded exercise and involve varying distances depending on the sport (Table 1/10.6), see p. 228). Laboratory and field tests mutually complement each other and are necessary together. Field tests can be carried out more frequently but are subject to external disruptive factors so that the conclusions about performance can be uncertain. Also, the measurement factors that can be applied in field tests are limited. The important parameter oxygen intake usually cannot be measured. Portable measuring systems for this are still in development and are too expensive.

An exception among the field tests is the swimming graded exercise test. It can be carried out under relatively constant conditions in indoor swimming pools. The specific swimming ergometer is the current channel.

In laboratory tests, constant loading conditions are ensured, and through the use of several measurement factors more reliable information is possible. It is not recommendable to make changes to training purely on the basis of lactate measurements. Under ideal external conditions the results of treadmill and field tests are identical with regard to HR and lactate regulation (see Fig. 1/10.5.2).

Summary

Competitive training is planned and orientated to the performance structure of the particular sport. The central elements of training regulation are the duration of load and velocity as well as maintaining rhythms of loading and unloading. Training analysis is often neglected, yet it is of great significance for recognising the causes of success or failure. As sports-methodological loading guidelines are not fixed points but are graded in intensity (load) areas, to ensure the right training load it is useful to additionally use biological measurement factors. The measurement factors heart rate (HR), lactate, serum urea and creatine kinase (CK) are preferred for daily load control and with their varying findings help differentiate adaptations to training load. The level of adaptation achieved can be tested periodically using complex performance diagnostics in the laboratory (CPD). In CPD usually sport-specific aerobic and anaerobic performance capacity and maximum oxygen uptake (VO_2 max) are ascertained. The development of performance capacity is related to the effects of training load. With very reliable sport-specific testing procedures, predictions of individual competition performance capacity are possible.

If the content of a training concept is not up to standard, no load control and sport-specific CPD will be able to compensate this.

CPD results serve the purpose of orientating either towards maintaining or changing training load. The structuring of training with effective stimuli has precedence over diagnostic measures, as the latter do not replace training. At the same time this means that measures of daily load control and medium-term CPD and/or field tests can provide well-founded arguments for further structuring of training.

10.7 Training at Measuring Stations

From what were once biomechanical sports-methodological measuring stations, practical training devices or training equipment have been developed. The sport-specific measuring station allows complex analysis of the carrying out of movement in a training or competition exercise. Thanks to computer technology, the necessary information is immediately available to coaches or athletes. Training is structured according to predefined parameters. The athlete can be directly involved in the cycle training-analysis-training. He can focus his inner model of movement and gain understanding of the amount of effort needed for training and performance motivation (Table 1/10.7).

Sport	Measuring Station	Influence
Swimming	Current channel, rope pulling ergometer	Prognosis demands, arm strength development and influencing of structure of pull
Cycling	Cycle ergometer, braked rolling	Specific strength capacities of the legs
Running	Treadmill	Racing course, stride structure
Triathlon	Combination of rope pulling ergometer/current channel cycle ergometer/tippable treadmill	Triathlon-specific capacity development (coupled training), racing course, movement structure
Cross-country skiing	Rope pulling ergometer, tippable treadmill	Pull structure, simulation of competition distances

Table 1/10.7: Measuring stations and possibilities of deliberate influence on performance relevant parameters

Summary

In competitive sport, biomechanical measuring stations and equipment are being used increasingly for monitored training. The carrying out of movement is directly presented with the help of computers and can be used immediately for analysing load. In measuring station training, the development level of capacities is comprehensible and can be influenced towards the desired adaptation. Preferred measurement stations with sport-specific loading simulation are the cycle ergometer and the rope pulling ergometer.

11 Training Structure with Courses

Training courses are a regular feature of top sport. In all endurance sports, the number of courses is increasing and these are being extended over the whole training year.

As opposed to home training, training at courses offers the following advantages:

- Suitable training conditions for peak load in the sport. In top sport loading of 35 to 45 hours/week is usual.
- Prerequisites for better regeneration, supported with physiotherapy and medical care. In case of incorrect loading and injuries, action can be taken immediately.
- Through group training the quality of load increases. Competition variations can be tried out with partners (relays in cycling, training starts in triathlon and cross-country skiing, training competitions etc).
- Expert advice in training control and teaching of self-regulation. Interdisciplinary coaching team helps appraise training. Recording of extensive performance-physiological and biomechanical measured data; carrying out of field tests.
- Technical support for training devices and technological exchange of information (e.g. bicycle mechanics, ski technicians).
- Exchange of information and opinions between athletes and the possibility of team formation.
- Material and technical service in training analysis and ensuring training is carried out (making of videos, accompanying vehicles, transport services to and from training etc).
- Advice on sports nutrition and possible supplementation.
- Further education on training methodology, performance physiology, sports nutrition etc.
- Training motivation through pleasant climatic condition and experience of nature.

In recent years more and more competitive athletes and fitness athletes have been making use of training camps in combination with vacations. The number of expertly qualified offerers of courses in climatically pleasant parts of the world is increasing. Group training creates more enjoyment and stimulates training commitment. For these athlete groups, too, the relationship between increasing training load (volume) and performance development is reliable. The training camps are deliberately used for individual peak performances. It should be noted that this load needs to be prepared for training methodologically. It can often be observed that training in the first days is too hard. The muscle glycogen cannot regenerate any more, current performance capacity goes down early. Overestimating performance capacity leads to not achieving the course goals.

This means that training camps require sound preplanning and well-thought out classification of the contents in individual annual performance development (see chapter 9).

As in training camps, strongly and more poorly performing athletes train together. Distinctions should be made in structuring training contents. This means that:

- There should be clear differences in training velocities and total volume.
- The proportions must be right in performance development (general performance prerequisites, BE and CSE).
- The rhythms of load and unloading must be kept to.
- The proportion of training means within total volume should be considered.
- The use of general, semi-specific and specific training means must depend on periodisation in the training year and
- camp training and any altitude training should be fitted into proportionality within total load.

This list already indicates the complexity of performance training and more or less excludes camps used by chance (Fig. 1/11).

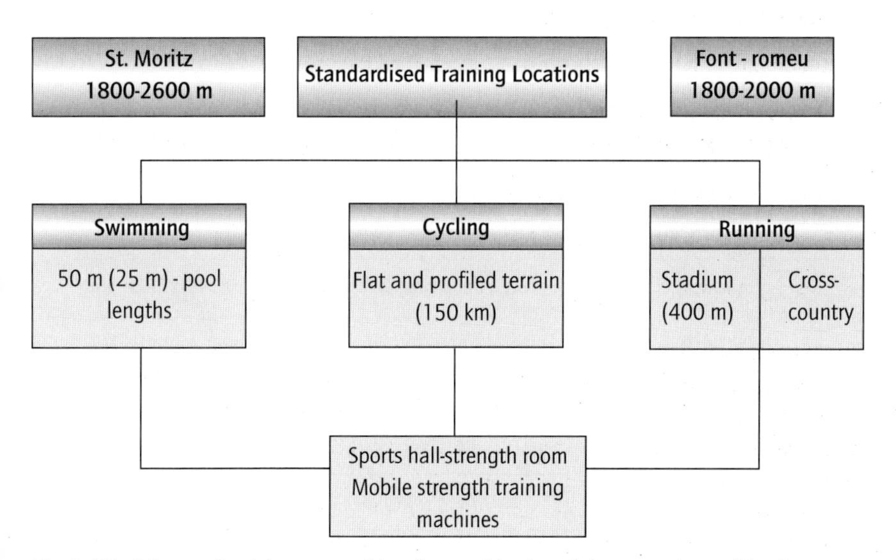

Fig. 1/11: Scheme of training prerequisites for an altitude training camp in combination sports (e.g. triathlon)

	Course location	Country	Month	Altitude	Content	Peculiarities
1	Lanzarote	Spain	December	0–300 m	Swimming, running	Very prone to wind
2	St. Moritz Oberstdorf	Switzerland Germany	January	1800–2200 m 840–1100 m	Skiing training Cross-country skiing	Altitude training NN
3	Stellenbosch	South Africa	February	0–100 m	Swimming, running	No time difference
4	Lanzarote	Spain	March	0–300 m	Swimming, running	Very prone to wind
5	Teneriffe	Spain	April	0–2300 m	Complex training	Partially altitude conditions
6	Majorca	Spain	March-May	0–500 m	Cycling training	Climatic adjustment
7	Font-Romeŭ	Frankreich	Mai	1800–2100 m	Complex training	Altitude training
8	St. Moritz	Switzerland	June	1800–2600 m	Complex traininig	Altitude training
9	Lanzarote	Spain	Sept.-Oct.	0–300 m	Cycling training	Very prone to wind

Table 1/11: Selected course locations for climate and altitude training in triathlon

Parameters	Top sport	Competitive sport
Training velocity	daily	daily
Training heart rate	daily	daily
Lactate	main training sessions	graded exercise test
Serum urea	daily early	after peak exertion
Creatine kinase (CK)	daily early	after unaccustomed exertion
Resting heart rate	daily early	daily early
Subjective body feeling	daily early/evenings	daily early/evenings
Body weight	weekly	weekly

Table 2/11: Parameters for daily training control

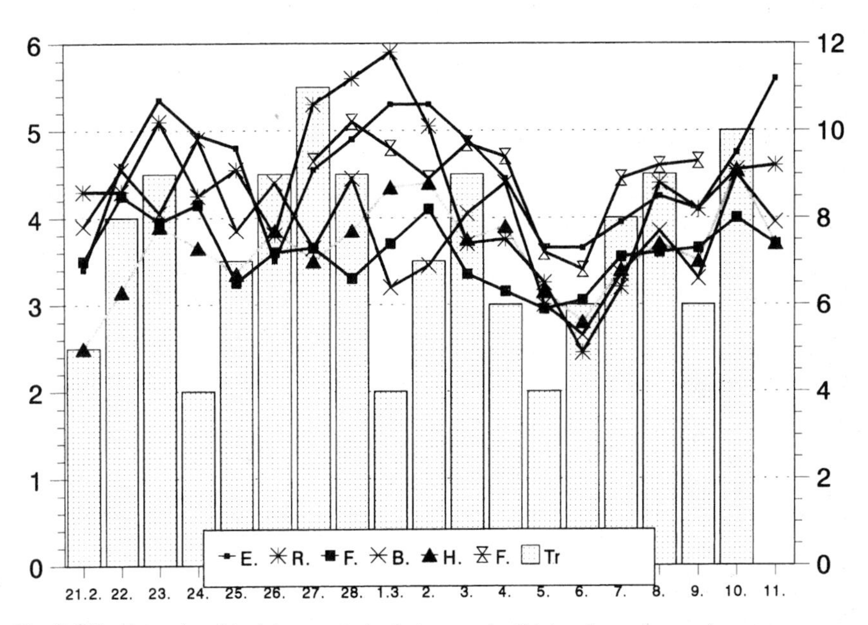

Fig. 2/11: Example of training control of six squad athletes through morning serum urea measurement. The individually different protein catabolism is reflected in the basic dynamics of load and unloading, mainly in a 3:1 rhythm.

The expense and the selection of camps depends on the sport. The most demanding are the combination sports such as duathlon, triathlon, biathlon etc. A triathlon camp should have an indoor swimming pool (25 or 50 m lengths), a traffic-free and profiled cycling course and various running courses (also 400 m synthetic track). In Europe for example the training locations listed in Table 1/11 are well-suited for diverse preparatory training in competitive sport.

Often climatic factors, good training conditions and group training lead to training euphoria. The consequences are overestimation of one's abilities and load at too high a level. Therefore training load must be adapted to real performance capacity. Aids here are course plans, daily monitoring of keeping to training areas as well as loading control with biological measurement factors (see chapter 10). Training control factors need to be used differently according to performance state and performance goals (Table 2/11). Despite keeping to a 3:1 load-unloading rhythm in a training camp, the use of protein metabolism (protein catabolism) varies among individual athletes, but they all react to a reduction in training load (Fig. 2/11).

Summary

Training courses are a regular part of performance training and are increasingly used by top athletes as well as fitness athletes. In addition to pleasant climatic and landscape conditions, course training has advantages over home training. These are: group training, qualified coaching, support in training regulation, physiotherapeutic and medical care, technical assistance, nutritional advice, further education, comprehensive communication and exchange of opinions, etc. These optimal loading conditions in the group often lead to training euphoria combined with overestimation of one's own performance capacity. In order to limit overtaxing, realistic and precise training planning which corresponds to one's performance state is necessary in the course.

12 Regeneration in the Training Process

It is a characteristic of training that re-loading takes place when regeneration is incomplete. The not yet completed regeneration is, however, the prerequisite for triggering adaptations in the body. After load the taxed functional systems vary in the time they need to return to their starting state (see Table 1/2). Because some functional systems reach their original state in one or two hours already, multiple loading in one day is possible.

The key prerequisite for re-loading is sufficient refilling of the emptied glycogen stores in the muscles and the liver.

The central element for assessing regeneration has proved to be the breaking down and rebuilding (catabolic and anabolic) functional state taking place in metabolism. This state can be registered by determining the insulin level and the cortisole concentration. When the insulin level rises and the cortisole concentration decreases, there is an increase in the anabolic state after great load (Table 1/12, see p. 238). After extreme endurance load as is currently increasing in a number of sports, there is such a strong catabolic metabolism situation that the sexual hormone testosterone, which has a strongly anabolic effect, decreases for a longer period of time (Fig. 1/12, see p. 239). This also means a reduction in male sexuality.

A further circumstance that has a major effect on the duration of regeneration is the level of training-methodological preparation for performance. Overestimation of one's own competition performance capacity in leisure and competitive sport objectively leads to longer regeneration time. The result is lengthened catabolic metabolism regulation in the muscles (Fig. 2/12, see p. 239).

The change from catabolic to anabolic metabolism is decisive for re-loading after great sporting load. Re-loading applied too early can increase or lengthen the still present catabolic state.

12.1 Sport-methodological Measures

In competitive training regeneration is almost as important as training itself. Orderly regeneration helps to process load better and allows re-load soon. The continuation of training at a high level of quality is the basis for personal top performances. Load breaks as a result of injury which are not connected with normal regeneration diminish the reaching of high total load. In the regeneration period the body is given a chance to transform load stimuli into adaptations. The body processes the training load in a self-regulating way; regeneration serves to ensure that the body is not disturbed too much while processing load.

Characterisation of Catabolic and Anabolic Metabolism after Major Endurance Load*	
Catabolic metabolism (dominance of breaking down regulation)	
Insulin	⇓
Cortisole	⇑
Serum urea	⇑
Creatine kinase	⇑
Amino acids	⇓
Ammoniac, uric acid	⇑,⇑
Immunoglobulins, acute phase reaction	⇓
Anabolic metabolism (dominance of building up regulation)	
Cortisole	⇓
Insulin	⇑
Testosterone (if dropped)	⇑
Serum urea	⇓
Creatine kinase	⇓
Amino acids	⇑
Immunoglobulins, acute phase reaction	⇑,⇑

** Changes can continue one to five days after load.*

Table 1/12: Characterisation of catabolic and anabolic metabolism after great endurance load

Sports-methodological measures to support regeneration are important and do not mean "filling in training".

It is proven practice that directly after great intensive load or competitions, motor post-loading in the same sport at a low level of performance or velocity occurs. Well-known terms for this are cool-down jogging, spinning down, cool-down swimming, rowing etc. The aim of these training forms is to loosen the muscles, break down high muscle tone and begin psychological untensing (Table 1/12.1, see p. 240). This first regeneration load should be limited to 20 to 30 minutes so that there is no further energy consumption from the emptied stores.

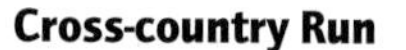

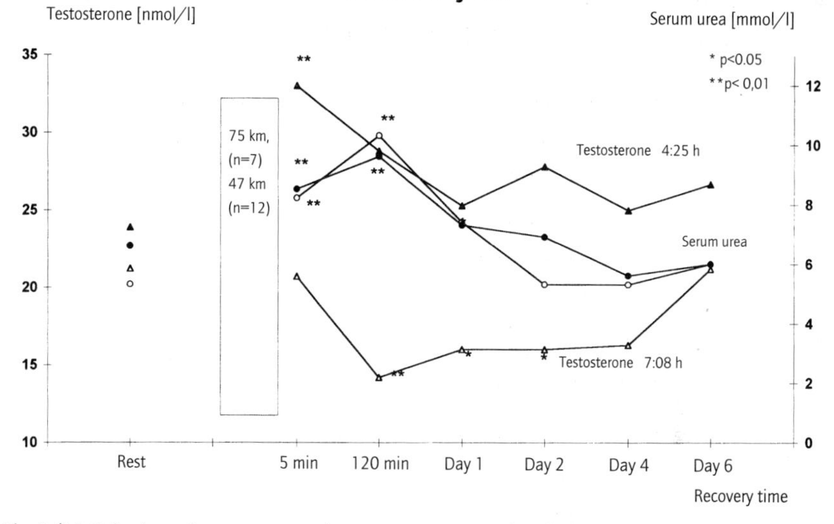

Fig. 1/12: Behaviour of testosterone and serum urea concentrations before and after a long cross-country run (uphill race). After the 75 km distance there was a decrease in serum testosterone for several days.

100 km Running

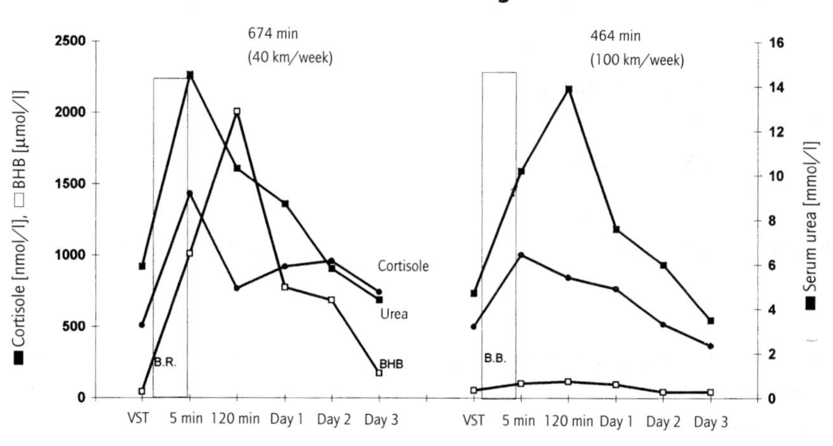

Fig. 2/12: Comparison of the change in cortisole, serum urea and betahydroxybutyrate (BHB) in a 100 km run of two athletes with different performance capacities. When there was considerably less load (40 km/week) there were considerably higher demands on the body and delayed regeneration.

Measures to Support Regeneration after Great Training Load (Camps), Competition Sequences and Long Duration Competitions					
Regeneration phases	Sports-medicine objectives	Training	Nutrition	Physiotherapy	Biopsychosocial evaluation
Early phase of regeneration (hours)	Compensation of fluid deficit, refilling of energy stores	Sport-specific or unspecific short load to relax and loosen up the muscles (up to 30 min)	Ample intake of liquids and electrolytes, early consumption of carbohydrates (50 g CH/h in first two hours)	Massage to loosen up and reduce tiredness, relaxing bath, hot and cold showers	Emotionally emphasised actions, current success or failure assessments, first psychosocial processing of performance, attempt at psychological relaxation
Middle phase of regeneration (1st to 3rd day)	Limiting of muscular structural and functional disturbances, preparation of muscle re-loading	Sport-specific or unspecific compensation training or sport-specific load break (load duration up to 60 min)	Carbohydrate-rich (6-8 g/kg) and protein-rich (1.5 g-2.5 g/kg) food. Supplementation with amino acids, minerals, vitamins (antioxidants), intake of active substances (L-Carnitine, immune stimulants)	Massages, in some cases electrotherapy, sauna, sleep	Evaluation of success or failure, processing of social assessments, derivation of action programmes
Late phase of regeneration (4th day to weeks)	Dealing with muscular disturbances, taking up performance training again	Aerobic training over short distances, initial resistance-orientated (strength) training	Sports nutrition adequate to load, continued intake of active substances	Individual physiotherapeutic measures	Development of motives for performance training, formulation of goals of action

Table 1/12.1: Measures to support regeneration after great training load

It must be considered that after competition the feeling for velocity is irritated and often regeneratively too much post-loading is applied. A monitoring factor is the HR, it should not exceed 120 bpm. Post-loading in aerobic metabolism accelerates lactate breakdown. The lactate is broken down more quickly by post-loading than by rest.

After very tiring muscle use, on the following day or in the following days, separate regeneration training, also called compensation training, should be carried out. Compensation training should be done sport-specifically or better yet sport-unspecifically or semi-specifically. Its duration should be limited to about 60 min. On beginning compensation training the day after a competition, lactate has been fully broken down, but not the products of muscular cell dissolution and the substrates of catabolic metabolism. In the case of muscle soreness, compensation training in aerobic metabolism is the best "cure". Muscle soreness is a sign of mild traumatisation in the contractile structures of the muscle. The swelling (edema) used by the body in the destroyed muscle fibres to eradicate the structural destruction causes the pain. This is best broken down through a low dosage of aerobic compensation training and the increase in blood circulation it triggers. In one to three days all forms of sore muscles have been removed by compensation training. The HR used to regulate compensation load should not exceed 120 bpm. In the late phase of regeneration, aerobic basic endurance training is the method to choose. All forms of intensive load which lead to lactate concentrations of over 5 mmol/l should be treated carefully; sports-methodologically they are not typical for regeneration training.

Summary

All intensive training load and competitions require sports-methodological follow-up work. The first regeneration load comes directly after the competition or training. Compensation training in aerobic metabolism can be carried out for a limited period of time as a separate training session.

12.2 Sports-medicine Measures

For a long time sports medicine rarely paid much attention to regeneration. The gradually decreasing loss of strength after hard load (especially after competitions) was considered a consequence of general tiredness. The causes of the tiredness problems in the muscles which athletes spoke of were not really known. Experienced coaches were aware of the loss of muscular strength and they compensated this empirically with sports-methodological measures.

Meanwhile the support of regeneration in the sport-specific muscles has become an important task of sports medicine care.

It has now been established with the help of muscle bioptic tests that unaccustomed and great load can lead to massive muscle fibre tearing and destruction of cell membranes. The mildest form of this disturbance is muscle soreness. This has nothing to do with overacidity of the muscle, because it also occurs during purely aerobic endurance load.

The consequence of muscular structural destruction or also of energetic bottlenecks during load is an increase in cell-based creatine kinase (CK) in the blood. Not all rises in CK, however, are an expression of ultra structural muscle destruction, especially when it is only four or five times average training values. The collapse of cell membrane stability in the case of an energy deficit already leads to CK moving from the inner cell space to the space between cell. The CK is then slowly transported via the lymph stream into the blood.

The greatest muscular functional and structural breakdown is caused by unaccustomed eccentric muscle load, such as fast running on hard ground and especially fast running down hill (Fig. 1/12.2, see p. 243). When running down hill, the cushioning of body mass occurs against the usual contraction direction of the muscle, resulting in greater structural destruction. The breakdown products of mechanically destroyed contraction proteins appear in the blood with a delay. This applies to the myosin heavy chain fragments and to troponin I. These muscle fibre breakdown products reflect the continuance of tiredness and the not yet complete performance state of muscle strength. Extreme running load (marathon, ultra triathlon, 100 km run, multiple Ironman etc.) also disrupts the aerobic energy potential in the mitochondria. This leads to changes in the form of the mitochondria, density changes in the inner space of the mitochondria as well as dying of mitochondria as a result of continuing lack of energy. Regeneration time after such long duration load is considerably longer than the time needed for refillment of the glycogen stores.

Refilling of the glycogen stores after endurance load takes longer than generally accepted; after marathon runs it can take several days (BLOM et l., 1986; SHERMAN et al., 1983).

The feeling of success after a competition must not be allowed to hide the fact that after extreme individual load the muscle is less loadable. After marathon runs or an ultra triathlon, a minimum muscle regeneration time of five to ten days must be reckoned with. In this time under no circumstances should further competitions be planned or carried out. Athletes who competed again too early after overestimating their abilities spent months afterwards trying to get back to form. They greatly delayed the regeneration of their muscle structure. If an athlete reaches the finish in a state of hypoglycaemia and is disorientated, he should be given glucose quickly. If he can still drink unaided, any kind of drink containing glucose is useful. In this state the safest thing is a glucose electrolyte infusion. If only a physiological saline infusion is given the state of hypoglycaemia does not end.

Through the intake of glucose the hypoglycaemic athlete is usually fully capable again within an hour; the blood sugar concentration rises above resting value (Fig. 2/12.2, see p. 244).

From a sports medicine perspective, measures to support regeneration, especially for the support apparatus and locomotor system, must always be seen in their complexity and structured on a long-term basis (FRÖHNER, 1995). Electrotherapy has great importance within the framework of physiotherapeutic measures, especially in supporting muscle regeneration and in treating local complaints (GILLERT et al., 1995). The main aim of all measures to influence regeneration is to reach re-loading tolerance for accustomed training load.

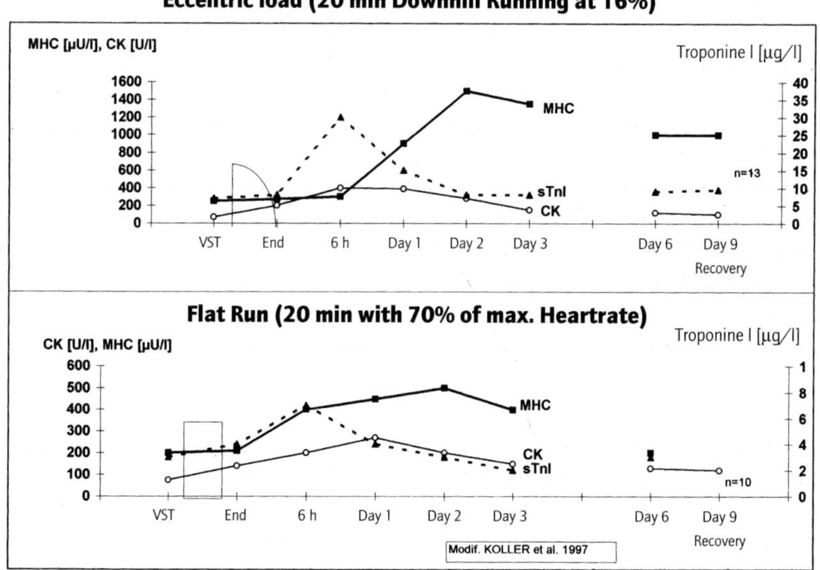

Fig. 1/12.2: Comparison of two forms of treadmill load at 4 mmol/l lactate and 20 min duration. Load was carried out as downhill running (eccentric load) and level running. Running downhill led to a longer lasting increase in myosin heavy chain fragments (MHC), of troponin I (sTnI) and of creatine kinase (CK). Data modified after KOLLER et al. (1997).

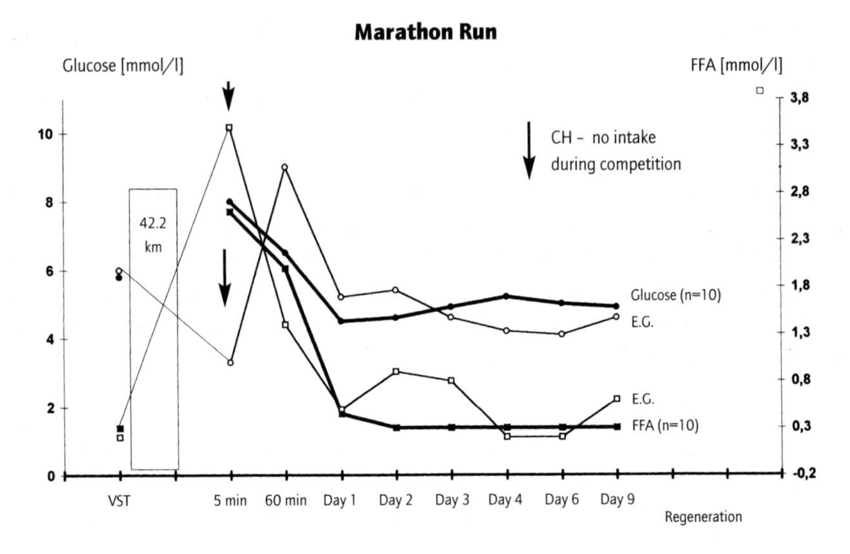

Fig. 2/12.2: Behaviour of glucose and free fatty acids (FFA) before and after a marathon run. The athlete e.g. did not consume any carbohydrates (CH) during the run and reached the finish in a state of hypoglycaemia. As compensation his FFAs were up greatly, in comparison to the average value of the group (n = 12). After CH intake at the finish his blood sugar was back to normal after 60 min.

Summary

Major sports medicine measures to encourage regeneration are:

- Quick refilling of energy reserves and supplementation with proven means (vitamins, minerals and other active substances) (see chapter 13).
- Making use of physiotherapeutic measures (including electro-physiotherapy).
- Long-term exercise programmes to overcome weaknesses in the support apparatus and locomotor system.
- Moving of psychologically demanding tasks from the high loading phases to the later regeneration phase.

12.3 Dietary Measures

The main dietary measures for accelerating regeneration are listed in chapter 13.

After sporting load the fluid deficit must first be balanced. Of the many options for fluid intake, sodium-rich mineral waters have proven convenient. Potassium-rich fruit juices and very sugary (sweet) solutions are not so good. Meanwhile a number of manufacturers have produced drinks based on scientific findings which meet the requirements of fast water intake, optimal electrolyte composition and a balanced amount of carbohydrates (Table 1/12.3, see p. 246). The alternative to their use is the cost factor.

After major dehydration (over 3% of body weight) it must be reckoned with that 24 hours will be needed to rebalance fluids. Only after this time are the dehydrated subcutaneous fatty tissue and the muscles in all their space structures again sufficiently filled with fluid.

After balancing fluids, refilling the glycogen stores has precedence in regeneration. With normal basic endurance load the glycogen stores are refilled after 20 hours; after fast long duration load (e.g. marathon run) refilling the stores takes up to a week.

The most effective method for accelerated glycogen store refilling is to exploit the increased rate of glycogen resynthesis, which is 7-8 %/h immediately after load. If the normal rate of glycogen resynthesis is 5-6 % (IVY et al., 1988), this means an increase in glycogen refilling of 20 %. The activity of glycogen synthetase is especially high for about two hours after load (Fig. 1/12.3, see p. 246).

In connection with fluid and food intake after load the state of the digestive system must be taken into consideration. The normal rate of stomach evacuation is not influenced at an intake of 30 to 80 g of carbohydrates/litre (3-8 %) (BROUNS, 1993). Mixtures of carbohydrates, fluids and common salt are absorbed most quickly.

The common brands of electrolyte carbohydrate drinks fulfil these requirements. By making your own water-salt-sugar solutions you can save costs. A mixture of three to six dessert-spoons of sugar to 1 l of water (= 45-90 g saccharose or 4.5-9 %) together with an additional teaspoon of common salt (= 1.2 g sodium/l) creates a wholesome hypotonic drink for about five cents.

Further intake of minerals, vitamins and trace elements depends on the extent of sweat loss and the duration of load. Because an insufficient supply of individual active substances is not immediately recognisable, preparations with a comprehensive spectrum of such substances should be given preference.

After major loss of sweat and major mechanical load (hill runs, marathon) the supply of magnesium is important. In this case the additional intake of 0.5 g of magnesium per day for several days is recommendable. By buying magnesium citrate as a powder from the chemist or having it prescribed by the family doctor costs can be saved. The consumption of water with a high magnesium content is useful for ensuring a supply of the substance. A normal blood concentration of magnesium (0.75 to 1.4 mmol/l) is not yet evidence of an undersupply, for only 1 % of the body's magnesium is contained in the blood. More credible evidence of a magnesium deficit are cramps or disturbances of feeling (paraesthesia) in the muscles.

Requirements of an Optimal Drink to Support Rehydration and Regeneration*	
• Carbohydrates	60-80 g/l
• Sodium	0.4-1.0 g/l
• Chloride	< 1.5 g/l
• Potassium	< 225 mg/l
• Calcium	< 225 mg/l
• Magnesium	< 100 mg/l
• Osmotic ability	200-300 mosmol/l
• Degree of acidity (pH)	> 4.0

** Figures according to BROUNS/KOVACS (1996). These requirements are met e.g. by Isotar® and Gatorade®.*

Table 1/12.3: Requirements of optimal drinks for support of rehydration and regeneration

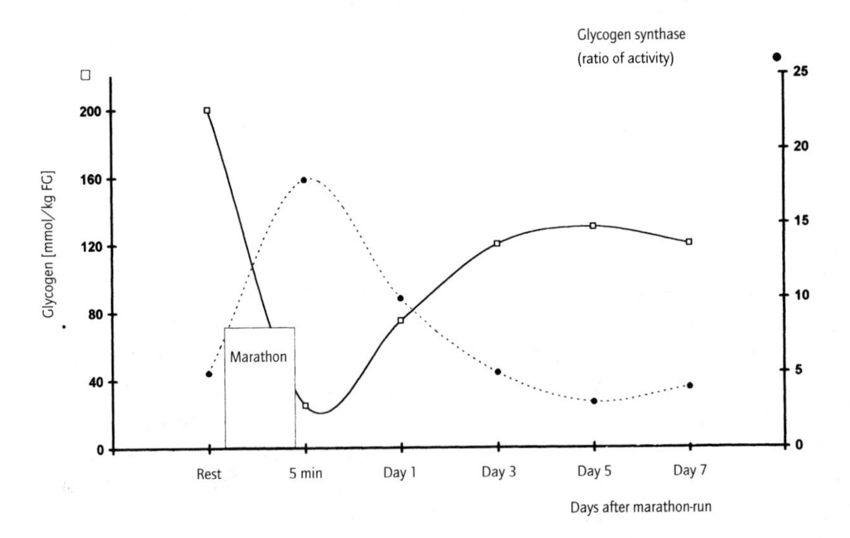

Fig. 1/12.3: Behaviour of muscle glycogen and activity of glycogen development enzyme (glycogen synthetase) before and after a marathon run. Data according to WILLMORE/COSTILL (1994)

Substances Aiding Regeneration	
Function	**Substances**
• Energy metabolism	Complex carbohydrates, creatine, branch chain amino acids (BCCA), medium-chain fatty acids (MCT)
• Micro-nutrients	Magnesium, zinc, selenium, chromium, vit. C, omega 6 fatty acids
• Cell protection • Antioxidants	L-carnitine, vit. E, selenium, vit. C, beta carotine
• Anti-catabolics	Glutamine, branch-chain amino acids, betahydroxybeta-methylbutyrate (BMB), arginine, ornithine, carbohydrate protein mixture
• Immune stimulants	Red sunhat (echinacea), L-carnitine, artemisia abrotanum, mistletoe, camomile, arnica, salicylic acid, green tea

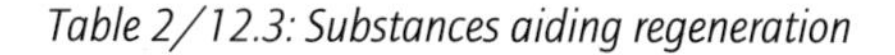

Table 2/12.3: Substances aiding regeneration

Vitamin C, a very effective antioxidant, can also be taken several times a day in amounts of 0.5 to 1 g after great load. Vitamin C also aids the immune system. If citrus fruits are not sufficiently available, vitamin C can be taken in tablet form or as ascorbic acid (low in price) (Table 2/12.3).

As for other vitamins, taking vitamin E in higher doses (100 to 400 mg/day) is useful for strong muscle pains or strained muscles.

Summary

After great training load, regeneration is almost as important as training itself. In aiding regeneration the emphasis is placed on sports-methodological, sports medicine, physiotherapeutic and dietary measures. Compensation training has a central role for the regeneration of tired muscles which are expressed in the form of loss of strength and endurance. Major supportive measures are balancing fluids, early carbohydrate consumption and the additional intake of vitamins, minerals and other active substances. Disregard of regenerative measures and participation in competitions during the regenerative process are often causes for stagnation of performance and conditions for overtraining. The decisive element in regeneration is fast restoration of muscle load tolerance.

13 Sports Nutrition

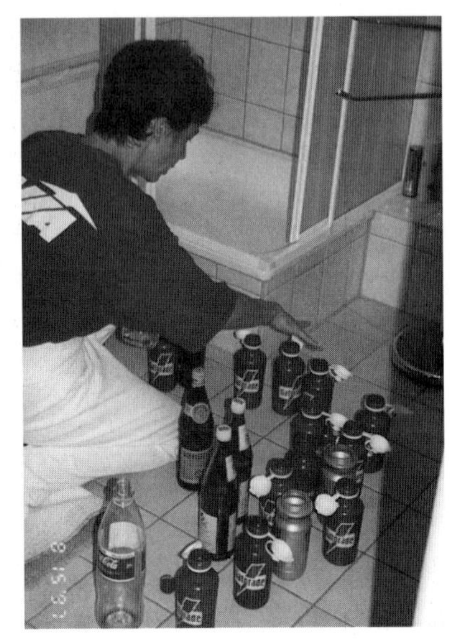

Careful preparation of provisions for a 100 km run.
Photo: Georg Neumann, Leipzig

When sports training is taken up it is advisable to make changes in dietary habits. It is not so much additional calorie intake which is important, rather the quality in nutrition and the distribution of nutrients. In contrast to usual nutrition it has generally proven helpful to increase the proportions of carbohydrates in endurance sports and protein in strength sports (Fig. 1/13, see p. 250). Alternative forms of sports nutrition are not very helpful in competitive training. The practising of certain sports forces athletes to depart from normal guidelines in nutrition by supplementing the increase or decrease in calories strived for with nutrients and active substances necessary for life, especially proteins (Table 1/13, see p. 250). In this chapter nutritional guidelines in sport are only briefly presented. For readers who wish to go into more detail there is a wide range of literature available (GEISS/HAMM, 1990; WEBER, 1988; HOLTMEIER, 1995; KEUL/WITZIGMANN, 1988; KONOPKA, 1994; NEUMANN, 1996; WORM, 1992 and many others).

The following pages cover recommendations with a direct relationship to sports training and load.

13.1 Energy Requirements and Loading

Energy requirements in sport are dependent on load. With weekly training load of two to six hours, one's customary diet need hardly be changed. At moderate load intensity 500-700 kcal are used per training hour. The energy intake of an untrained person with a body weight of 60 to 80 kg is 2500-3000 kcal per day. Energy requirements are a combination of basic use, digestive use and performance use. Basic use to maintain normal living ability is 1500-1700 kcal per day. An additional amount of about 10 % of energy intake is required for digestive processes (Fig. 1/13.1, see p. 251).

With abundant and protein-rich food consumption in warm surroundings, heat from digestion makes itself noticeable through sweating. For everyday load and a lifestyle with little exercise 500 to 1000 kcal are needed daily.

A small amount of 100 to 200 kcal per day more energy intake than is needed will unnoticeably lead to an increase in body weight in a few weeks.

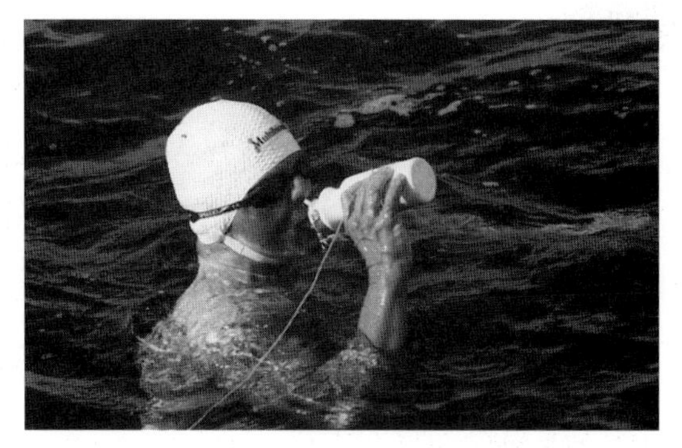

Food consumption during swimming of the English Channel by K. Stutzer in 1997 (14 h 9 min) at a water temperature of 16° C. (Photo: Klaus Stutzer)

Meanwhile, 30 % of people of adult age are overweight. That is an expression of food consumption beyond personal needs. Taking up sporting activity is a useful alternative for breaking down excessive nutritional energy. Interrupting load and maintaining the accustomed level of food consumption soon leads to increased body weight. The calculation of energy use is based on determining oxygen intake.

Energy requirements in sport are dependent on which metabolism state a person is in (ratio of carbohydrates, proteins and fats consumed) (Table 1/13.1, see p. 252).

In competitive sport, determining oxygen intake is an important diagnostic measure. Energy consumption is made up of the proportions of carbohydrates, fatty acids and proteins used. These metabolism proportions in energy consumption can be worked out from the level of oxygen intake and the RQ (respiratory quotient) measured with it.

By measuring oxygen intake, it is possible to ascertain total energy consumption during shorter or longer periods of load. The speed of forward motion influences energy consumption (Fig. 2/13.1, see p. 252).

To date, the greatest energy consumption per day was measured in professional road cyclists during the Tour de France. During this tour, an average energy consumption of 6500 kcal/day was established (SARIS, 1989). The top values were recorded in the mountain stages at 9500 kcal/day. In comparison, for a marathon run in 130 min about 3000 kcal are needed. The energy consumption of top runners is 1300 kcal/h. Slower running competitive or fitness athletes use about 850 kcal/h. Because they run longer, however, their total consumption over four hours rises to 3400 kcal.

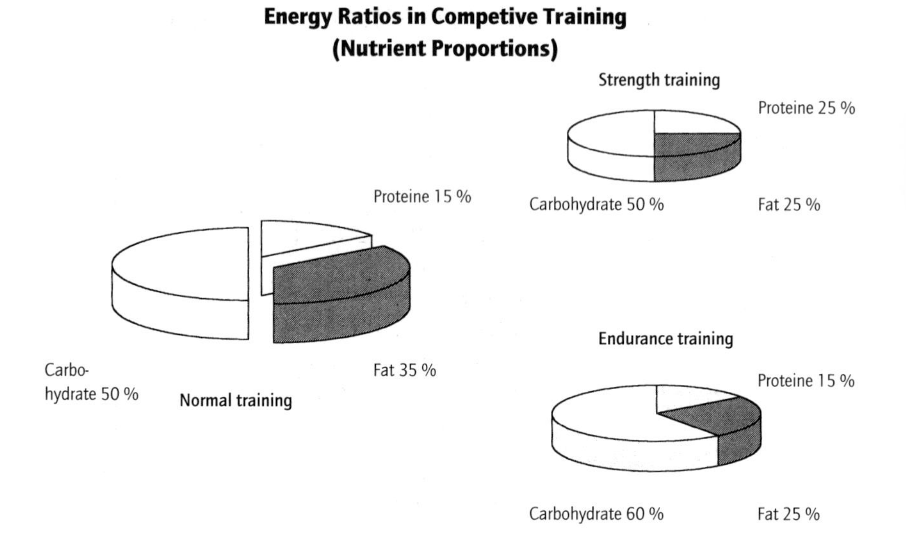

Fig. 1/13: Nutrient regulation in normal, endurance-oriented and strength-oriented training

Risk Groups of Energy Intake in Competitive Sport		
Advantages	**Sports**	**Nutrition**
Maintenance of low body mass and ensuring of load tolerance	Gymnastics, ballet, rhythmical sports gymnastics, figure skating	Low calorie diet over longer periods is compensated for with protein concentrates, vitamins and minerals.
Development of large muscle mass with little fat	Body building, weight lifting	Protein-rich diet (up to 3 g/kg). Deliberate intake of arginine, ornithine, glutamine and trytophane to develop muscles.
Development and maintenance of muscle strength endurance, ensuring of muscular regeneration after high demands	Cycling, running, swimming, rowing, canoeing, triathlon etc	Doubling of energy intake (4500-6500 kcal/day). Increased protein consumption (12-17 % of nutritional energy or 1.5 to 2.5 g/kg). Supplementation of carbohydrates, vitamins, minerals and active substances to develop performance and secure regeneration.
Rapid change in body weight, start in lower weight class	Wrestling, judo and boxing	Repeated drastic changes in energy and fluid consumption. After food restriction deliberate consumption of fluids, carbohydrates and protein in a short period.

Table 1/13: Risk groups of energy intake in competitive sport

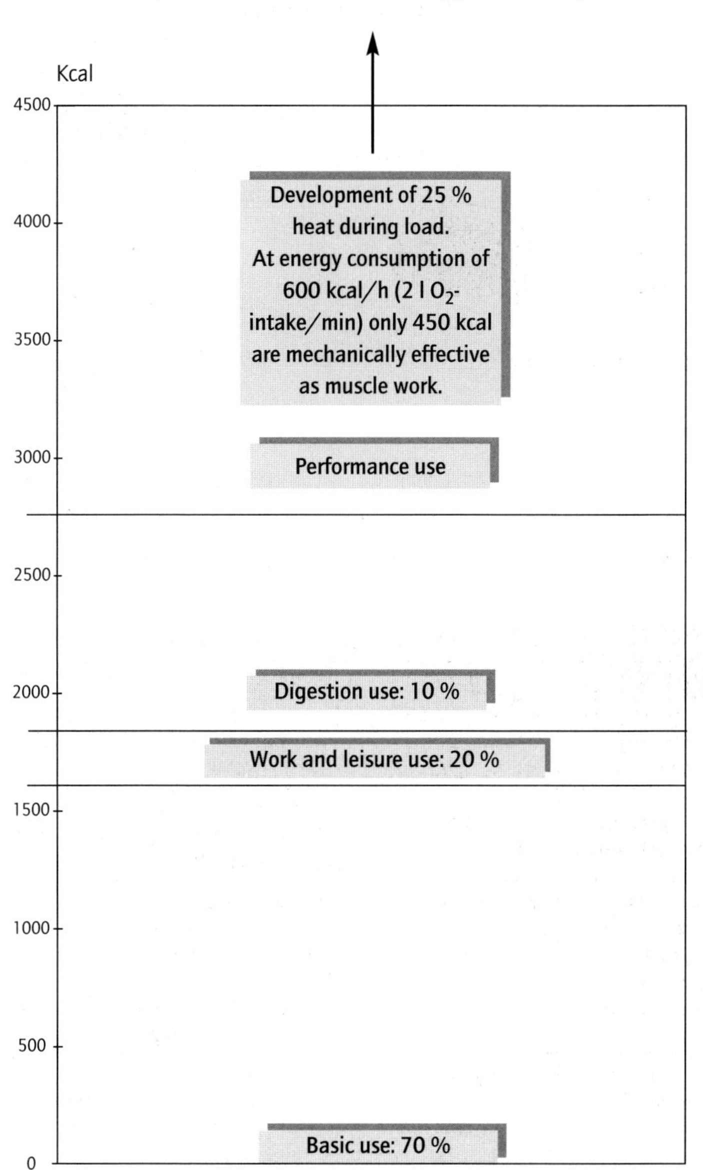

Fig. 1/13.1: Proportions of energy consumption at rest, work and practising sport

Energy Equivalents to Oxygen Uptake of 1 l/min in Various Metabolism States		
Respiratory quotient (RQ)	Metabolism state (Transformation of energy)	Energy equivalent from burning of oxygen
RQ 1.0	only carbohydrates (CH)	5.05 kcal (21.2kJ)
RQ 0.9	CH/fatty acids	4.93 kcal (20.7 kJ)
RQ 0.8	fatty acids/CH	4.81 kcal (20.2 kJ)
RQ 0.7	only fatty acids	4.69 kcal (19.7 kJ)

Table 1/13.1: Energy equivalents to oxygen uptake of 1 l/min in various metabolism states

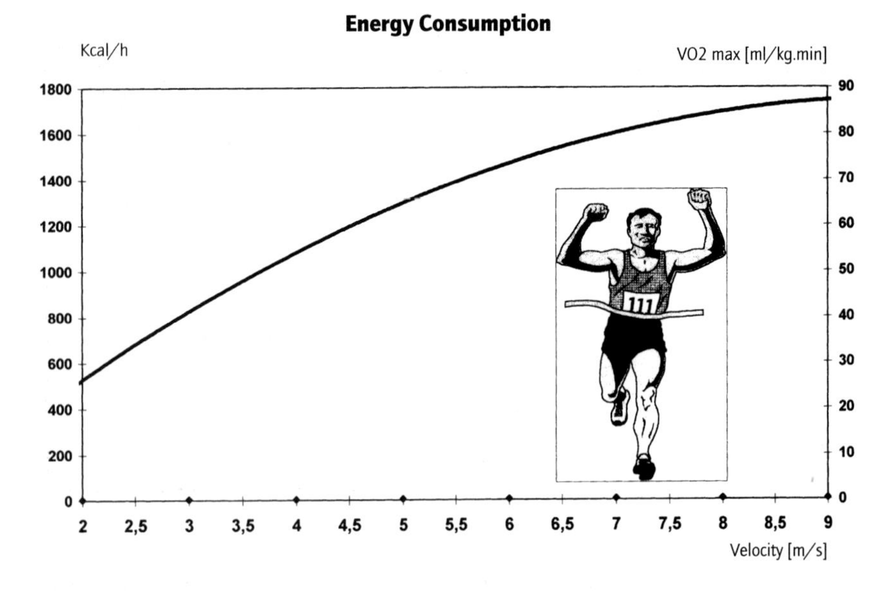

Fig. 2/13.1: Relationship of energy consumption to performance capacity

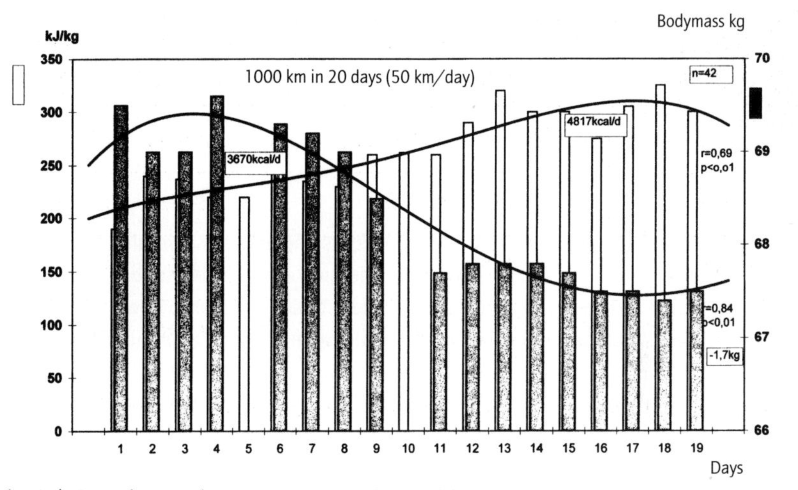

Fig. 3/13.1: Changes in energy consumption and body weight during an extreme endurance run over a total of 1000 km (data according to RASCHKA/PLATH, 1997)

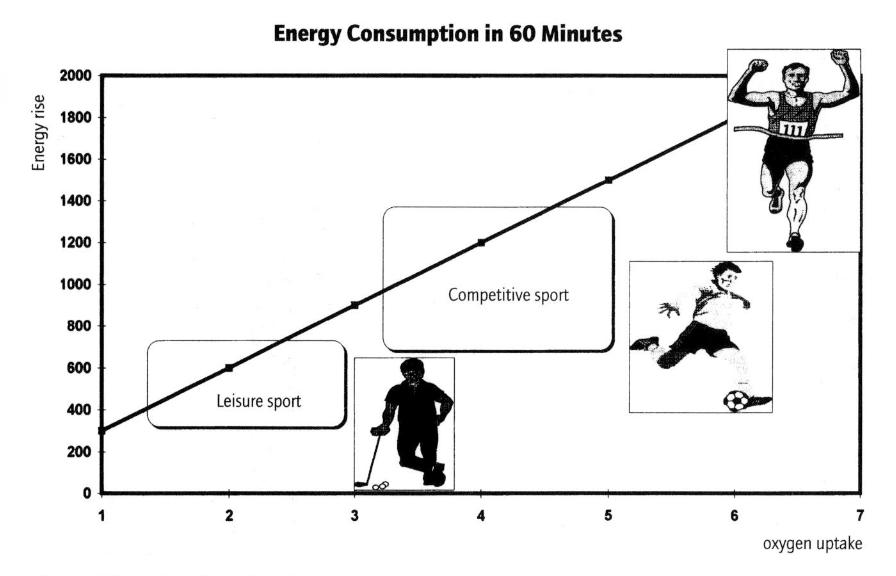

Fig. 4/13.1: Relationship of energy consumption to the increase in oxygen uptake during training in fitness sport and competitive sport

In cases of extremely long duration load, energy requirements go up considerably in the course of the days of load while body weight goes down (Fig. 3/13.1, see p. 253). With long lasting load, consideration must be given to the increase in food consumption coupled with increasing muscle tiredness and decreasing performance if one has to carry one's own provisions.

In daily training, energy use is about 500 kcal/h in fitness sport and 700-1000 kcal/h in top sport (Fig. 4/13.1, see p. 253). In individual cases of heavier people these values can be higher.

Daily energy intake should be oriented to load-linked consumption. If, as a result of great load, an energy deficit of 7700 kcal developed over a longer period, as compensation 1 kg of fatty tissue or 3 kg of muscle mass or a combination of these tissues are broken down as weight is lost. This decrease in mass can occur when there are digestion problems and thus a decrease in energy absorption during training. 80 % of short-term weight loss after training is loss of water.

The ratios of carbohydrates and fatty acids used in energy metabolism changes with increasing performance capacity. As a rule, the proportion of fatty acids used increases in endurance training.

13.2 Carbohydrates

13.2.1 Carbohydrate Metabolism and Loading

In short and medium duration sporting load, carbohydrates (CH) are the substrates mainly used for generation of energy. In all intensive and longer lasting load, CH must be constantly consumed in varying forms over 90 min duration. CH or glucose intake is important for two reasons. Firstly, the brain cannot cope with hypoglycaemia, and secondly, fatty acids can only be burnt when CH metabolism is functioning.

Going under a blood sugar concentration of 3.5 mmol/l (63 mg/dl) is a state practically all training athletes know as a disruptive occurrence. The limits of performance drop from hypoglycaemia vary individually (NEUMANN/REUTER, 1993).

Glycogen is only consumed in muscle groups included in the sport-specific movement programme. Muscles not loaded keep their glycogen. This regulation is used by triathletes, who activate three different muscle programmes.

Training stimuli which lead to exhaustion of the glycogen stores are the basis for increasing activity of the glycogen building enzyme glycogen synthetase. Increased activity of this enzyme is the prerequisite for triggering glycogen overcompensation. Athletes who only train short distances with moderate total load do not achieve the effect of glycogen overcompensation after increased carbohydrate consumption, or else only to a limited extent (BLOM et al., 1987).

For the muscles, continuation of load when the glycogen stores are exhausted means an energetic emergency situation. The main form of help is through the breakdown of double chain amino acids. This redevelopment of sugar from the amino acids is supported by increased releasing of adrenaline and cortisole. Through gluconeogenesis the liver can release 0.9 g of glucose per minute or 54 g per hour. Liver glycogen, however, is exhausted after two hours of aerobic load; after very intensive load earlier still. The branch chain amino acids (valin, leucin, isoleucin) provide the carbon framework for pyruvate development. From 1 g of amino acids 0.6 g of glucose can be made. In a state of glucose shortage the proportion of fat metabolism in energy transformation increases. With the major increase in fatty acid combustion, however, forward motion velocity or performance decreases because from fat combustion less energy per time unit can be won than through carbohydrate combustion (see chapter 4.5)

The glucose from gluconeogenesis is not sufficient to compensate for the lack of glucose so that additional quantities of carbohydrates (CH) must be consumed at an amount of at least 30 g/h. The amount of CH consumed during load holds the balance in maintaining endurance performance. If carbohydrate intake is insufficient, forward motion velocity drops or there is an early end to loading.

The feeling of hunger is unreliable during load. In the case of load, over several hours the necessary food consumption must occur according to factors of reason, not feeling.

13.2.2 Carbohydrate Intake before Loading

Full glycogen stores before important competitions help performance. Better performance can be expected from normal or increased glycogen stores than if they are incompletely filled. For a long time, filling the glycogen stores above their normal state was considered an important performance reserve. Current knowledge relativises this statement. Through plenty of eating alone without appropriate training the glycogen stores cannot be filled above normal.

Glycogen overcompensation as proposed by HULTMAN (1974), through a special low carbohydrate and high fat and protein diet before competitions as a measure to improve performance, is no longer usual in the classic form in competitive sport. These are the reasons:

To achieve glycogen overcompensation, while consuming high protein and low carbohydrate foods, one must train for several days. In this time athletes feel weak and can also have diarrhoea.

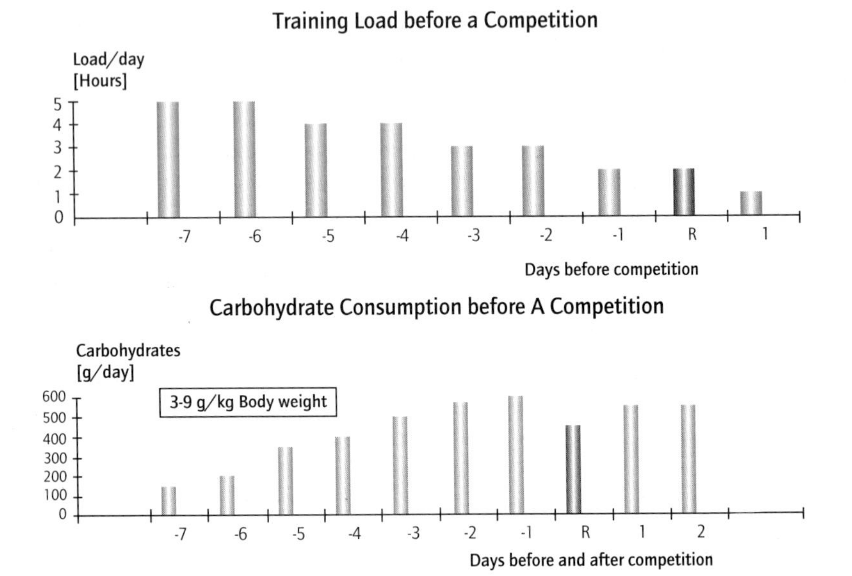

Fig. 1/13.2.2: Structuring of "modern" glycogen overcompensation in competitive training before a race. Training load is gradually reduced and carbohydrate consumption increased.

Nutrition Before Competitions
1. Several days filling the glycogen stores with abundant carbohydrate consumption (CH) before the competition (C). Seven days before is best.
2. Basic principle: increased CH intake and decreased load (reduction in volume while ensuring training quality).
3. Glycogen overcompensation is possible when the CH amount is increased to 600 g/day (maximum 10 g/kg body weight), in the last 2-3 days before a competition.
4. In addition, two days before the C plenty of fluids should be drunk (preferably easily digestible electrolytes).
5. Reduce fibre and fatty foods in the last days before C.
6. Directly before C (2-3 hours) lots of CH can be consumed additionally (if possible in fluid form), in this way safe filling of liver glycogen is achieved.
7. Shortly before load lasting several hours or C, solid CH can again be consumed (light or white bread, energy bar with low fat and protein).
8. To avoid hypoglycaemic regulation before the start when consuming concentrated CH, this should only take place 5-10 min before the start (absorption then occurs in loading time and the glucose is immediately used by the muscles).

Tab. 1/13.2.2: Nutrition before competitions

At today's performance levels athletes can barely afford arbitrary training breaks of 3-7 days before important competitions, and from a sports-methodological point of view this method is considered risky.

The alternative to classic overcompensation is that before major competitions, training load is gradually reduced and at the same time carbohydrate intake is increased (Fig. 1/13.2.2, see p. 256). One week before the competition (C), daily load reduction and daily CH consumption increase begin. The amount of CH should increase from 6 to 10 g/kg body weight per day. 600 g CH per day is enough, however; greater amounts are of no additional value for filling the stores (BURKE et al., 1993).

Directly before a longer competition (over two hours duration) a small CH meal is useful to fill up liver glycogen (Table 1/13.2.2, see p. 256). Competitions under 60 minutes duration need no special CH consumption. Easily digestible CH in the form of energy drinks or bars is sufficient, especially when there is not much time before the start. Competition performances of up to 90 min duration are powered from available glycogen reserves anyway, so that a start on an empty stomach is possible.

13.2.3 Carbohydrate Intake during Loading

The breakdown speed of glycogen is dependent on load intensity. With load in aerobic metabolism, it is slower than with anaerobic load. Long duration load with over 4 mmol/l lactate leads to early exhaustion of glycogen.

Lack of glycogen leads to gradual hypoglycaemia, especially when liver glycogen is exhausted and no CH food has been consumed yet. When blood sugar drops, motor drive of the cerebrum and the muscles drops and forward movement velocity goes down. The lack of energy is experienced by the athlete as an increasing feeling of tiredness in the working muscles, moving forward becomes more difficult. Strength decreases, the strides shorten. These are first signs of a loss of overview regulation of the central nervous system for movement propulsion. The only remedy when hypoglycaemia threatens is immediate intake of carbohydrates in any available form. In this energetic emergency situation it does not matter which sugar is consumed. The amount that leads to a rise in blood sugar is decisive (Fig. 1/13.2.3, see p. 260).

Disaccharides and monosaccharides have proven quickly effective. These pass into the digestive system and reach the muscles via the blood in only five to seven minutes. CH intake during load needs to be estimated by athletes beforehand. In particular this applies to training state, load intensity and duration of load in competitions. In the endurance sports or in load lasting more than an hour, the glucose used comes from food consumed during load. The level of the oxidation rate of glucose from carbohydrate intake is indirectly derivable from the respiratory quotient (RQ). Water intake during endurance load places higher demands on fat metabolism (drop in RQ), but leads to a drop in velocity or to stopping before completion of the course (Fig. 2/13.2.3, see p. 260). One high CH intake during load causes an increase in blood sugar of about 60 min and an extension of cycling time of 20 % (Fig. 3/13.2.3, see p. 261).

CH intake can be constant or in larger servings at once. Constant glucose intake leads to a slight increase in blood sugar, but also to a performance improvement (see Fig. 1/13.2.3). Both procedures raise blood sugar. In general, constant intake is given preference where competition tactics allow it.

Consumption of 30 to 80 g CH per hour (after 70 minutes load) improves performance capacity considerably. The additional oxidatable glucose makes it possible to maintain velocity by an average of 20 % longer load duration without a drop in velocity. CH consumption spares the glycogen stores.

The timing and the amount of CH consumption are dependent on load duration and performance capacity. CH intake during load should only take place after 60 min. In competitions over 60 min or training over 90 min duration, CH intake is always useful. In case of doubt it should be considered whether performance capacity or the load intensity to be maintained require additional CH consumption. All competitions between 90 to 120 min or training between 120 min and 150 min duration are borderline situations for the availability of glycogen. Practice shows that blood sugar can also drop 5 to 10 min before the finish, combined with a dramatic drop in velocity or the impossibility of a burst.

Because of limited absorption capacity, not more than 60 g CH/hour can be absorbed. Timing of the first intake of CH should be about 70 min into the competition so that beforehand CH and fat metabolism can regulate themselves. Preference should be given to complex CH, which contain glucose, maltose, saccharose, glucose polymers and soluble starch.

It should be noted that fructose, galactose and insoluble starch (unripe bananas) are absorbed more slowly. The ripeness of bananas decides on the proportion of absorbable starch and sugar. While yellow-green bananas have about 40 % starch and 45 % sugar, when they are fully ripe (yellow with many black patches) the ratio changes to 5 % starch and 85 % sugar. Fully ripe bananas are best from a nutritional-physiology point of view.

Ideas on fructose consumption have changed. Because fructose intake does not provoke a rise in insulin, it was thought it was the optimal carbohydrate for load. It was not considered that the intake of high concentrations of fructose is not well handled by the gastro-intestinal tract and causes diarrhoea in many athletes. Because fructose can only be split into glucose in the liver, it reaches the muscles via the blood later. In concentrations of over 3.5 % , fructose causes gastro-intestinal problems and diarrhoea. Consuming it alone should be avoided. Fructose can be consumed in low doses together with glucose.

In competitive sport, the combined carbohydrate-electrolyte drinks and energy bars are currently the preferred carbohydrates consumed during load. Mixtures of oatflakes or other grain products and water are also easily digestible and work longer thanks to their physiologically favourable CH composition.

The digestibility of CH and food supplements should always be checked before consumption in competitions (Table 1/13.2.3, see p. 261).

During load the consumption of food rich in fibre and protein should be avoided. A new recommendation is to also consume certain amino acids during load. To diminish the carbohydrate deficit, branch-chain amino acids in particular can be consumed during long duration load (see chapter 13.4).

The digestibility of carbohydrates depends on their composition and their concentration. During load, CH concentrations of 6 to 8 % should not be exceeded, i.e. 60 to 80 g CH to one litre of fluid. When taking the usual kinds of sports drinks, which generally contain 3-6 % carbohydrates, the amounts should be limited to 0.7 to 1.0 litre of fluids per hour of load. Higher CH concentrations are absorbed too slowly and a feeling of fullness in the stomach and intestines arises. A CH concentration of over 16 % is very likely to cause problems with digestion and digestibility. Malt sugars are an exception which can be consumed in high concentrations because of the smaller molecule size.

CH consumed during load spare the glycogen reserves because this glucose is oxidised first. Muscular tiredness cannot be hindered just by CH consumption because performance capacity is also influenced by non-dietary factors.

During load consumption, CH with a high glycaemic index is preferable, i.e. those CH which because of low fibre content lead to a rapid rise in blood sugar concentrations. Endurance load is also possible for athletes with diabetes or diabetic metabolism. During load, insulin requirements drop. The diabetic's higher resting glucose disappears during load. The blood sugar reaches the muscles via insulin-independent glucose receptors (Gluc 4 transporters) (Fig. 4/13.2.3, see p. 262). By observing certain basic dietary rules, diabetics can practise competitive sport without problems.

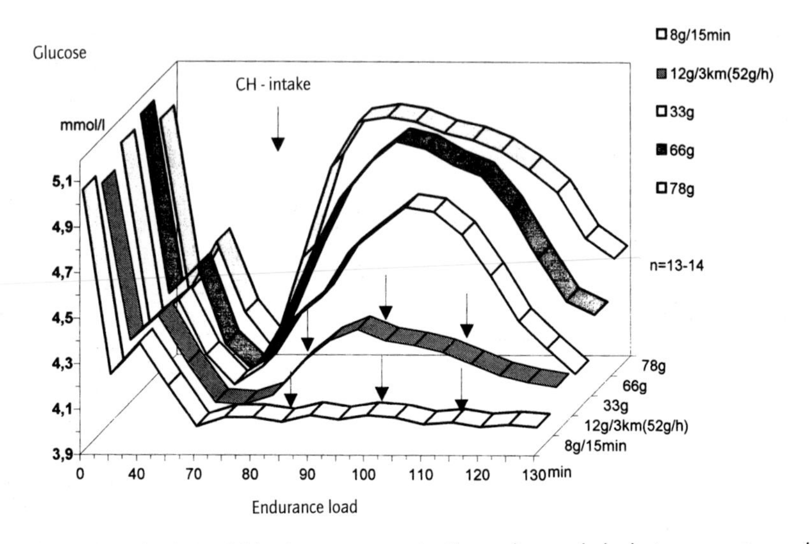

Fig. 1/13.2.3: Behaviour of blood sugar concentrations when carbohydrates are consumed once in a larger amount and constantly in smaller amounts.

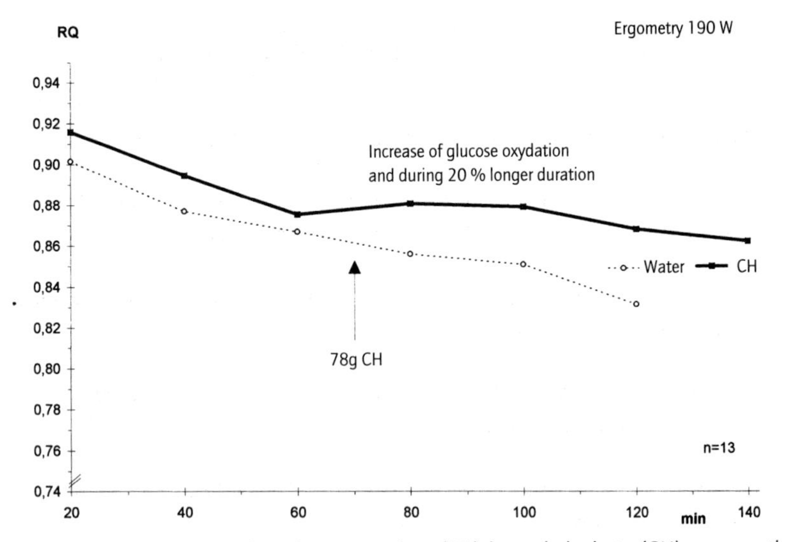

Fig. 2/13.2.3: Influencing of respiratory quotient (RQ) by carbohydrate (CH) consumption in comparison to water intake during ergometer endurance load. When CH are consumed the RQ rises as a sign of increased glucose use.

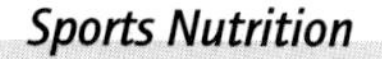

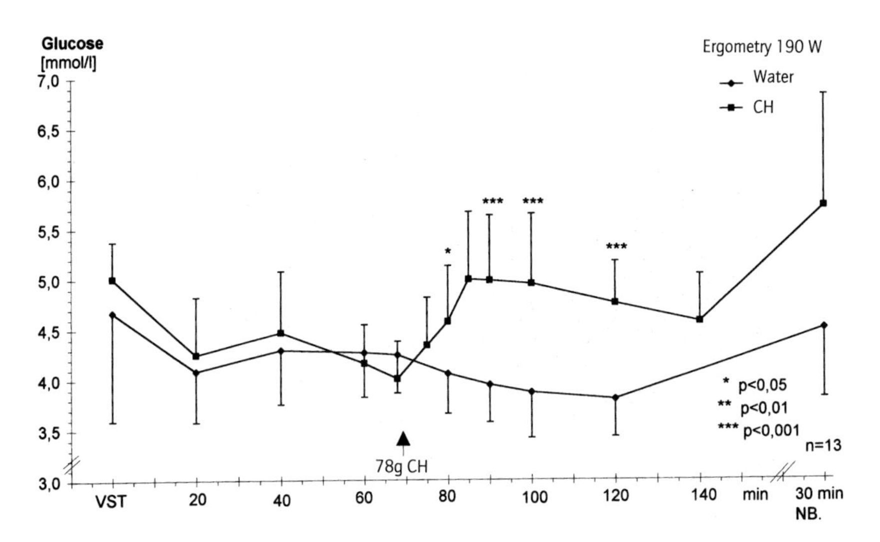

Fig. 3/13.2.3 Behaviour of blood sugar during a cycling continuous test (190W). In the first test the athlete took up just water. in the second test in the 70 th minute 78 g carbohydrates. During carbohydrate-uptake the load deration increased by 19 %.

Carbohydrate (CH) Consumption during Loading

1. During load under 45 min there is no objective need for CH consumption.
2. The first CH consumption in competitive sport takes place after 60 min load (but fluid intake earlier!). Exception: early CH consumption during load of several hours!
3. From the 2nd hour of load onwards 40 to 60 g CH/h is sufficient. Consumption in several small servings if possible.
4. During load consumption of glucose, maltose, saccharose and glucose polymers is preferable. Fructose alone is less effective.
5. Solid CH are absorbed and oxidised more slowly in the intestines. For very intensive load liquid CH are better.

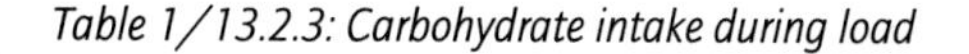

Table 1/13.2.3: Carbohydrate intake during load

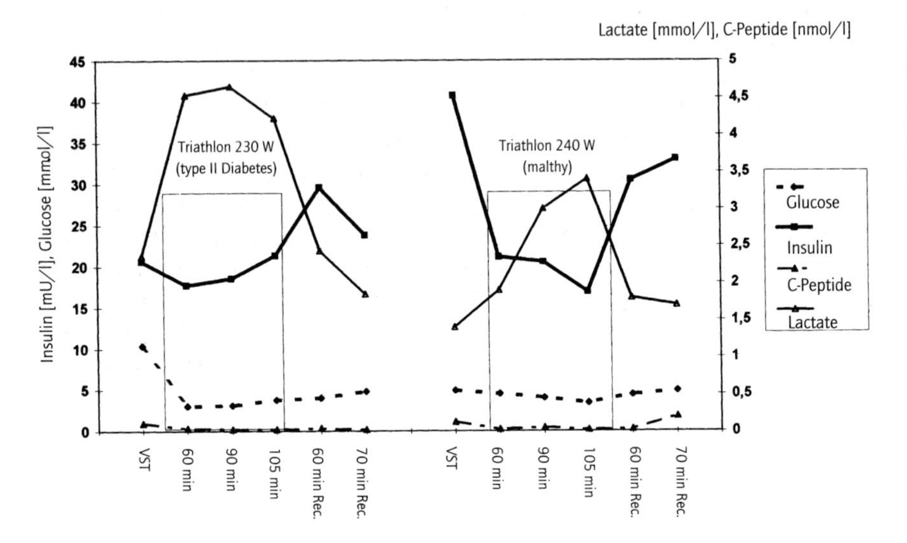

Fig. 4/13.2.3: Comparison of metabolism measurement factors during ergometer load of a sportingly active diabetic (type II diabetes) and a healthy athlete. For the diabetic the insulin concentration during load remains unchanged and blood sugar drops from the resting value of 10 mmol/l (180 mg/dl) to 3.5 mmol/l during load.

13.2.4 Carbohydrate Intake after Loading

Directly after load the activity of the glycogen developing enzyme (glycogen synthetase) increases (see chapter 12, Fig. 12.3, see p. 246).

In the early stages of regeneration the consumption of larger quantities of carbohydrates leads to about 20% accelerated muscle glycogen development.

For this reason, after training or a competition of several hours, in addition to fluids, CH should be consumed as quickly a possible. CH consumption must take place independently of hunger feelings. Directly after load the beginning metabolism anabolism must be exploited. Glycogen redevelopment is determined by the quantity, type and timing of food consumption. The glycogen synthesis rate during the first hours after load is 7-8 %. On the average 5 % of used up glycogen is refilled per hour. This happens only if 8 to 10 g/kg of carbohydrates per day are consumed.

In the first hour of recovery 25-30 g of easily digestible CH or 50 g spread over two hours are to be consumed. CH absorption is aided by the use of 0.6-1.0 g of common salt (NaCl) per litre of fluid. At the following meal salt should be put on food. After a competition or strenuous training about 600 g CH should be consumed within 24 hours. After average training load in aerobic metabolism, one day later the muscle glycogen stores are filled up enough for normal training to carry on. After strenuous competitions lasting several hours, however, refilling of the glycogen depots is considerably delayed. After long duration competitions (e.g. marathon, ultra triathlon, 100 km run, multiple ultra triathlon etc) refilling of the mucle glycogen stores can take several days or up to a week. Destruction in the muscles probably prevents orderly glycogen refilling. By reducing training load the glycogen stores can be refilled more quickly. If the carbohydrates consumed have a high glycaemic index, glycogen repletion is aided. Major consumption of fruit sugars delays glycogen resynthesis; because of the low glycaemic index of fructose, glycogen development is only half as fast.

Summary

Sports training increases energy requirements. Carbohydrates (CH) are important components of sports nutrition. They are the vital energy supplier for all forms of intensive load. The glycogen stores in the liver and the muscles allow intensive load for up to 90 min and training load for up to 120 min without food intake. For longer endurance load constant CH intake of 30 to 60 g per hour is necessary. Through endurance training the glycogen stores in the muscles can be enlarged quite considerably, in extreme cases they can double in size. All endurance load with lactate concentrations under 2 mmol/l spares the glycogen stores. Load with lactate development over 4 mmol/l leads to faster breakdown of glycogen. When there is a shortage of carbohydrates the fat metabolism proportion of energy use rises. CH consumed during load are oxidised first, in this way the glycogen stores are spared. Consumption of carbohydrates before and after load has clear advantages for performance. After load, early and plentiful CH consumption accelerates regeneration.

13.3 Fatty Acids

13.3.1 Fat Metabolism and Loading

The free fatty acids (FFA) are the main substrates for energy transformation for all long duration load. Fat metabolism only becomes fully effective for energy transformation when load is long enough and coupled with lactate development of 2 mmol/l. In all loads over several hours (running, cross-country skiing, cycling, swimming), up to 70 % of energy is won through combustion of free fatty acids. The fatty acid reservoir is large and even under extreme sporting load it is practically inexhaustible. From the fat depots of 6 to 8 kg usually found in competitive athletes, theoretically an energy equivalent of about 70,000 kcal could be released. With that 23 marathons could be run. Use of fatty acids does not occur in isolation, it is always linked with an intact carbohydrate metabolism state. If there is a carbohydrate deficit, fat combustion is incomplete; large amounts of ketone bodies (betahydroxybutyrate, acetone, acetacetate) are created. Quantitatively betahydroxybutyrate (BHB) dominates, see Fig. 3, chapter 4.5.3.

Two substances hinder use of fatty acids - insulin and lactate. As long as the insulin level is still high during load, only a limited amount of FFA can be metabolised. This is the case with all intensive short duration loads up to 30 min. Insulin encourages glucose use by allowing sweeping of glucose into the muscle cell at rest. Only after longer load (from 30 min. duration onwards) does the insulin concentration drop considerably. Blood sugar then gets into the muscles during load through the insulin-dependent receptors (glucoreceptors). This is the reason diabetics should also be active in endurance sports (see chapter 12.3.3, Fig. 4). They need no increased insulin secretion during load. The hormonal counterpart of insulin, glucagon, aids use of fatty acids. The second disruptive factor for fat metabolism after insulin is lactate. Increased lactate concentration has a great effect on FFA use. Too much lactate in the blood restricts the release of FFA from the fat cells. If lactate concentration exceeds 7 mmol/l, lipolysis is greatly limited through the restriction of triglyceride lipase (see Fig. 1/4.5.3). This means that training which is too intensive suppresses the development of fat metabolism in favour of CH metabolism.

13.3.2 Fat Intake before Loading

Before load, consumption of FFA is not necessary. Firstly, the fat stores are so abundant that they are inexhaustible, and secondly, abundant fat consumption before training or a competition start would strain the stomach. By consuming easily digestible food about two hours before a competition this experience is taken into account. Whether and how much can be eaten beforehand is always decided by the type of sport and the duration of load. The shorter and more intensive the load, the less food with fat proportions should be consumed. A completely fat free diet is hardly possible because many products popular in sport contain hidden fats.

13.3.3 Fat Intake during Loading

When the consumption of energy suppliers during loading was begun, the emphasis was originally on fatty acids. Fats have the greatest energy content of all foods. The intake of fatty acids during load has become greatly reduced to extreme load. For intensive endurance load of under three hours no fatty acids should be consumed. During longer load foodstuffs with low fat dosages in hidden form (e.g. biscuits, waffles) are eaten. The disadvantage of fatty acid consumption is difficult digestion. They stay in the stomach longer. In the meantime it is common practice to consume fatty acids for hour-long or repeated long duration load, e.g. multiple ultra triathlons, stage cross-country races (50 to 100 km/day) or up to 4700 km in a row. Apart from anything else, fats are preferred for taste reasons as sweet carbohydrates are no longer wanted or can no longer be digested. The low velocity of forward movement in extreme competitions allows the intake of solid and fatty foods during load also or else during short breaks. The digestibility of the fatty acid mixture and also the amounts the stomach can process should always be individually tested before competitions. Disregarding this simple rule has caused the failure of many a sporting undertaking.

Independent of the sport, long duration training leads to enlargement of the intramuscular neutral fats (triglycerides). After long duration load, a decrease in triglycerides in the blood can always be established as a sign of their increased use. During long lasting load the combustion of fatty acids is dependent on carbohydrate availability. If CH consumption is too abundant, these are burnt first and the breakdown of the FFA, as well as of glycogen, is spared.

Greater fatty acid breakdown can be supported with a number of practical tricks, firstly through training without breakfast for 60 to 90 min duration. A further possibility is to keep CH intake low during load and only consume 20 to 30 g CH per hour. Additionally the flooding of long and medium chain fatty acids into the mitochondria can be increased through intake of 1-2 g of L-carnitine. L-carnitine is a component of a fatty acid transport system into the mitochondria and can increase fatty acid use.

The advantage of increased fatty acid combustion during load is the sparing of the glycogen stores. Loading intensity can be maintained for longer and protein breakdown is delayed. Decisively for training fat metabolism there is little lactate. At 4 mmol/l lactate already the use of fatty acids and carbohydrates is reduced by half (see Fig. 2/4.5.3). Omitting fat metabolism training hinders the development of the stability of endurance performance capacity and reduces load tolerance.

13.3.4 Fat Intake after Loading

Fatty acid intake after load should be delayed initially. First carbohydrate intake has absolute precedence. Consumption of mixed foods too early after training exhausts the glycogen stores and considerably delays glycogen refilling.

About two hours after the end of exhaustion, the accustomed meal containing greater quantities of fats and proteins can be begun. Before this, CH with a high glycaemic index should be given preference (see chapter 13.2.4).

Summary

The free fatty acids (FFA) are the vital energy suppliers for long duration load. Through deliberate long duration endurance training, the intramuscular fat stores grow and total body fat decreases. Long-distance athletes have a fat reserve of 6 to 10% of body weight. These stores are practically inexhaustible. A great deal of body fat is ballast for endurance athletes.

Through endurance training the proportion of FFA in energy use is increased. Long duration load is secured energetically by 60 to 70 % through fatty acid combustion. Use of FFA only functions if the supply of carbohydrates is intact. If there is a carbohydrate deficit, the fatty acids are not broken down completely and ketone bodies are created. Through the high use of FFA during load, sport-specific aerobic load tolerance increases; a greater volume of training can be coped with energetically. Through the increased use of fatty acids, the glycogen stores are spared and protein breakdown is delayed.

Training of fat metabolism is hindered during short duration load with lactate development over 4 mmol/l, and at over 7 mmol/l it is suppressed.

Through the intake of L-carnitine, the utilisation of the long and medium chain fatty acids in the mitochondria is increased, so more FFA can be used.

13.4 Proteins

13.4.1 Protein Metabolism and Loading

Normally protein consumption increases with increasing energy consumption. In usual mixed food there is 12 to 15 % protein. Competitive athletes expand their energy consumption during load by a factor of 3 to 5 and with it their protein requirements. Every form of competitive sports training increases protein requirements as a result of protein breakdown in the exerted muscles. For training of less than six hours/week, normal food intake is sufficient. Only when weekly training load exceeds fifteen hours is it necessary to check one's diet with regard to protein content. This especially applies to vegetarian athletes. Protein requirements are related to the volume of weekly training.

In competitive sport there are four risk groups with regard to energy and protein intake (see Table 1/13). These concern protein deficit when calorie supply is too low (female dancers and gymnasts), increased requirements of strength sports (body builders, weight lifters) as well as endurance sports and muscle strength regeneration in weight class sports (wrestling, judo).

The reserves of freely available proteins are limited in the form of amino acids. If broken down completely, the pool of 110 g of amino acids would theoretically provide energy generation of 450 kcal.

The essential amino acids have a central position in the protein balance, they have to be constantly consumed with food because the body cannot make them. In competitive sport, states of protein deficit in nutrition do not occur, but an unbalanced ratio of amino acids in food intake can delay muscle regeneration. Because amino acid requirements and also their availability at any time are not known exactly, athletes consume these in excess. The additional intake of amino acids or predigested protein hydrolysates is being practised increasingly. This procedure has not yet been supported by scientific findings. Highly exerted top athletes say that through deliberate amino acid intake their regeneration proceeds better and their strength comes back sooner. Excess protein or amino acid consumption is not harmful to healthy persons, with the exception of when someone has a kidney illness.

13.4.2 Protein Intake before Loading

Ensuring protein consumption before loading goes back to a longer-term effect of the protein ratio in nutrition. This means that the amounts of protein consumed in competitive sport should be higher than the recommendations of the German food authorities for untrained persons (DGE 1991). These recommendations are orientated to protein intake of 0.8 to 1.2 g/kg body weight. With this the requirements in sport are not taken into account at all. The data gained from untrained persons on protein intake cannot be applied to competitive athletes. The recommendations, based on socio-political interests, are suboptimal for competitive athletes (LEMON, 1994). With increasing energy utilisation, protein requirements also go up; they are usually twice that of untrained persons. With normal mixed food, training load of over 20 h/week cannot be kept up over longer periods of time without sufficient protein supply. The consumption of proteins, protein hydrolysates and amino acids is meanwhile a normal nutritional requirement in competitive sport. The reasons for the additional consumption of dietary products with protein in sport are:

- **Reduction of protein catabolism caused by load.**
- **Acceleration of muscle regeneration after strength and strength endurance loads.**
- **Aiding of muscle development (muscle fibre hypertrophy) in certain training phases.**
- **Increasing or maintaining sport-specific muscle strength and strength endurance.**
- **Protection against overloading (overtraining).**
- **Reduction of states of energy deficit as a result of load and increasing of load tolerance.**

Results can hardly be expected from a brief increase in protein intake before load. Protein consumption must be long-term and correspond to the speed of muscle development. The amino acids arginine and ornithine aid competitive training by increasing the supply of fatty acids to the muscles, aiding rebuilding of destroyed muscle cell structures, supporting the immune system and greatly activating the growth hormone. They have a building-up effect in metabolism.

13.4.3 Protein Intake during Loading

Extreme sporting performances can no longer be achieved with usual nutrition. Long duration load provokes hunger states and these increase amino acid absorption in the intestines (FRICKER et al., 1991). In addition to the amino acids the protein hydrolysates are easily digestible. Protein hydrolysates are created by industrially carried out "predigestion" of proteins. Hydrolysates and amino acids are both absorbed as quickly as carbohydrates so that their consumption during load causes no problems with digestion. During long duration load it can certainly be useful to consume amino acids. Especially suitable here are branch-chain amino acids (valin, leucin, isoleucin). Their consumption reduces protein catabolism caused by load (BLOMSTRAND et al., 1991). In the breaks between training sessions competitive athletes training four to nine hours a day cannot eat as accustomed. Difficult to digest meat meals with protein and fat consumption are not possible any more on the day of training. The alternative for athletes is to take predigested proteins (hydrolysates) and individual amino acids. In this way the dietetic protein hydrolysates and amino acids become important components of snacks between meals in modern competitive training. The choice of proteins depends on the intended effect in the sport.

13.4.4 Protein Intake after Loading

The legitimacy of increased consumption of amino acids is to be found in the greater degree of protein catabolism in competitive sport. After competition load, there is an increase in serum urea lasting over four to six days (see Fig. 3/4.5.3). Thus additional protein intake, especially after training camps, cycling tours, competition series and extreme load is useful for low complication and undelayed regeneration (see chapter 12). While in strength athletes the amino acids are used in the regeneration period for muscle development, in endurance athletes the influencing of regeneration of muscle cell destruction through load is in the foreground. The detoxicative by-product of protein broken down in metabolism is urea. This appears in the blood before leaving the body via the kidneys. The level of serum urea concentration shows the degree of protein breakdown and under this aspect justifies the deliberate consumption of protein in regeneration.

Summary

With increasing energy utilisation in competitive sport, average protein requirements can double. For vegetarian athletes the increased consumption of nutritional proteins, protein hydrolysates and/or amino acids is of long-term significance for ensuring load tolerance. The justification for additional protein intake in competitive sport derives from the following indications:

- Reduction in protein breakdown through load.
- Acceleration of regeneration in the muscles after strength and strength endurance training, aiding of muscle build-up (muscle hypertrophy).
- Maintaining and increasing sport-specific muscle strength.
- Stabilisation of the immune system and protection against immune cell breakdown.
- Ensuring of daily load tolerance and re-loading tolerance in competition series (competitions in stages).
- Higher concentrations of absorped mixtures of arginin and ornithin increase the release of the growing hormone and act physiologically anabolic on the change of regeneration.

The consumption of amino acids in the physiologically effective L-form is without risk healthwise. Overdoses are unknown.

14 Substances Influencing Performance

The desire to influence performance capacity with nutrients or certain substances is an old virtue of mankind. Numerous examples from the ancient Olympic Games have been recorded. After appeals to keep to the rules and to fairness in the modern Olympics bore no fruit, the International Olympic Committee (IOC) decided on the recommendation of the Medical Commission 1964 to prohibit the use of certain drugs or substances at the time of the competition. With this the list of banned substances was drawn up. It was assumed that the active substances in the list had a performance-enhancing effect. Independent of the doping list, numerous physiological substances were tested which can have an effect on sporting performance capacity. This development was supported by industry. The indications and effects of vitamins, minerals and other substances listed by manufacturers do not always correspond to reality or are often one-sided.

On the following pages a selection of active substances is described which can be useful for athletes from a certain level of load onwards. Their use should be checked individually. This applies to vitamins, electrolytes, carbohydrate mixtures and substances with an immune-modulating effect among others.

It should be noted that the consumption of medicines or drugs during illness also has effects on sporting performance capacity and especially in competitions can make itself noticeable negatively. For this reason intensive loads or starts in competitions while taking medicines (also antibiotics) should be avoided.

14.1 Ergogenic Substances

For performance-enhancing substances not on the doping list, the term ergogenic substances or active substances has become accepted (Table 1/14.1).

With normal nutrition, today's competitive training can no longer be carried out successfully or with few complications. To aid regeneration and maintain load tolerance, numerous possibilities based on scientific findings have become available.

Most active substances are declared as food supplement substances and are thus subject to the foodstuffs laws. Through enrichment by the manufacturers these can be absorbed in greater quantities than in a natural diet. The following performance-enhancing active substances are allowed which are not substances in the sense of doping:

Performance-enhancing Ergogenic Substances	
• Carbohydrates (CH)	40-80 g/h CH during the competition (C). Before C 3-6 g/kg CH.
• Caffeine	200-500 mg before C. At 9 mg/kg the doping limit is reached. (Drinking coffee contains 50-90 mg of caffeine in 100 ml.)
• Creatine (CR)	Altogether 30-100 g in five days is enough to fill the muscle depots; 2 g/day is a maintaining dosage for a limited time. In 20 % of athletes CR has no effect.
• Sodium bicarbonate (citrate)	0.3-0.5 g/kg in one litre of water (usually indigestible)

Table 1/14.1: Performance-enhancing ergogenic substances

Caffeine

Caffeine is the active substance in coffee, tea and guarana. Caffeine is regularly taken by many people as a luxury foodstuff for mental and physical stimulation and when tired. Caffeine activates the central nervous system and the sympathetic nervous system. Through the activation of the catecholamines by caffeine, more free fatty acids are released and their utilisation increased. Thus glycogen breakdown is also restricted. Performance-enhancing effects have only been scientifically proven by intake of pure caffeine, but not through coffee. The effect of caffeine depends on the dosage.

Amounts of 300 mg improve reaction time and motor co-ordination. When 6 mg/kg (about 350-400 mg) is consumed, a positive influencing of endurance performance can be expected. The greatest caffeine consumption is required for influencing strength and short duration endurance, here quantities of over 7 mg/kg are assumed.

Because with higher doses of caffeine, in principle, a performance-enhancing effect is possible, in sport it was decided that the excretion of a quantity of 12 μg/ml of caffeine in urine constitutes a doping offence. This border amount can already be reached by drinking more than four cups of strong coffee. The individual differences are great. A normal coffee contains 300 mg/l (or 120 mg per large cup) and a strong coffee or espresso contains 500-600 mg/l of caffeine. There are obviously great differences in the digestibility and the breakdown of caffeine. The caffeine doping limit is certainly reached when more than 9 mg/kg body weight of caffeine or caffeinated products is consumed. That means more than five cups of coffee for a person weighing 70 kg. Care should be taken when consuming carbohydrate and caffeinated brain drinks (disco drinks) which are now available as "Red Bull" or "Flying Horse". 250 ml cans of both German-made products contain 320 mg caffeine and thus the equivalent of three cups of coffee. Austrian products contain considerably more caffeine!

If taking 2-3 cups of normal coffee two hours before the start there is no danger of exceeding the urine limit of 12 μg/ml.

Creatine

Creatine is a physiological active substance which is indispensable for muscle contraction. From the amino acids arginine, glycine and methionine the body can create 1-2 g of creatine daily. A further 1 g/day is consumed with food, mainly through meat and fish. Vegetarians consume very little creatine through vegetable nutrition. As a result they have smaller creatine stores.

In the muscle cell only 30 % of total creatine is stored as free creatine. Most of it is bound to phosphate and creates the energy-rich compound creatine phosphate (CP). CP is the alactic energy store (see chapter 4.5.1). The creatine used up by muscle contraction is swept out of the cell as creatinine and excreted via the kidneys. The necessary creatine is replaced from the bloodstream by special transporters.

When the CP stores are full, creatine can increase alactic performance capacity and is therefore included among the ergogenic substances. In its utilisation the CP store comes before the glycogen store. The CP stores increase through alactic performance training. Through additional consumption of 10 to 20 g of creatine daily for five days, the muscle CP stores can increase by about 20 %. Once full, CP stores stay up for about 14-21 days. The full state of the CP stores can be maintained for a longer period by taking about 2 g/day of creatine.

The result of increased CP stores is both an increase in alactic performance capacity and faster regeneration of the alactic potential after strength or short duration interval training. Possibly competition performance capacity is improved in its alactic components. Reports on increased performance capacity in competitions after taking creatine are contradictory. It should be noted that about 20 % of athletes do not react to creatine intake, they are so-called non-responders. Endurance performance capacity is probably not increased by creatine consumption.

Amino Acids

During endurance load there is a great deal of protein breakdown and protein restructuring. This means it is necessary to consume protein additionally to normal meals.

Because proteins are of central significance to metabolism and the development of muscles, their additional consumption for high training and competition load is justified. For the consumption of protein hydrolysates (predigested proteins) and amino acids there are the following arguments, for the acceptance of which each athlete must decide for himself.

The intake of increased protein quantities of 1.5 to 2.5 g/kg body weight as natural protein in meat, fish and plants and also as amino acids or protein hydrolysates has the following effects:

- Reduction of protein breakdown after long duration load.
- Accelerated regeneration of intensively used muscles (especially after strength training).
- Aiding of muscle development.
- Protection of muscles from overloading.
- Aiding of glycogen development and gluconeogenesis.

Overdoses in the consumption of amino acids are unknown. If an athlete decides in favour of additional amino acid consumption, then qualified advice is necessary. This applies to the necessary amount, composition and favourable timing of consumption. It should be taken into account that deliberate amino acid consumption is very expensive. Beforehand it should be checked whether the desired effect can be achieved by taking biologically highly valuable natural proteins or protein hydrolysates. For risk groups in sports nutrition or in energy intake, knowledge about additional protein consumption is useful (see Table 1/13).

L-Carnitine

L-carnitine is a substance with a wide spectrum of effects and has no direct influence on sporting performance capacity. Through its diverse physiological functions, L-carnitine works to ensure load tolerance in sport. In this sense it is not an ergogenic substance (see Table 2/12.3, see p. 247).

In an unloaded state the body creates 20 % of its L-carnitine needs from methionine and lysine. The greater part of the L-carnitine is taken in with food. Mutton has a high carnitine content. In sport people became aware of L-carnitine when its function of sweeping fatty acids into the mitochondria was proven. After that numerous useful side-effects were discovered.

In competitive athletes an undersupply of L-carnitine is possible. This applies to low meat and vegetarian diets.

Additional L-carnitine consumption, especially in cases of high training load, has the following physiological effects:

- Increase in the utilisation of long and medium chain fatty acids by sweeping these into the mitochondrium space and breakdown via beta oxidation.
- Increasing of pyruvate dehydrogenase flow in carbohydrate metabolism through activation of the pyruvate dehydrogenase complex (increase in pyruvate oxidation).
- Increase in glycolysis (greater lactate development) through stimulation of the glycolytic key enzyme phosphofructokinase.
- Aiding of alactic energy transformation by transporting long chain fatty acids out of the mitochondria.
- Activation of cells in the immune system and thus general immune stimulating effect.
- Stabilisation of cell membranes and cell protection by transporting away the acryl groups (fatty acids) that have been taken up by them and development of an antioxidative effect.

The additional intake of L-carnitine ensures load tolerance, especially when training load is maintained at a high level for a longer period of time. If loading rises to 25 to 40 h/week, then additional L-carnitine consumption is advantageous for ensuring load tolerance. Many top athletes in the endurance sports base their load tolerance on L-carnitine.

For fitness athletes in their middle years and also for older athletes, L-carnitine consumption is also justified at relatively low levels of load. Because of the lower training state as a result of age, normal sporting load is already felt to be high psychophysically.

The following dosages are currently accepted:

- Before intensive long duration load (2-3 hours before a competition of several hours) 2-4 g of L-carnitine can be taken.
- In phases of very high training load 1-2 g/day should be taken over several weeks. Higher dosages are not advisable as the substance is excreted.
- To cover muscular L-carnitine requirements competitive endurance athletes can take 0.3-0.5 g/day for a longer period.
- For highly-exerted fitness athletes and older athletes irregular consumption of 0.2 to 0.5 g/week can be advantageous.

In times of reduced loading L-carnitine intake should be stopped. This ensures that the body's own production remains active. Undisturbed self-synthesis is only possible if the co-factors of L-carnitine biosynthesis (lysine, methionine, niacine, vitamin B_6, vitamin C and iron) are available in sufficient quantities. After longer breaks in consumption a higher dosage can be chosen for a week. Obviously 30 to 50 mg/kg body weight (or 2-4 g of L-carnitine) is enough to increase the receptor density of the slow twitch muscle fibres (STF) again. Via more receptors a greater amount of free L-carnitine gets from the blood to the muscle cells, where it works.

In competitive sport the additional intake of L-carnitine does not directly influence performance capacity. Abundantly available L-carnitine does, however, influence the load tolerance conditions of the heart and skeletal muscles positively. On the whole the abundant supply of L-carnitine to the muscles allows an increase in ability to handle load, stimulation of the immune system and increased cell membrane protection.

The consumption of L-carnitine is not a "doping activity"; in clinical medicine it is also considered a valuable medicine for numerous illnesses of the nervous system and the heart muscles.

Summary

As a matter of principle, sporting performance capacity can only be improved by training. To aid load tolerance and regeneration, the consumption of physiologically active substances or ergogenic substances is advantageous. Sporting performance capacity can be influenced by the taking of medicines to treat illnesses. Because performance restrictions are possible, e.g. through taking of antibiotics, their consumption before or during a competition or training should be discussed with a doctor.

All active substances or medicines/drugs which have a clear performance enhancing or performance influencing effect and thus give individual athletes advantages are on the doping list. Their consumption is a health risk and unethical.

14.2 Doping

Over the years the term doping has changed in meaning. The consumption of certain drugs and active substances is not necessarily doping.

For the authorisation of consumption of certain drugs in performance sport the stipulations of the Medical Commission of the IOC are binding. All active substances from which a direct influencing of performance capacity is known are on the doping list. The doping list was introduced in 1964. In it are listed all substances and methods not allowed in competitive sport. The "doping list" can be changed at short notice if there is a reason for this (Table 1/14.2, see p. 276).

Banned Substances and Manipulations in Competitive Sport*	
Effect Group	Effects
1. Stimulants (amphetamines, ephedrine, cocaine, fencamfamine, fenetylline, pemoline)	Major activation of the central nervous system, removal of tiredness; moving of performance limits
2. Narcotics (morphine, pentazocine, pethidine)	Euphoria, suppression of pain, especially in the muscles; further load free of pain
3. Anabolic substances (clostebol, mesterolon, nandrolon, stanozolol, testosterone, clenbuterol)	Muscle development, fibre hypertrophy, euphoria, mascularisation of women, impotence in men; increased strength, great training enjoyment
4. Diuretics (furosemide, hydrochlorothiacide, spironolacton, triamteren)	Major urine excretion, urine dilution; dehydration in weight class sports; start in lower weight class in competition
5. Peptide hormones and analogues (growth hormone (STH), erythropoietin (EPO), corticotrophin (ACTH))	Muscle growth and whole body anabolism through STH and ACTH, increase in erythrocytes (haemoglobin increase) through EPO; increased strength, faster anabolism, increased oxygen transport capacity (EPO)
6. Analogue active substances (chemically and pharmacologically related compounds of 1-5 above)	Similar effect strived for to the compounds under 1-5.
7. Banned methods (pharmacological, chemical and physical manipulation of urine tests, blood doping)	Disguising or greatly diluting active substance consumption; increased oxygen transport capacity through increase in haemoglobin
8. Substance groups with restrictions (alcohol, beta blockers, local anaesthetics, asthma drugs, corticosteroids, marijuana)	Consumption or application notifiable. Banned in certain sports (e.g. alcohol and beta blockers for shooters)

** Refusal of doping tests in training or after competitions is considered a positive finding.*

Information on active substance consumption: Anti-Doping Commission DSB and NOK, Otto-Fleck-Schneise 12, D-60528 Frankfurt/M., Germany

Table 1/14.2: Banned substances and manipulations in competitive sport

On the basis of the stipulations of the Medical Commission of the IOC the German organisation Deutscher Sportbund (DSB) created a valid list for all sports associations. Consumption of banned substances, manipulation of urine tests and refusal to take urine tests are punished with bans on participation in organised sport (squad athletes in top sport). Recently warnings have also been issued in the case of first evidence of certain substances (e.g. caffeine, ephedrine). Findings of anabolic steroids result in immediate suspension, which for first offenders is no longer for four but for two years. Competition suspension is only applied in competitive sport when the A and B tests have identical results.

In addition to competition checks, a comprehensive system of training checks has been established in Germany. In Germany there are internationally accredited doping laboratories in Cologne and Kreischa (Dresden). The IOC has recognised 25 doping laboratories around the world. Of 90,000 tests per year 1.6 % were positive.

As a matter of principle the consumption of drugs and substances on the doping list should be avoided, for ethical and moral reasons, out of fairness to sporting rivals and also because of the proven health risks. It is a fact anyway that real increases in performance are only possible through appropriate training.

Banned substances in sport include:

1. Stimulants

These remove tiredness and activate the central nervous system. The stimulants include amphetamines, caffeine, cocaine and ephedrine. Caffeine consumption is allowed in certain dosages. Practically it is possible to drink 3-4 cups without exceeding the caffeine dose limit of 12 µg/ml.

2. Narcotics

These include morphine preparations which remove great pain.

3. Anabolic Steroids

These protein building substances are the most abused substances in sport. They include the androgenic anabolic steroids with a testosterone effect and recently also further active substances with anabolic effects. The finding of the asthma drug clenbuterol in sprinters created a stir. Clenbuterol is a long-lasting asthma drug with obviously anabolic side- effects.

4. Beta Blockers

The drugs classified as beta blockers (e.g. propranolol) calm and stabilise motor activities. They are abused by shooters. Taking beta blockers in endurance sport on the other hand is pointless because they restrict performance by lowering the heart rate and blood pressure.

5. Diuretics

Diuretics (furesimide, spironolacton) lead to dehydration and dilute the urine. They are mainly abused by weight class athletes for fast dehydration and to get into lower weight classes in competitions.

6. Peptide Hormones

These include the growth hormone (STH) and erythropoietin (EPO). STH has a general anabolic effect. Erythropoietin increases blood development and thus raises oxygen transport capacity. Because proof in urine is not yet certain, indirect procedures to prove blood thickening are used for the protection of athletes. The international cycling association (UCI) has haemocrit (HC) checked and for values over 50 % places a competition ban of fourteen days. The international ski association, on the other hand, (FIS) orientates itself to haemoglobin (Hb) measurement and considers an Hb over 18.5 g/dl for men and over 16.5 g/dl for women to be too dangerous for a race. In practice, however, the values laid down are disputed as there are athletes who for hereditary reasons already reach Hb values of 19 g/dl or an HC of over 50 %.

7. Blood Doping

Transferring of one's own or someone else's blood increases oxygen transporting capacity and improves endurance performance capacity. Blood transfers are therefore banned in competitive sport and apart from that they are very risky healthwise.

8. Manipulation of Urine Tests

Through dilution of the urine, the abuse of banned substances can be covered up or proving their consumption made more difficult. Providing urine from another person is banned.

9. Substance Groups with Restrictions

Some drugs may only be taken in certain forms, these include e.g. asthma drugs of the type beta 2 mimetics. The briefly working substances salbutamol, terbutaline and salmeterol may only be used as a spray. The taking of these sprays must be notified before competitions. The same applies to sprays based on cortisone. Taking these substances as tablets counts as doping.

In case of doubt, a doctor should always be consulted before taking medical drugs during training and before competitions. The DSB has made a list of allowed medicinal drugs, which include, e.g. all common rheumatism and pain drugs. Codeine, which stems coughing, was taken off the doping list. Uncertainties arise during training checks and especially when a squad athlete is ill and is being treated with medicines. The treating doctor should at least point out the possibility of training checks and must keep a written record of the therapy.

Summary

Doping is the use of substances from the banned active substance groups and the use of banned methods. The doping list can be changed at short notice if there is a reason for this. Proven consumption of banned substances (positive result of both A and B urine tests), manipulation of the urine test and refusal to provide urine are punishable. Efforts to expand testing to blood are being made or have already been introduced in certain circumstances by some associations. In Germany training checks have proven to be an effective measure. Internationally the training checking system is not yet applied everywhere.

15 Physiological Performance Reserves

The most important performance reserve is training itself. Through training the physiological possibilities of the individual situation and adaptability are exploited. The reserves mentioned here are supportive measures for reaching qualitatively higher training load.

Training conditions in Europe are greatly influenced by climatic factors. This applies especially to cycling, cross-country skiing and to a certain extent running. For cyclists it has become normal to go to warmer climate zones from February onwards after compensation sport on snow. Preferred destinations are the Mediterranean countries, Mediterranean islands (e.g. Majorca) and the Canary Islands for spring training in the preparatory period. Cross-country skiiers extend their specific training opportunities in summer and autumn with visits to the polar region or on glaciers. Glacier training has the side-effect of altitude training for cross-country skiers. There is no ideal altitude training for all endurance sports, training is done with climatically induced restrictions. The third variation in addition to climate and altitude training is training in a different time zone on the northern or southern side of the equator. Training in different time zones is influenced by the adjustment to the natural day-night rhythm. For athletes, the period of the return journey is strenuous because after journeys in the opposite direction of the course of the sun (from west to east), often several days are needed to adjust to the time difference. Not taking into consideration adjustment periods after time zone changes of over six hours has caused many an athlete to lose their chances of success. For two hours of time difference at least one day for readjustment of the day-night rhythm must be planned for.

15.1 Training in Warm Climate Zones

The physical weather factors: air temperature, humidity (steam pressure of the air), ray temperature and wind speed influence how one feels during training. The outside temperature has the greatest influence on performance capacity. The medium and lasting state of these physical weather factors is known collectively as climate.

In autumn, winter and early spring it is now common to transfer training for some summer endurance sports to warmer climatic zones. As in warmer climatic zones the outside temperature is usually higher than desired, there can be acclimatisation problems. This also applies when competitions (e.g. marathon run, triathlon) take place in another time zone and in heat.

Heat Acclimatisation

The regulatory adjustment and adaptation of the body to high outside temperatures is known as acclimatisation. Heat acclimatisation does not occur during body resting. It requires a certain period of time and is linked to load in heat. The prerequisite for heat acclimatisation is the increase in body core temperature through repeated load in heat. Under this aspect, normal endurance training is already a mild form of heat acclimatisation because here body temperature rises (Fig. 1/15.1, see p. 284).

The increase in body core temperature through muscle work to 39°C is the physiological prerequisite for heat acclimatisation. If an athlete is subjected to heat of over 30°C for three to four days, an increase in the rate of sweating occurs already at 1-2 hours of training load per day. The sweat glands produce more sweat per unit of time. Through the increase in reabsorption they may hold back more minerals; the salt content of sweat goes down considerably. Sweat on the skin is no longer so salty. The body protects itself against increased loss of minerals by diluting the sweat.

The main physiological change through heat acclimatisation is the lowering of body core temperature by 0.5°C or more. This inner shifting of the "set point" has the effect that the heat centre in the hypothalamus reacts more sensitively to outside temperatures. The temperature gradient between body core temperature and skin temperature increases. The increase in the difference between body core and outside temperature is the main cause of earlier sweat development in heat. When temperatures are high, athletes acclimatised to heat react earlier under load by sweating than do non-acclimatised athletes. Sweating earlier causes sweat evaporation and associated cooling down to take effect more quickly.

Adaptation to higher outside temperatures leads to adjustments in the cardiovascular system (Fig. 2/15.1, see p. 285). Plasma volume goes up, the blood gets thinner. Under load, rises in heart rate (HR) and body core temperature occur with a delay. The initially higher oxygen uptake also goes back to its starting level. These signs indicate that heat is being coped with better.

After about five days of training in heat, about 70 % of the necessary functional adjustments have begun and after ten days the athlete's heat acclimatisation is finished. Endurance-trained athletes cope with load in heat considerably better than untrained persons. As already mentioned, endurance training is already a mild form of acclimatisation training. This means that preparation for tropical heat can begin at home already by beginning with more intensive endurance training over shorter distances. Ability to cope with heat is not the same for everybody. Women, children and older people handle heat less well. The sometimes temporarily lower heat tolerance of women has hormonal causes. The luteal phase in the second half of menstruation leads to an increase in core temperature of 0.3-0.6° C. This removes the temperature difference which makes up the physiological background of heat acclimatisation. Young female athletes who have not begun menstruating or in whom menstruation is centrally suppressed (amenorrhoe) have better heat tolerance. This can make itself positively noticeable in marathon runs in high temperatures.

In comparison to men, adult women sweat less and have less blood in their skin. Children also sweat less. The causes lie in the hormonal balance of woman and growing children. Lower concentrations of aldosterone and testosterone mean that the sweat glands are smaller and shorter and thus cannot release so much sweat. In older people testosterone development decreases and with it training of the sweating mechanism through increasing lack of exercise. They like to move in the neutral temperature zone and are thus unprepared for temperature adjustments.

Structuring of Acclimatisation Training

To make training in heat more comfortable there are a number of influencing options (Table 1/15.1, see p. 284).

A moderate training dosage of 60 to 120 min duration per day helps the body prepare for heat better than short and intensive training. To ensure that regeneration is not unnecessarily prolonged after load in heat, the training session can also be divided up. The guideline for running load in heat (over 30°C) is 40 to 70 min load duration per session. By limiting load duration, the increase in body core temperature to 39 to 40°C is limited. On the other hand, however, this core temperature increase is necessary to trigger acclimatisation.

A further factor influencing the delay in the temperature rise is the degree of energy utilisation. Energy utilisation is mainly influenced by load intensity (e.g. running velocity). Therefore, running in heat should be considerably slower than usual in order to delay the rise in core temperature. Measurements of body core temperature at the end of marathon runs showed that those runners who increased velocity in the last third of the competition had the greatest rise in body core temperature and also dehydration at the finish (NOAKES, 1992). The main danger of long running in heat is the increase in body core temperature through running too fast at the beginning. The increase in body core temperature is a greater health risk than a fluid loss of 3 to 4 %. Training should be shifted to times of the day when the additional sunshine is low. The early morning hours are most suitable. In high outside temperatures intensive training quickly leads to a rise in core temperature to 39°C. Sweat does not have an effect if it flows too quickly and drops off.

The dangers of training and competitions in heat lie mainly in the uncontrolled rising of body core temperature to over 40°C. Through this various forms of heat illness occur (Table 2/15.1, see p. 286).

Abundant fluid intake is of central importance when training in heat. Drinking must take place rationally even if it does not correspond to the natural feeling of thirst. Daily checking of weight is a good way of estimating the state of hydration. In addition, the ratio of solid and fluid blood components can be measured as haematocrit. Values of over 50 % point to a fluid deficit. A reduction in body weight of over 4% in a short time is an indication of fluid deficit and should cause one to deliberately consume fluids to reduce the strain.

In a state of dehydration both plasma volume and heart volume per minute go down; a characteristic of this state is an increase in heart rate under load.

The fluid deficit which arises during competitions cannot be compensated even by drinking a lot. During load, in heat the fluid loss via sweat is greater than possible compensation by drinking. In a warm humid climate, (over 30°C) 1 to 2.5 l sweat/h can be produced in every hour of training or competing. The greatest fluid losses occur during longer and very intensive load (Fig. 3/15.1, see p. 287).

During load, fluid intake is limited by the state of the stomach. In training and competition practice of running, up to 700 ml of fluids per hour has proven to be manageable. In cycling more can be drunk, about 1000 ml/h. Under certain conditions of long-distance running the "overdrinking phenomenon" can occur (NOAKES, 1992). This can develop during running load of several hours at low velocity and with simultaneous high water consumption. In order for the intestines to absorb the large quantities of water, the body has to temporarily diffuse sodium ions into the intestines. The water can only be absorbed with the help of salt. The sodium and chloride ions released by the bloodstream into the intestines reduce their concentration in the blood. The result is that the sodium concentration in the blood drops considerably. Hyponatriaemia develops. Such hyponotriaemias were originally found in over 30 % of tested starters in the Hawaii ultra triathlon. A drop in sodium is also possible in the 100 km run in heat. When the sodium concentration in the blood drops under 130 mmol/l, it leads to disorientation during the competition and afterwards to serious brain function disturbances which can lead to brain oedema. As a preventive measure under these conditions, fluids to which only salt has been added should be taken (about 0.5-1.0 g/l). Pure water can be harmful because it is low in salt.

Protection against Overheating

The decisive measures during load in heat are reducing load intensity and drinking plenty of fluids before, during and after load (Table 3/15.1, see p. 287). When training in heat load, intensity should be kept low and 75 % of best performance should not be exceeded. During heat load athletes should always have the feeling of still having sufficient reserves.

Heat acclimatisation

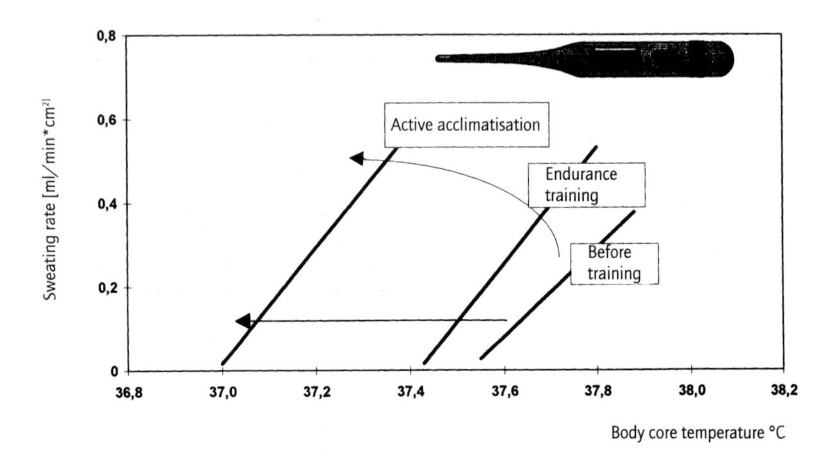

Fig. 1/15.1: Shifting body core temperature in endurance and heat training. By lowering body core temperature the sweating rate can be increased when the outside temperature rises.

Sports Medicine Recommendations for Heat Training (Outside Temperature over 27°C)

- Before training already drink plenty of fluids (0.3-0.5 l).
- Drink early during load (after 20 min).
- If load lasts over 60 min, it is preferable to drink electrolyte solutions with 5-8% carbohydrate mixtures.
- Carry out endurance training with especially low intensity (velocity) (fitness athletes < 60% and competitive athletes < 70 % of personal best performance).
- Limit load duration to 90 min in running and if over 30°C to 60 min. Cycling training is possible over longer distances if there is plenty of cooling wind from movement.
- Monitor load intensity by measuring HR. The heat HR should only be 10 bpm higher than normal, otherwise reduce intensity.
- Adapt clothing to outside temperature, sunshine, air movement and air humidity. Light coloured cotton clothing (T-shirt, string vest). If sun intensity allows, it is possible to train without a shirt. Wear light-coloured head gear (baseball cap). Synthetic sports clothing cools well, but during long loads it leads to high sweat loss.
- Immediately after load ends drink plenty of fluids (electrolytes) and consume carbohydrates.

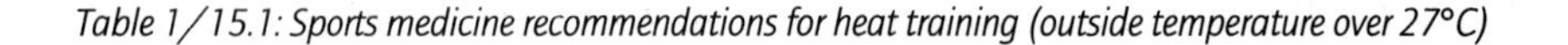

Table 1/15.1: Sports medicine recommendations for heat training (outside temperature over 27°C)

Acclimatisation to Moist Heat

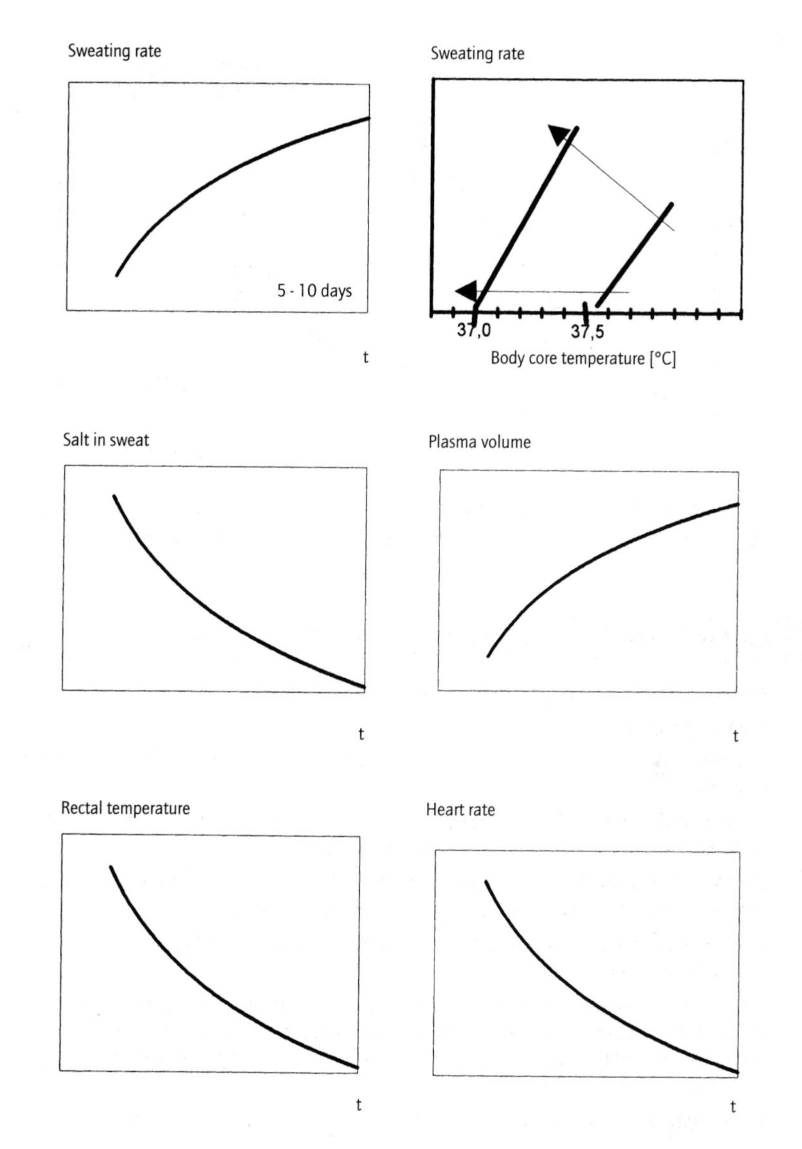

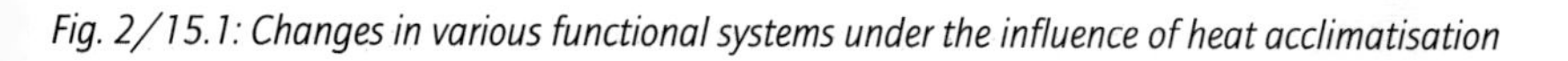
Fig. 2/15.1: Changes in various functional systems under the influence of heat acclimatisation

	Heat Illnesses in Sport		
Forms	Symptoms	Causes	Treatment
Heat cramps	Aching muscle pain, cramps of individual muscle fibres and muscle groups.	Local disturbances to blood circulation and mineral metabolism by dehydration.	Consumption of drinks containing salt and magnesium.
Sunstroke	Restlessness, nausea, dizziness, stiff neck. Under load heatstroke is possible.	Longer sun exposure on unprotected head. Irritation of brain surface.	Keep in shade, cool down, cover head, rest.
Heat breakdown	Paleness and equilibrium disturbances when upright, usually directly after finishing.	Major loss of fluids; rush of blood to leg muscles.	Lie flat in shade, put legs up (auto-transfusion), cooling, drinking.
Heat exhaustion	Great loss of sweat (cold sweat), headache, tiredness, disorientation. Major drop in performance. Low blood pressure, high heart rate. A difference is made between minor, serious and very serious forms.	Major dehydration and rise of body core temperature above 40° C.	Lie flat, cooling of any kind, call doctor, infusion of salt solutions with glucose, if necesary hospitalisation.
Heatstroke	Most of serious form of heat illnesses, disturbances in motor activity, disorientation, warm, dry skin, major drop in performance. Breakdown with unconsciousness.	Major dehydration with rise of body core temperature above 41 °C. Disturbances of overview regulation in the cerebrum and of motor activity regulation in the cerebellum.	Lie flat and drastic cooling measures (water, ice, wet towels), infusion, measure temperature (rectally), call a doctor, transport to hospital in accompaniment of a doctor.

Table 2/15.1: Heat illnesses in sport. The current view is that heat cramps and sunstroke no longer count among the heat illnesses because they can also occur without heat or movement.

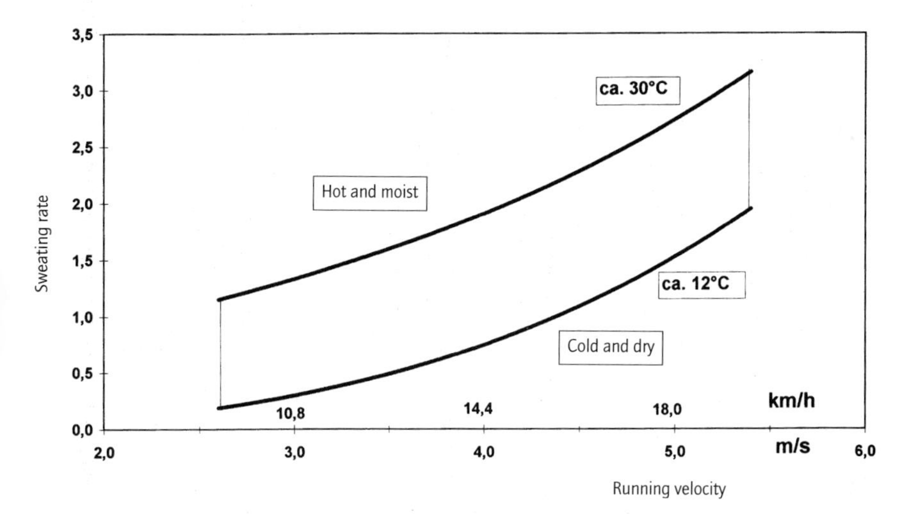

Fig. 3/15.1: Increase in sweating rate in relation to running velocity in heat

Advantages of Fluid Consumption in Heat
• Orientation amount for fluid consumption is 500-700 ml/h. Drinking should be begun earlier than eating (after 20 min of load).
• Endurance and strength endurance performance (velocity) can be maintained longer at the desired quality level.
• The heart rate rises later during load.
• The lactate concentration increases with a delay during load, muscle oxygen supply remains stable longer.
• The rise in body core temperature is delayed.
• Skin circulation is not cut back because of body stress.
• "Thickening" of the blood (haemo-concentration) happens more slowly and at less than 4 % weight loss remains in the physiologically tolerable region.
• If load lasts more than 60 min, carbohydrate mixtures should be drunk in addition to the electrolyte solution.
• Common sports drinks combine both requirements, i.e. they contain electrolytes and carbohydrates. The digestibility of sports drinks should be tested before competitions.

Table 3/15.1: Advantages of fluid consumption in heat

In competitions it is useful to observe a number of behavioural rules. The aim is to delay heating up of the whole body. This means limiting heat before the start or staying in air-conditioned rooms until just before the start. During a longer duration endurance competition (e.g. marathon run), the pace should be consciously kept low to begin with to delay the rise in core temperature. The worse an athlete's state of preparation is, the more important it is to reduce load intensity. Running velocity has a decisive effect on the release of heat, independent of the level of performance. According to research by NOAKES et al. (1991), increasing speed still had an effect on the rising of body core temperature in the last 6 km of a marathon run. The degree of dehydration played a secondary role in this connection.

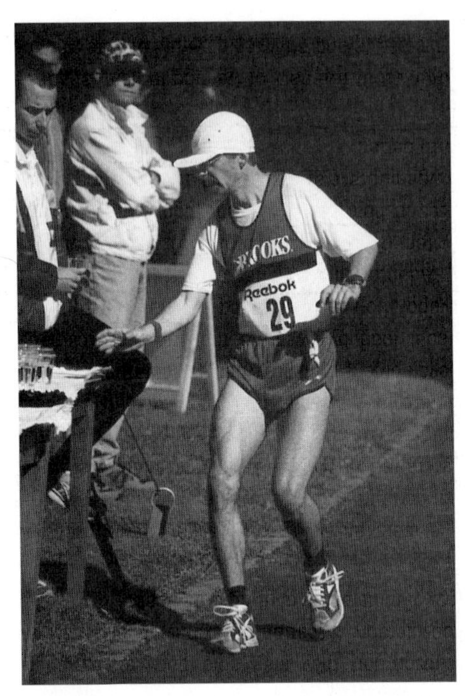

Reaching for water during a 100 km run (Photo: Georg Neumann, Leipzig)

Under heat load, water or sweat evaporation creates the most effective cooling. For this reason, further cooling should be caused by using wet sponges or tipping water over one's head.

Drinking during competitions can be a problem if the organisers provide fluids that are too cold or which are not known to the runner. Stomach cramps are usually caused by consuming fluids which are very rich, hyperosmotic or too cold. Not all commercially available drinks meet physiological requirements or are individually digestible in heat. Important characteristics of fluids are details about particle density (osmotic ability), salt content and mineral content (see Table 1/12.3). The carbohydrate components should be checked whereby one should especially look for a lack of or low fructose content (see chapter 13). The drinks offered during races should be checked beforehand if possible to see if they are digestible during load. In the past, drinks consumed that were too cold have already "deactivated" experienced elite athletes through gastro-intestinal discomfort. If the drinks are handed out from a freezer then they should be carried for a while, warmed up with body heat and only consumed in small amounts at a time.

Summary

The body can acclimatise to increased outside temperatures in a very short time. For this, training load of five to ten days in heat (27°C) is necessary. When the body is resting no acclimatisation occurs. In heat acclimatisation the body shifts the regulatory area of the body temperature centre in the brain towards a lower body core temperature; at the same time blood circulation in the skin and sweat production during load are increased. The low salt and finely distributed sweat leads to effective cooling through evaporation. Heat-acclimatised athletes react more sensitively to increases in outside temperature, they sweat earlier and more than untrained persons. Important precautionary measures for load in heat are conscious reduction of loading intensity as well as early and abundant drinking.

15.2 Altitude Training

Altitude training has now become an internationally recognised way of preparing for sporting performance peaks. The idea of altitude training came from the 1968 Olympic Games in Mexico City at an altitude of 2240 m. Many endurance performances over 2 min duration at these Olympic Games showed a drop in performance of 2-8 %. In order to prevent the drop in performance, preventive altitude training in endurance sports was introduced. It was found that training at altitudes between 1800 and 3000 m can be helpful for performance development in endurance sports. The positions on altitude training are contradictory. This has been contributed to by failures resulting from structuring of loading methodology and not attributable to altitude. It is a fact that in comparison to sea level, being at an altitude of 750 m already leads to certain physiological adjustments. These increase at 1500 m. Training as it is understood from a performance-physiological point of view begins at 1700 m and higher and ends for the moment at 3200 m. Top athletes find altitudes of 1700-2000 m barely noticeable and exert themselves as usual. Compensation of hypoxia begins via increased lactate production of 1-2 mmol/l in comparison to normal altitude at sea level (NN). Only at altitudes above 2200 m do corrections need to be made to velocity in running in particular, which are in the area of minus 0.2 to 0.4 m/s in the individual training areas. Despite the corrections in the velocity of running training, the lactate concentration of 1.0 to 2.0 mmol/l is higher than below NN.

When taking up altitude training, observing certain training-methodological prerequisites and conditions is of great significance for one's success.

Training-methodological Prerequisites for Altitude Training

Before travelling to medium altitude areas, athletes should already have several years of performance-oriented training with over 20 hours of load per week behind them. Stable sport-specific basic aerobic performance capacity is necessary for altitude training. If there are deficits in sport-specific aerobic performance foundations, no altitude training should be carried out, as this is not a training form for catching up. Altitude training is effective through repetition ("altitude chains"). This is the form in which it should be fitted into total performance development. Altitude training which is too short (less than 13 days) is not advantageous; altitude training is only effective adaptively after three weeks.

Training load for altitude training must be carefully preplanned and also controlled. Not observing training control can easily lead to overloading (see chapter 10). When performance is down, after illnesses or directly before important competitions, it is not helpful to do altitude training for the first time.

If the preconditions mentioned are observed, then altitude training will seldom cause sports-methodological disturbances or individual overloading.

From a training-methodological point of view, altitude training is an intensive form of endurance training. Through reduction of the partial oxygen pressure of breathing air (oxygen deficit), the stimulus effect of load increases by 3 to 4 % without having to increase velocity. In order to ensure load tolerance, especially in the more intensive training sections (BE 2 or CSE), running velocity is usually reduced by 0.2 to 0.3 m/s. In swimming or cycling training no major velocity concessions are needed. Control of recovery is done through structuring of the breaks.

On snow, lowering velocity is not without problems as the varying gliding conditions make it more difficult to categorise skiing velocity and the load intensity control. Monitoring load intensity using biological measurement factors is very important in cross-country skiing altitude training.

If an athlete has no stable aerobic performance capacity at the beginning of altitude training the risk of overloading increases. The result is that after altitude training there is a longer period of performance stagnation and the effect is considered negative.

Maximum oxygen intake can be used as an orientation indicator for the level of aerobic performance reached before altitude training. For men this should be at least 65 ml/kg • min and for women 60 ml/kg • min.

A summary of the sports-methodological altitude training experience of German athletes can be found in FUCHS/REISS (1990) and in MARTIN et al. (1996).

Physiological Effect of Altitude Training

Adaptation to oxygen deficit (hypoxia) at medium altitudes only takes place through sport-specific training load. Resting stays or sleeping at higher altitudes do result in mild physiological altitude regulation, but this has no influence on performance capacity. In academic literature, the findings of LEVINE et al. (1997) caused a lively discussion. In a solid study he found that the athlete groups (runners) who trained at 1250 m and lived at 2500 m were 13 s faster in the following 5000 m run at altitude than those who trained and lived on the flat . These results led to the recommendation to sleep at a high altitude and train at low altitude ("sleep high - train low").

Mountaineering at altitudes over 5000 m triggers various physiological adjustments and adaptations such as improvement in breathing and increased oxygen transporting capacity (BÖNING et al., 1996; STEINACKER et al., 1996; MAIRBÄURL et al., 1986 and others). Adaptation for the requirements of performance sport, however, barely takes place at all through mountaineering at great altitudes.

Changes in Air Pressure and Oxygen Concentration at Increasing Altitudes		
Altitude (m)	Air pressure (Torr)	Oxygen concentration (%)
0	760	20.9
500	716	19.7
1000	674	18.4
1500	634	17.2
2000	596	16.1
2500	560	15.1
3000	526	14.1
3500	493	13.1
4000	462	12.2
4500	433	11.3
5000	405	10.5
8872 (Mount Everest)	240	5.9

Table 1/15.2: Changes in air pressure and oxygen concentration at increasing altitudes

Examinations of expedition members (Himalayas) found that there was even a loss of muscle as a result of relative lack of movement due to the extreme oxygen deficit (HOPPELER et al., 1990).

Internationally the physiological effects of hypoxia on sporting and physical performance capacity have been shown many times (BERGLUND, 1992; BÖNING, 1997 and others). At medium altitudes the lack of oxygen is caused by the drop in partial oxygen pressure and thus of oxygen concentration in the atmosphere (Table 1/15.2, see p. 291). At an altitude of 2000 m there is 5 % less oxygen in the air breathed in. The oxygen deficit increases the body's own releasing of erythropoietin and strongly activates the development of blood in the bone marrow. A similar effect is achieved through erythropoietin consumption in top sport, which is a clear case of doping.

The altitude effect can also be created artificially. Technologically there are two variants for this. Firstly, hypoxia is possible by lowering the air pressure in specially constructed well-sealed chambers (hypobar hypoxia). Such a chamber was used in the GDR in Kienbaum (Berlin) until 1990. The other variant is to put nitrogen into room air. This way hypoxia can also be achieved (normobar hypoxia). Currently skiiers in Scandinavian countries are gathering experience with normobar hypoxia. In central Finland (Vuokatti) a 1.25 km long skiing tunnel has been built to allow imitation of altitude training all year round on artificial snow. Although the effect of artificial or naturally hypoxy on the body is the same in principle, top athletes find training under natural altitude conditions more pleasant psychologically and prefer it.

Oxygen Supply

During the first stay at high altitude there are major adjustments in breathing, the cardiovascular system and in metabolism. The body uses all of its functional options to compensate the undersupply of oxygen during load. This happens mainly through increased breathing and cardiovascular work. In the blood the oxygen compound curve moves to the right. In this way the oxygen taken in gets into the blood more easily and can be better diffused from the blood into the muscle tissue. Only when these adjustments during training under hypoxia are maintained for three weeks do first adaptations begin. These are caused by the increase in oxygen transport capacity to the needy muscle tissue and the improved processing of oxygen.

Under the influence of hypoxia stress, the hormone erythropoietin developed by the kidneys and the liver is released in greater quantities. Erythropoietin reacts very sensitively to differences in the oxygen provision to the blood. In case of hypoxia this hormone triggers the development of new erythrocytes in the blood. More erythrocytes increase the oxygen transporting capacity of the blood. In order to release the oxygen from the haemoglobin of the erythrocytes to the tissue more easily, there is a simultaneous increase of the enzyme diphosphoglycerate (2,3 DPG) which works in the erythrocytes. 2,3 DPG allows easier detaching of the oxygen from the haemoglobin and thus improves the release of oxygen to the muscles. In order to increase oxygen transporting capacity altogether the erythrocyte ratio (total amount of haemoglobin) in the blood must increase. Because the concentration of haemoglobin (Hb) in the blood remains constant as a result of the additional increase in plasma volume, normal haemoglobin measurement is not a useful method for assessing oxygen transport capacity through altitude training. Only through complicated measurement of total haemoglobin can the haemoglobin increase be measured. Usual Hb measurement only allows rough information about the Hb increase and should be supplemented with haematocrit measurement at the same time. A high haematocrit reading (> 50 %) impedes the flowing properties of the blood and reduces performance because the release of oxygen to the tissue is hindered.

Through altitude training the increase in the number of erythrocytes is compensated by the simultaneous increase in plasma volume, as a result the haematocrit value remains almost unchanged. Through the haematocrit remaining the same or going down, "thickening of the blood" is avoided physiologically. If the haematocrit is over 52 % and especially if it is over 55 %, dangerous capillary blockages can occur. In comparing altitude training with training at low levels, it can be ascertained that hypoxia training increases the number of erythrocytes (rise in haematocrit) and NN endurance training on the other hand leads to an increase in blood volume, i.e. the haematocrit goes down.

With altitude training there is also a loss of water through the respiratory tract so that it is important to drink plenty of fluids. If sufficient fluid consumption does not take place then the blood fluid is reduced and the haematocrit rises over 50 % even without an increase in haemoglobin. The upper physiological haemoglobin concentration for men is about 18 g/dl and for women on average about 2 g/dl less, i.e. 16 g/dl. Higher haematoglobin concentrations are rare, but possible.

In competitive sport the main effect of altitude training is an increase in the oxygen transporting capacity of the blood and a better supply of oxygen to loaded muscles. Thus similar adaptations take place to those after endurance training, but at a level of load with a higher stimulus effect.

In order to avoid altitude training or to acquire forbidden performance advantages in oxygen transport at normal altitudes some athletes in top sport have taken the hormone erythropoietin. The thickening of the blood is a health risk which can lead to thrombosis or embolism. If the haematocrit value of competitive athletes who have no fluid deficit rises quickly to over 52 %, then the haematoglobin value is probably 18 g/dl for men and 16 g/dl for women.

To protect athletes, since 1997 haemoglobin testing has been carried out in winter sports before international races as an "additional doping test".

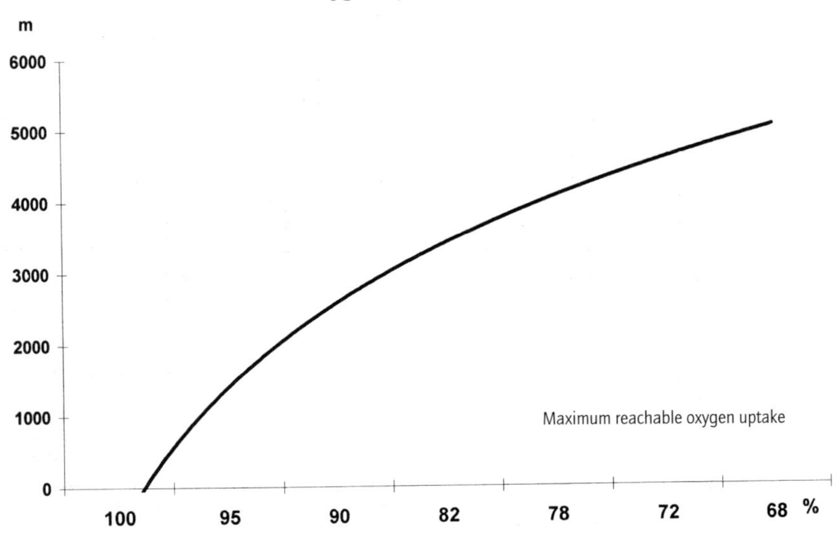

Fig. 1/15.2: Decrease in maximum oxygen uptake at high altitudes

A competition ban is imposed if for men the haematoglobin reading exceeds 18.5 g/dl and for women if it is above 16.5 g/dl. In cycling the haematocrit value is used. If the haematocrit rises over 50 % a 14 day competition ban is imposed. Increasing the body's own erythropoietin using injections is a form of doping which is extremely dangerous to health.

Energy Metabolism

The lack of oxygen at high altitudes also influences energy metabolism. Carbohydrates need less oxygen for their combustion than fatty acids so that they are utilised first at high altitudes. During altitude training, metabolism shifts in the direction of increasing carbohydrate breakdown. In training control the favoured carbohydrate breakdown can be ascertained through the higher lactate development. In altitude training, lactate development is considerably higher than at sea level at the same running velocity. The oxygen deficit is compensated for by increased glycolysis, but with earlier exhaustion of the glycogen stores. In the course of altitude training, disturbances in substrate regeneration occur more quickly. The chronic glycogen deficit during competitive altitude training forces the body to constantly develop new glycogen. This is linked with a breakdown of proteins. Balanced nutrition with an emphasis on carbohydrates is important for ensuring performance and aiding regeneration in altitude training.

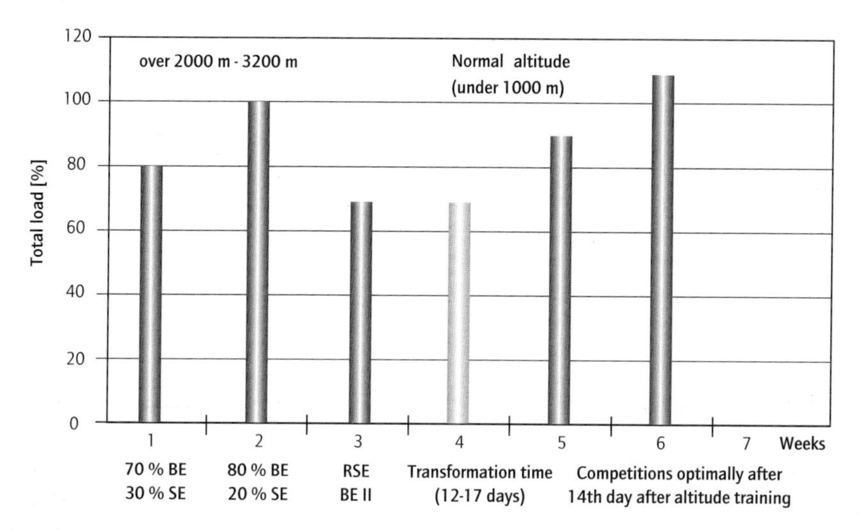

Fig. 2/15.2: Example of a possible structuring of load at an altitude training camp

To avoid a glycogen deficit or too much protein catabolism, loading intensity should be lowered or the break extended at the first sign of overloading.

Because of the low training velocity, only limited demands are placed on maximum oxygen intake capacity. Reducing loading intensity during altitude training above 2500 m is also necessary because the absolute level of maximum oxygen intake goes down considerably in comparison to sea level (Fig. 1/15.2). Thus lower maximum performances are possible and maximum lactate development is lower when stretched to the limit. Lower lactate concentration after brief maximum load at high altitudes has, however, only been found in averagely trained persons. This finding has been described as "lactate paradox". Because, however, maximum lactate development is always dependent on absolute performance (or velocity), it must be lower under hypoxia loading. It should be noted that lactate mobilisation always depends on the individual aerobic performance level and is lower the lower performance capacity is.

In top athletes, the lactate concentration is dependent on the availability of sport-specific motor performance capacity; as a rule this is not lower during altitude training. Altitude training can also be used to create stimuli for the development of aerobic mobilisation if this were necessary as a content of training. In this case, however, the duration of load should be reduced considerably. Lower air resistance is favourable to sprinting performance.

From a scientific point of view it has been attempted to assess the effect of altitude training using the criterion of the increase in maximum oxygen uptake (VO_2 max). Because its increase does not occur or cannot be ascertained immediately, altitude training was considered as dispensable for this. In the application of scientific assessment criteria of altitude training, however, training reality was not considered. The contradiction to training arises from the fact that under hypoxia only the submaximal part of aerobic performance capacity is trained and the maximum part only to a very limited degree. In altitude training, basic endurance training in its lowest velocity proportions is favoured which initially has an effect on the development of VO_2 max. Thus VO_2 max is not an objective criterion for assessing the effectiveness of altitude training. If there is an increase in VO_2 max, then only after at least three weeks of transformation training with higher intensity proportions at normal altitudes (Fig. 3/15.2, see p. 298).

Sports-methodological Structuring of Altitude Training

The idea of carrying out endurance and strength endurance training at high altitudes comes from the experience that when maintaining usual velocity there can be an increase in load stimulus in the range of 5 to 10 % at altitudes of 2100 to 2500 m. Thus altitude training has the effect of being a very intensive variant of endurance training.

In order to ensure re-loading tolerance during several weeks of altitude training, it is, however, usual practice to reduce accustomed training velocity in running by 5 to 10 %. This definitely applies to altitudes above 2200 m. If, on the other hand, the training location is only at an altitude of 1700 to 1800 m (e.g. St. Moritz/Switzerland), top athletes load themselves at the velocities they are used to at normal altitudes. At this altitude they can cope with daily re-loading or else compensate regeneration deficits with longer breaks. In swimming and cycling, at this low altitude load intensity hardly needs to be reduced at all. High levels of training load with effective stimulus function are compensated by extending regeneration.

As a rule, two to three (4-6) altitude training camps per year are planned and carried out. This corresponds to recommendations for structuring "altitude training chains" (FUCHS/REISS, 1990). In the practical utilisation of load at medium altitudes many variants are possible, which are influenced by local conditions and the weather. In winter sports these are additionally characterised by the amount of snow or glacier conditions. Another factor is that cross-country skiing is trained at altitudes from 1800 to 3200 m (glaciers). After training they can move to valley stations at 600 to 1000 m. In this way regeneration is aided.

The following is an example for planning the timing of altitude training, which in concrete cases can always be varied. If, for example, the performance peak is in July, then altitude training can be spread over the months following:

1. Altitude training in February
2. Altitude training in April
3. Altitude training in June (as DCP).

The first three altitude camps should be used to develop basic aerobic performance capacity. At the first camp, load can be structured semi-specifically or even sport-unspecifically. For summer sports, cross-country ski training is possible here. If the performance peak is earlier or later, the timing must be altered. Altitude chains have the advantage that the body is pre-adapted and can adjust its regulation to hypoxia more quickly. Through repeated altitude training, both the individual athlete and the coach gather experience about reactions and ability to handle load. In order for the triggering of stable adaptation to occur, the stay at high altitudes should be extended to three weeks. Tests have shown that at least four to six weeks of effective load stimulus are necessary for the achievement of structural adaptations (NEUMANN/BERBALK, 1991). Three weeks of altitude training are justified in so far as the 4th week can or should be used for transformation back at the normal altitude. Three weeks of altitude training are a minimum prerequisite for the triggering of adaptation to a higher level of load. Successful endurance athletes (e.g. marathon runners) have meanwhile moved their place of residence to medium altitudes. The successful east African runners live at medium altitudes and train higher still. They achieve their best performances at low altitudes. Just living and training at medium altitudes is no guarantee of sporting success and does not protect one from sports-methodological faults.

For the relevant sports, in the coming years the duration of altitude training will probably be extended further still. For very active fitness and competitive athletes, altitude training for longer periods is a financial problem.

In those places where local conditions allow (funicular), athletes can commute between a training location at a higher altitude and a place of residence in the valley (NN). For younger athletes, fitness athletes or women, at the beginning of competitive training it is possible to train at a higher altitude (e.g. glacier) and sleep under NN conditions. Through easier regeneration, load tolerance is increased.

From the experience of combination sports it is known that strenuous altitude training leads to disturbances in the (mental) regulation area of concentration. Thus intensive motor activity training (tempo runs over 200 to 400 m) at higher altitudes would be advantageous because of reduced air resistance, but the athlete's mental drive for this can be reduced.

The variant brought into scientific discussion of training in the lowlands and sleeping at high altitudes ("sleep high, train low") is not recommendable because no altitude adaptations that aid performance occur during sleep or inactivity. Even mountaineering at great heights is an unsuitable measure for endurance training and cannot be compared with it because of the slow pace of movement.

For endurance training at higher altitudes the following basic variant can be applied (Fig. 3/15.2, see p. 295): basic endurance (BE), strength endurance (SE), competition-specific endurance (CSE).

1st week: BE and SE training
2nd week: BE and SE training with increase of 20 %
3rd week: After a regenerative break, CSE and BE 2 training
4th week: Travel home and regeneration with major reduction of load
6th week: Emphasis on CSE training with compensation
7th week: Begin with first competitions (optimal: 17th day)

In altitude training, the volume of total load that can be expected of an athlete depends on his level of performance and the length of regenerative breaks after individual training sessions. If the recovery time necessary after a training session in the lowlands is taken as an individual yardstick, then this can more or less be kept to in BE and SE altitude training.

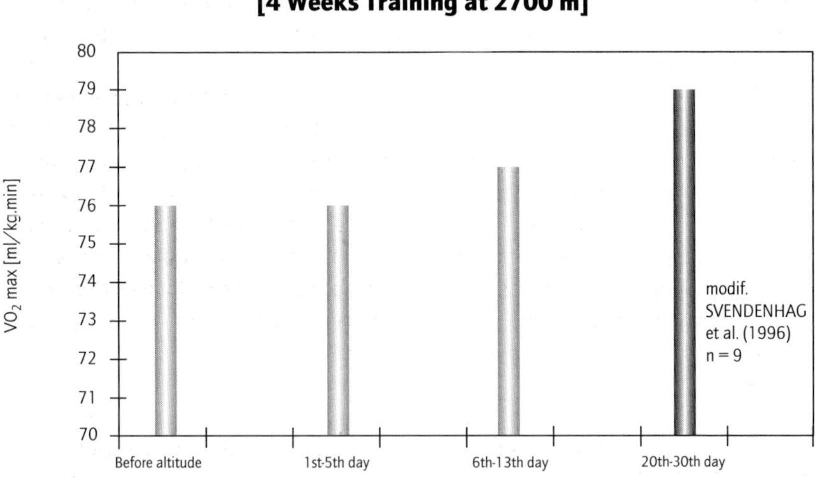

Fig. 3/15.2: Changes to maximum oxygen uptake (VO_2 max) in top athletes and after altitude training (modif. from SVEDENHAG et al., 1996). Only 3-4 weeks after the altitude training camp did VO_2 max increase.

The more intensive BE 2 training requires a longer break (about 15 %). Even longer recovery times are needed by competition-specific training and brief competitions, the lengthening of the breaks should be 40 %. Splitting the training day with longer recovery periods is necessary for regeneration of the energy stores and for psychological relaxation. If regeneration time is ignored, processing of training takes longer. Faulty or overtraining can be the result. Competitions at medium altitudes obligatorily require "altitude chains" for their preparation and presence on location for several weeks beforehand.

Transformation Time after Altitude Training

The structuring of training load after the return to the lowlands (NN) is the core of post altitude training activity. All load blocks in competitive training require a longer period for processing. This also applies to altitude training. The main cause of sporting failure lies in the ignoring of longer regeneration periods after altitude training. After altitude training with effective stimuli, temporary instability of performance is normal and requires appropriate methodological conclusions.

The effect of altitude cannot be confirmed directly or a few days afterwards by sporting performances. In this period, performance is reduced in about 70 % of athletes. Maximum oxygen uptake is also temporarily lower through training. Experience with structuring the transformation time after great load says that at least two weeks must be allowed for this. If the altitude training camps are considered a 3:1 load-unloading cycle, then there should be a marked reduction in load in the 4th week in the lowlands. Because altitude training is intensive endurance training, one week of regeneration is not sufficient. The safest period for top sporting performance is between the 14th-17th day after normal altitude training. The greatest probability of performance failing is between the 4th and 10th day after returning to NN. In this period of post-processing of altitude stress the immune system is also weakened. The risk of health instability is greater than usual in this period. If altitude training is carried out with too low sport-specific aerobic performance capacity, then the transformation time lasts well over two weeks. Participation in an important competition at NN before the third week after returning from medium altitudes is not recommendable.

In exceptional circumstances it is possible to compete immediately after altitude training, i.e. on the 1st to 3rd day. At this early point in time the body is not yet subject to general altitude stress regulation and in this functional state it is still capable of greater performance. With this "early start" it should be noted that the regeneration time or the transformation lasts longer. If an immediate start is necessary after altitude training, there is the alternative of reducing total load at higher altitude earlier than usual.

If altitude training is done with a very high volume of training or if the athlete's performance state is average, then processing of load takes over three weeks.

In altitude training the individual performance prerequisites of the athletes must be considered more closely than in lowland training. There is obviously varying ability to cope with hypoxia stimuli, the reason for which is unknown. Before altitude training the blood picture and iron metabolism should be examined. States of iron undersupply should be registered by monitoring storage iron (ferritin) and/or the serum iron concentration. Altitude training is not experimental training before performance peaks, it should be built up on secured experience of coaches and athletes.

Control of Altitude Training

The main methodological aim of altitude training is the further development of sport-specific aerobic performance capacity, whereby the emphasis is on BE and SE training. A criterion for orientation for load intensity is lactate concentration. During most BE sessions this should not be too much over 2 mmol/l. At the beginning of altitude training in the adjustment period, lactate concentration can be 2 or 3 mmol/l higher than usual. In the case of continued high lactate concentration, load intensity should be reduced in the following days or else running velocity should be reduced in the range of 0.2 to 0.4 m/s. If, as a result of his low aerobic performance level, an athlete cannot reduce load-induced lactate concentration very much, then longer recovery breaks must be taken between training sessions.

A sure method for self-checking of loading intensity is measuring the heart rate (HR). The guideline figures for the HR vary individually and should build on experience at low altitudes. As a rule, BE training is done at an HR of 130 to 150 bpm. In BE 2 or SE training HR values in a range of 160-180 bpm are possible. Independent of the individual HR level it should be noted that an increase in HR of more than eight bpm already shows that a higher level of load has been reached. In altitude training it is important to monitor recovery capacity. This can be done by ascertaining the resting HR and/or recovery HR about 1 min after the particular training session. Normally the HR goes down by about 30 bpm in 1 min.

By measuring the "resting pulse" each day while still in bed, recovery capacity and the ability to cope with load can be estimated. If the HR rises more than 6 bpm above the individual level it is a first indication of increasing tiredness. A rise in HR of over 10 bpm usually means the beginning of a health disturbance and should cause one to take a break or reduce load.

By determining the serum urea concentration the level of total load can be assessed (see Fig. 2/11). With increasing protein breakdown and a reduction in the ability to cope with load the serum urea concentration rises. Serum urea should be measured early, before training. Training load is too high if at rest the serum urea concentration is over 10 mmol/l for several days in a row. Effective stimulus load is being applied if the serum urea concentration at rest is between 7 to 9 mmol/l in men and between 6 to 8 mmol/l in women. A daily increase in serum urea by 0.5 to 1 mmol/l is an indication of increasing protein catabolism. By taking a half day break and consuming plenty of carbohydrates the rise in serum urea can be interrupted. Under hypoxia conditions breathing is increased, more water is released through the respiratory tracts. Linked with this is a greater loss of water, but not a mineral deficit. In altitude training, plentiful fluid consumption must be ensured. The most simple monitoring measure is daily weighing. A weight reduction of more than 2 kg in altitude training calls for a check on diet, fluid consumption and load. A rise of the haematocrit over 50 % indicates a fluid deficit.

Summary

Course training at medium altitudes of 1800 to 2500 m is a variant of endurance and strength endurance training being increasingly used in endurance sports. Altitude training assumes a high level of aerobic performance and should only be used by performance-oriented healthy athletes who have already been training with over 20 h/week of load. In order to trigger effective adaptations for an increase in oxygen transporting capacity, altitude training of three weeks duration is necessary. Training of intensive endurance sessions should take place below NN, but not at higher altitudes. Altitude training leads to increased glycogen consumption, lactate development is greater than under NN.

After altitude training, the majority of athletes experience instability of performance between the 4th and 12th day, so that only after the 14th day increased performance capacity under lowland conditions can be reckoned with. Observing this transformation time is a major factor of successful altitude training.

Ideally altitude training camps of three weeks duration should be carried out three to four times a year, collectively referred to as "altitude chains". Altitude training should be fitted sports-methodologically into endurance training and considered a more intensive form of load. The timing of altitude training should be oriented to preparation of individual performance peaks. Through altitude training sport-specific submaximal aerobic performance capacity is developed and not maximum oxygen uptake (VO_2 max). An increase in VO_2 max only occurs after three weeks of lowland training after the altitude training.

16 Overtraining and Faulty Training in Performance Sport

Overtraining is an often overworked term in competitive training which is interpreted in varying ways. Overtraining is a particular form of faulty training which can appear both through sport-specific load overloading and through one-sided underloading. In training practice, deteriorating performance capacity or stagnating performance development when training is continued are interpreted as overtraining. In most cases the reason for the state of falling performance capacity and willingness to train is unphysiologically structured training load. The basic rules of sports-methodological load structuring have not been observed (Table 1/16, see p. 304).

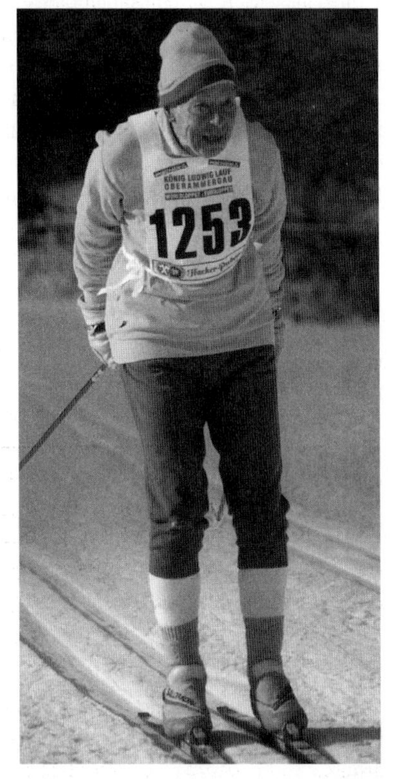

Swedish cross-country skiier AK 80 during 50 km event.
(Photo: Georg Neumann, Leipzig)

Overtraining is usually preceded by long lasting states of muscular tiredness which can no longer be compensated for by normal recovery between training sessions. Overtraining is probably a form of muscular overloading which has become chronic and which cannot be overcome even by central nervous system and hormonal aids. The most obvious characteristic is the loss of muscular strength and endurance, especially at higher velocities and resistances.

Greatly delayed regeneration after training or competitions can have its origins in destroyed contractile functional proteins and mitochondria of the muscle. This state alone needs several weeks or months to overcome it. Possibly there is a connection between muscle structure destruction and overtraining. These could arise if an athlete tries to continue load in spite of muscle disturbances to muscular functions. A typical example is the continuation of usual training after a strenuous marathon. If training is continued in a situation of long-lasting high protein catabolism and mineral shortage, overtraining can follow (Fig. 1/16, see p. 305). Training with major muscle tiredness triggers system stress, only in this "state of alarm" is it possible to continue load.

Efforts to explain the causes of overtraining scientifically have not been very successful. Nevertheless, numerous theoretical approaches to overtraining have been developed (LEHMANN et al., 1993; NEWSHOLME, 1995; PARRY-BILLINGS et al., 1992 among others). The favourite explanation for overtraining is a far reaching disturbance in the hormonal axes hypothalamus-hypophysis-suprarenal gland cortex (Fig. 2/16, see p. 306).

Overtraining arises in sport-specific training when the basic principles of load tolerance of the body are violated. The muscle glycogen deficit arising in competitive training is not at all the cause of overtraining. The emptying of the glycogen stores is a normal physiological process which occurs after two hours of training load or 90 min competing. By the next day the stores are not yet fully refilled. The refilling of the glycogen stores can, however, take place without problems in 1-3 days through deliberate carbohydrate consumption and/or reducing load (see chapter 13.2).

In individual training overtraining seldom occurs in the endurance sports, more often it arises after group training. In group training individual performance capacity is frequently overloaded if basic training-methodological principles are not observed. In group training the person with the greatest performance capacity determines the intensity of load. Athletes who are in a weaker state of adaptation or have less training experience are constantly encouraged to manage load with 3 to 5 % higher biological effort. This often applies to ambitious and keen athletes in the first years of the men's class who go without a break in loading. In the course of several days or weeks, a central stress regulation is triggered in order to be able to handle the load under great muscular tiring or overloading. The highly-exerted muscles are supported by further functional systems in order to secure forward propulsion (Table 2/16, see p. 306). The cut-back in body functions is already an indication of advanced functional disturbance or overtraining. An attempt is made to protect the body from further load, in particular intensive load, through centrally triggered vagotonia.

This stress regulation to cope with muscle load demands leads to certain signs which are partially recognised by the athlete himself or confirmed when asked (Table 3/16, see p. 307). The main symptoms are disturbances in the vegetative nerve functions which already led ISRAEL (1976) to speak of a form of overexcitement (sympathicotonal overtraining) and a form of underexcitement (parasympathicotonal overtraining). The idea of central regulation is to protect the body from further load so that after initial activation and overexcitement gradually the braking function of the vagonal (parasympathicotonal) nervous system gains the upper hand.

Common Causes of Faulty Training

- Volume of training too low and one-sided application of continuous training method. Resulting insufficient development of aerobic performance capacity and maximum oxygen uptake.
- Intensity proportions too high when total load is low, e.g. over 30 % of specific load above lactate 3 mmol/l.
- Preference given to mixed training, no deliberate capacity training (endurance, strength endurance, speed).
- Not keeping to rhythms of load and unloading (optimal weekly load-unloading rhythm 3:1 or 2:1).
- Limited increase in load over the training year or methodologically unprepared increases in load.
- Group training with too much biological load effort among those with weaker performance (e.g. joint training of juniors and men).
- Spontaneous changes to training contents which do not belong together, such as e.g. blocks of intensive speed training in basic endurance training.
- Underestimating of unspecific strength training and general athletics as a prerequisite for securing load tolerance.
- Structuring training according to subjective feeling and dispensing with objective regulatory criteria such as velocity, heart rate, lactate, performance checks.

Fig. 1/16: Common causes of faulty training

The state of overexcitement and the high activity is hardly noticed by the athlete because he knows them as a typical precompetitive reaction. A major accompanying reaction when functions influencing performance are cut back is the disturbance of the biological defences. The consequences of weakened immune functions are unexpectedly occurring illnesses before important competitions or after training camps. The disturbed immune function can be well corrected by reducing load or taking a break of several days. If training is carried on despite indisposition or inefficiency, the energetic processes for securing load become ineffective. The high proportions of anaerobic metabolism lead to premature glycogen exhaustion. The body is forced to increasingly break down amino acids and proteins. The increased protein catabolism can be recognised through the high serum urea level and the increase in creatine kinase under relatively low load. Further indicators of faulty load are: increase in noradrenaline, decrease in testosterone, increase in cortisole, fall in iron level as well as in the level of plasma glutamine.

Tiredness after a Marathon Run

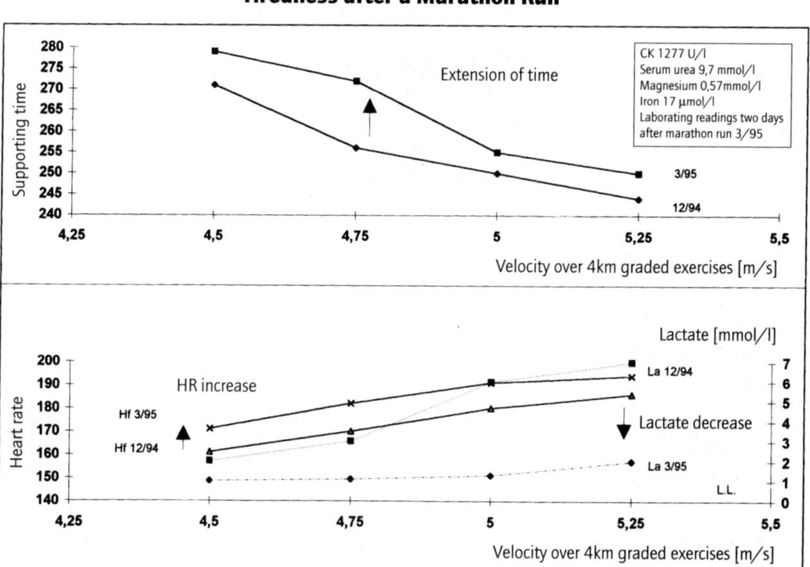

Fig. 1/16: Current state of tiredness of a top athlete after a marathon run. The disturbance in the release of performance showed up in the extension of supporting time, in the lactate decrease as a result of a glycogen shortage and in laboratory clinical readings. The performance diagnostics occurred through overestimation of the athlete's performance capacity; after five days normal performance capacity for training was reached.

The diverse, not easily classifiable signals in a state of reduced performance are also called staleness or burnout (LEHMANN et al., 1994). Increases in resting HR and/or HR during usual load should cause one to also think of the possibility of overtraining.

A state of stagnation or a deterioration in sporting performance capacity can be staleness or greatly disturbed regeneration. In the case of performance stagnation, appropriate sports-methodological and dietary measures must be taken (Table 4/16, see p. 307).

In every case of performance stagnation, training should be analysed and possible methodological faults in load structuring should be sought (see Table 1/16). Often it turns out that performance development was based on an aerobic performance foundation that was too weak and the following intensification of training, the increase in load or competitions lead to overloading. Training took place in a state of too much residual tiredness, resulting in permanent deterioration in performance.

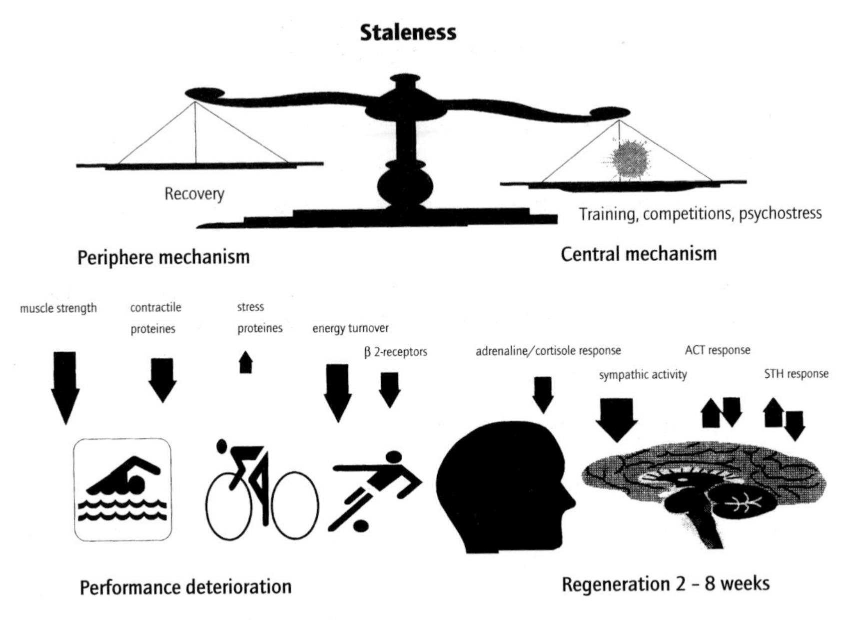

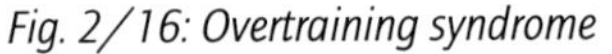

Fig. 2/16: Overtraining syndrome

Causes of Major Muscular Tiring

- Sport-specific disturbances of muscle functions in the contractile apparatus.
- Deteriorating impulse transmission to the final motor plate. In the case of an acetylcholine deficiency, nerval stimuli are incompletely passed on in order to protect the muscle.
- Interrupted release of calcium to the T channels and of CA^{++} intake in the sarcoplasmatic reticulum.
- Substrate exhaustion (creatine phosphate and glycogen).
- Disturbed flows of energy in aerobic and anaerobic metabolism (ratio of carbohydrate and fat metabolism shifted towards carbohydrates or increase in anaerobic glycogen breakdown).
- Central nerval tiredness through increase in seratonine in the brain (seratonine is a mediatory substance for tiredness during long duration load).
- Increase in free tryptophanes (fTRP) or rations of fTRP to branch-chain amino acids (BCCA). Increase in fTRP/BCCA favours seratonine increase in the brain and thus general tiredness with falling motor drive.

Table 2/16: Causes of major muscular tiring

Indications of Overtraining (Faulty Training)
• General performance drop-off despite training. Stagnation in the development of performance capacity. • Increasing tiredness and lack of interest in qualitatively high motor drive (inferior intensity training). • Conspicuous disturbances in well-being, especially in the vegetative functions (sleeping problems, lack of appetite, loss of libido, loss of weight). • Increasing number of banal infections and indispositions healthwise. • Rise in resting heart rate (HR) and also loading HR. • Higher lactate concentration under standard load and lower maximum values. • Rise in serum urea concentration and/or creatine kinase at rest or after load above individual values.

Table 3/16: Indications of overtraining

Measures to Overcome Faulty Training or Overtraining
• Temporary reduction in load or training break. • Analysis of training to date. New establishment of load-unloading rhythm (e.g. 3:1 rhythm). • Checking of laboratory findings, especially iron, magnesium and indicators of protein and muscle metabolism. • If necessary, change in diet and deliberate consumption of active substances (immune stimulants, L-carnitine, high dosages of vitamins: B_1, B_6, E and C. • Evaluation of the influences of the social environment. Removal of multiple stress (work-sport, family-sport, honorary function-sport). • Begin load with basic aerobic training for two weeks.

Table 4/16: Measures to Overcome Faulty Training or Overtraining

In a state of overtraining or faulty training the continuation of accustomed training load will be fruitless. In competitive training, a correction is only possible through a load break followed by long aerobic basic endurance training. Intensive training sessions and competitions should be refrained from.

If it is estimated that at least 4-6 weeks of training are needed to reach a higher state of adaptation, and muscular regeneration in the form of amino acid restructuring is only 2 to 6 % per day, then correctional training of at least one to two months is necessary to overcome a drop in performance as a result of faulty training (overtraining). Assuming 2 % restructuring in the muscles per day, after ten days only 20 % of muscle structure would be renewed. False training-methodological decisions are frequent in overtraining because often the courage to radically correct training is missing. Athletes know the consequences; failures mount up, the season is "over"!

Summary

Overtraining is a state of deteriorating performance capacity and declining willingness to train in competitive sport. The causes are still not certain. Overtraining is preceded by muscle overloading where usually training continues without breaks for recovery. Overloading in training while omitting regeneration leads to system stress with diverse indications. After initial overexcitement the body triggers a centrally working braking function to protect the muscles. Functional inhibition (vagotonia) dominates and thus load at higher velocities and greater resistances (strength endurance) is hardly possible any longer. Only a change in the structuring of training can help, after an appropriate break in load or a considerable reduction in load. The emphasis should be on basic aerobic training for at least two weeks together with dietary measures.

17 Bibliography

BERBALK, A/NEUMANN, G./PFÜTZNER, A. (1994). Triathlon - Kardiale Anpassung und Ausdauerleistungsfähigkeit. In: ENGELHARDT, M./FRANZ, B./NEUMANN, G./PFÜTZNER, A. (Hrsg.): Triathlon: medizinische und methodische Probleme des Trainings. Band 9. Hamburg: Czwalina.

BERBALK, A./NEUMANN, G./PFÜTZNER, A./ Große, St. (1995). Kardiale Anpassungsdiagnostik in den Ausdauersportarten - Grenzen der kardialen Adaptabilität durch Hochleistungstraining. In: ENGELHARDT, M./FRANZ, B./NEUMANN, G./PFÜTZNER, A. (Hrsg.): 9. Internationales Triathlon-Symposium 1994 Kiel. Band 10. Hamburg: Czwalina.

BERBALK, A. (1996). Sportherz des Nachwuchsathleten - Komplexe Anpassungen an Ausdauertraining. In: TW Sport + Medizin 8, 214-224.

BERBALK, A. (1997). Echokardiographische Studie zum Sportherz bei Ausdauerathleten.
In: Zeitschrift für Angewandte Trainingswissenschaft 4, 34-64. Aachen: Meyer & Meyer

BERGLUND, B. (1992). High-altitude Training. Aspects of Haematological Adaptation. In: Sports Med. 14, 289-303.

BERGSTRÖM, J. (1962). Muscle Electrolytes in Man. In: Scand. J. Clin. Lab. Invest. 68 (Suppl.), 1-110.

BLOM P./COSTILL D.L./ VOLLESTAD N.K. (1987). Exhaustive Running: Lappriate as a Stimulus of Muscle Glycogen Super-compensation. In: Med. Sci. Sports Exercise 19, 389-403.

BLOM P./VOLLESTAD N.K./COSTILL D.L. (1986). Factors Affecting Changes in Muscle Glycogen Concentration during and after Prolonged Exercise. In: Acta Physiol. Scand. 128 (Suppl. 556), 67-74.

BLOMSTRAND, E./HASSEN, P./EKBLOM, B./NEWSHOLME, E.A. (1991). Administration of Branched-chain Amino Acids during Sustained Exercise-effects on Performance and on Plasma Concentration of Amino Acids. In: Eur. J. Appl. Physiol. 63, 83-88.

BÖNING, D. (1997). Altitude and Hypoxia Training - A Short Review. In: Int. J. Sports Med. 18, 565-570.

BÖNING, D./MAASSEN, N./JOCHUM, F./STEINACKER, J/HALDER; A./THOMAS, A./ SCHMIDT, W./NOE, G./KUBANEK, B. (1997). After-effects of a High Altitude Expedition on Blood. In: Int. J. Sports Med. 18, 179-185.

BROUNS, F. (1993). Die Ernährungsbedürfnisse von Sportlern. In: Berlin: Springer.

BROUNS, F./KOVAC, E. (1996). Rehydratationsgetränke für Sportler. In: TW Sport + Medizin 8, 167-174.

BURKE L.M./COLLIER G.R./HARG, REAVES, M. (1993). Muscle Glycogen Storage after Prolonged Exercise: Effect of the Glycemic Index of Carbohydrate Feedings. In: J. Appl. Physiol. 75, 1019-1023.

CHAN, K.M./DIAMOND, P./LAW, C.K./HSU,S./LEUNG, P.C.,SO, S.Y./WANG, R. (1985). Case Study - Beijing to Hong Kong Super-marathon, Sports Medicine Research. In: Brit.J. Sports Med. 19, 145-147.

CLASING, D./WEICKER, H./ BÖNING, D. (1994). Der Stellenwert der Laktatbestimmung in der Leistungsdiagnostik (Hrsg.). Jena: G.Fischer.

CONVERTINO, V.A. (1991). Neuromuscular Aspects in Development of Exercise Countermeasures. In: Physiologist 34, S125-S128.

COSTILL, D.L./DANIELS, J./EVANS, W./FINK, W./KRAHENBUHL, G./SALIN B. (1976). Skeletal Muscle Enzymes and Fiber Composition in Male and Female Track Athletes. In: J.Appl. Physiol. 40, 149-154.

DECOMBAZ J.E./GMÜNDER, B./BIELINSKI, R. (1988). Nutritional Profile during a Transcontinental Run. In: Cand.J. Sport Sci. 13, 9-15.

DGE (1991). Deutsche Gesellschaft für Ernährung. Empfehlungen für die Nährstoffzufuhr. Frankfurt/M.: Umschau-Verlag.

DICKHUTH, H.-H./URHAUSEN, A./HUONKER, M./HEITKAMP, H./KINDERMANN, W./SIMON, G./KEUL, J. (1990). Die echokardiographische Herzgrößenbestimmung in der Sportmedizin. In: Dtsch. Z. Sportmed. 41, 4-12.

DOUGLAS, P.S. (1989). Cardiac Considerations in the Triathlete. In: Med. Sci. Sports Exerc. 21, 5 (suppl.), 214-218.

DUFAUX, B. (1989). Immunologische Unterscheidung von „Selbst und Nichtselbst" unter körperlicher Belastung. In: Dtsch. Z. Sportmed.40, Sonderheft 52-59.

ENGELHARDT, M./ NEUMANN, G. (1994). Sportmedizin. Grundlagen für alle Sportarten. München: BLV Verlagsgesellschaft.

FRANZ, B./PFÜTZNER, A. (1997). Entwicklungstendenzen der Trainings- und Wettkampfsysteme in den Ausdauersportarten mit Folgerungen für den Olympiazyklus 1996-2000. Beiträge Workshop Ausdauer. Institut für Angewandte Trainingswissenschaft Leipzig 1997.

FRICKER, P./BEASLEY, S./COPELAND I. (1991). A Preliminary Study on the Effects of Amino Acids, Fasting and Exercise on Nocturnal Growth Hormone Released in Weightlifters. In: Exel. Belconen 7, 2-5.

Fröhner, G. (1995). Einfluß des Triathlontrainings auf die Belastung des Stütz- und Bewegungssystems. In: ENGELHARDT, M./FRANZ, B./NEUMANN, G./PFÜTZNER, A. (Hrsg.): 9. Internationales Triathlon-Symposium 1994 Kiel. Band 10. Hamburg: Czwalina.

FUCHS, U./REIß, M. (1990). Höhentraining. Münster: Philippka.

GEIß, K.-R./HAMM, M. (1990). Handbuch Sporternährung. Reinbek/Hamburg: Rowohlt.

GILLERT, O./RULFFS, W./ BOEGELEIN, K. (1995). Elektrotherapie. 3. Aufl. München: Pflaum Verlag.

GLEDHILL, N. (1993). Hämoglobin, Blutvolumen und Ausdauer. In: SHEPARD, R.J./ASTRAND, P.O. (Hrsg.). Ausdauer im Sport. Köln: Deutscher Ärzteverlag.

Gohlitz, D. (1994). Bewertung integrativer Meßgrößen der Lauftechnik in der komplexen Leistungsdiagnostik des leichtathletischen Laufs und Triathlons mit Folgerungen für das Kraftausdauertraining. In: ENGELHARDT, M./FRANZ, B./NEUMANN, G./PFÜTZNER, A. (Hrsg.): Triathlon: medizinische und methodische Probleme des Trainings. Band 9. Hamburg: Czwalina.

HAMM, M./ WEBER, M. (1988). Sporternährung praxisnah. Weil der Stadt: Hädecke Verlag.

HARRE; D. (1986). Trainingslehre. 10. Aufl. Berlin: Sportverlag.

HASKELL, W.L. (1986). The Influence of Exercise Training on Plasma Lipids and Lipoproteins in Health and Disease. In: Acta Med. Scand. Suppl. 711, 25-37.

HECK; H. (1990). Energiestoffwechsel und medizinische Leistungsdiagnostik. Schorndorf: Hoffmann.

HOLLMANN, W./HETTINGER, TH. (1990). Sportmedizin - Arbeits- und Trainingsgrundlagen. 3. Aufl. Stuttgart-New York: Schattauer.

HOLLOSZY, J.O. (1975). Adaptation of Sceletal Muscle to Endurance Exercise. In: Med. Sci. Sports 7, 155-164.

HOLTMEIER, H.-J. (1995). Gesunde Ernährung von Kindern und Jugendlichen. 3. Aufl. Berlin: Springer.

HOPPELER, H./KLEINERT, E./SCHLEGEL, C./CLAASEN, H./HOWALD, H./KAYAR, S.R./CERETELLI, P. (1990). Muscular Exercise at High Altitude. II. Morphological Adaptations of Human Sceletal Muscle to Chronic Hypoxia. Int. J. Sports Med. 11, S 3-9

Hottenrott, K./ BETZ, M. (1995). Langfristiger Leistungsaufbau im Triathlon. In: ENGELHARDT, M./FRANZ, B./NEUMANN, G./PFÜTZNER, A. (Hrsg.): 9. Internationales Triathlon-Symposium 1994 Kiel. Band 10. Hamburg: Czwalina.

HOTTENROTT, K./ ZÜLCH, M. (1995). Ausdauerprogramme. Reinbeck/Hamburg: Rowohlt.

HOTTENROTT, K. (1996). Inline -Skating. Aachen, Meyer & Meyer.

HOWALD, H. (1982). Training Induced Morphological and Functional Changes in Skeletal Muscle. In: Int. J. Sports Med. 3, 1-12.

HOPPELER, H./LÜTHI, P./CLAASEN, H./WEIBEL, E.R./HOWALD, H. (1973). The Ultrastructure of the Normal Human Skeletal Muscle. A Morphometric Analysis on Untrained Men, Women and Well Trained Orienteers. In: Pflügers Arch. 344, 217-232.

HULTMAN, E. (1974). Diatary Manipulation an Aid to Preparation for Competitions. In: Procedings of the World Conference on Sports Medicine. pp. 239-265, Melbourne.

ISRAEL, S. (1976). Zur Problematik des Übertrainings aus internistischer und leistungsphysiologischer Sicht. In: Med. u. Sport 16, 49-53.

ISRAEL, S. (1995). Sport mit Senioren. Leipzig: Barth Verlag, Hüttig GmbH.

IVY, J.L./LEE, M.C./BRONZINIC, Jr., J.T./REED, M.J. (1988) Muscle Glycogen Storage after Different Amounts of Carbohydrate Ingestion. J. Appl. Physiol. 65, 2018-2023.

IVY, J.L/KATZ, A.L/CUTLER, C.L/SHERMAN, W.M./COYLE, E.F. (1988b). Muscle Glycogen Synthesis after Exercise: Effect of Time of Carbohydrate Ingestion. In: J. Appl. in: Physiol. 65, 1480-1485.

IKAI (1967) zit. bei PIEPER, S./ SCHARSCHMIDT, F. (1981).

KEUL, J./WITZIGMANN, E. (1988). Die Olympia-Diät. München. Heyne.

KOLLER, A./GEBERT, W./SORICHTER; J./MAIR, J./ARTNER, E./PUSCHENDORFER, B./RAMA, D./CALZOLARI, C: (1997). Troponin I a New Marker of Muscle Damage in Alpine Skiing. In: MÜLLER, E./SCHWAMEDER, H./KORNEXL, E./RASCHER, C. (eds.). Science and Skiing., London: E.& FN SPON.

KONOPKA, P. (1994). Sporternährung. 5. Aufl. München: BLV Sportwissen.

LEHMANN; M./DIMEO,F./HUONKER, M. (1994). Aktuelle Vorstellungen zu den Ursachen des Übertrainings. In: ENGELHARDT, M., FRANZ, B.

LEHMANN, M./MANN, H./GASTMANN, U./KEUL, J./VETTER, D./STEINACKER, J.M./HÄUSSINGER, D.(1993). Unaccustomed High-milage vs Intensity Training-related Changes in Performance and Serum Amino Acid Levels. In: Int. J. Med. 17, 187-192.

LEMON, P.W.R. (1994). Are Dietary Protein Needs Affected by Regular Exercise? In: News on Sport Nutrition Insider (Maastricht). 2, 1-4.

LEVINE, B.D./ STRAY-GUNDERSEN, J. (1997). „Living high - Training low": Effect of Moderate-Altitude Acclimatization with Low-altitude Training on Performance. In: J. Appl. Physiol. 83, 102-112.

MADER, A. (1994). Die Komponenten der Stoffwechselleistung in den leichtathletischen Ausdauerdisziplinen - Bedeutung für Wettkampfleistung und Möglichkeiten ihrer Bestimmung. In:

TSCHIENE, P. (Hrsg.): Neue Tendenzen im Ausdauertraining, Bundesausschuß Leistungssport, Informationen zum Leistungssport Bd. 12. Frankfurt.

MAIRBÄURL, H./SCHOBERSBERGER, W./HUMPELER, E./HASIBEDER, W./FISCHER, W./ RAAS, E. (1986). Benefical Effects of Exercising at Moderate Altitude on Red Cell Oxygen Transport and on Exercise Performance. In: Pflügers Archiv 406, 594-599.

MARTIN, D. (1991). Grundlagen der Trainingslehre. Schorndorf: Hoffmann.

MARTIN, D./KRUG, J./REIß, M./ROST, K. (1997). Entwicklungstendenzen der Trainings- und Wettkampfsysteme im Spitzensport mit Folgerungen für den Olympiazyklus 1996 bis 2000. In: Leistungssport 27, 25-31.

MARTIN, D./NEUMANN, G./PFÜTZNER, A./REIß, M. (1996). Höhentraining in den Ausdauersportarten – Aspekte zu Forschungs- und trainingsmethodischen Fragen. In: Zeitschrift für Angewandte Trainingswissenschaft 3, 127-137. Aachen: Meyer & Meyer.

MARTIN, D./ROST, K. (1996). Standpunkte zur Weiterentwicklung des Nachwuchstrainingssystems im deutschen Sport. In: Zeitschrift für Angewandte Trainingswissenschaft, 3, 6-29. Aachen: Meyer & Meyer.

MEDVED, R./PAVISIT, V./STUKE, K. (1975). Das größte gesunde Sportherz bei Frauen. In: Sportarzt und Sportmed. 26, 174-176.

NEUMANN, G./ PFÜTZNER, A. (Hrsg.) Triathlon: medizinische und methodische Probleme des Trainings. Band 9, 75-82. Hamburg: Cwalina.

NEUMANN, G. (1990). Die Leistungsstruktur in den Ausdauersportarten aus sportmedizinischer Sicht. In: Leistungssport 20, 14-20.

NEUMANN, G. (1991). Ausdauerbelastung. Ein sportmedizinischer Ratgeber. Leipzig-Heidelberg: J.A.Barth.

NEUMANN, G. (1991b). Zur Leistungsstruktur der Kurz- und Mittelzeitausdauer-Sportarten aus sportmedizinischer Sicht. In: Leistungssport 21, 29-31.

NEUMANN, G. (1991c). Erschließung von Anpassungsreserven des Organismus. Leistungsreserven im Ausdauertraining. In: REIß, M./ PFEIFFER, U. (Hrsg.) 34-39. Leistungsreserven im Ausdauertraining. Berlin: Sportverlag.

NEUMANN, G./STEINBACH, K. (1990). Veränderungen der verzweigtkettigen Aminosäuren Valin, Leucin und Isoleucin bei Marathon und 100 km-Lauf. In: Med.u. Sport 30, 249-253.

NEUMANN, G./FEUSTEL, G./SCHOBER, F. (1990). Zur Erhöhung der Reizwirksamkeit der Trainingsbelastung. In: REIß, M./PFEIFFER, U. (Hrsg.) Leistungsreserven im Ausdauertraining. S.145-160. Berlin: Sportverlag.

NEUMANN, G./ BERBALK, A. (1991). Umstellung und Anpassung des Organismus - grundlegende Voraussetzung der sportlichen Leistungsfähigkeit. In: BERNETT, P./JESCHKE, D. (Hrsg.): Sport und Medizin. Pro und Contra. München: W. Zuckschwerdt.

NEUMANN, G./PFÜTZNER, A. (1992). Leistungsstruktur der Langzeitausdauer im Triathlon. In: BREMER, D./ENGELHARDT, M./NEUMANN, G./WODICK, R. (Hrsg.). Band 6, 61-66. Hamburg: Czwalina.

NEUMANN, G./REUTER, I. (1993). Kohlenhydratbilanzierung beim Kurztriathlon. In: BREMER, D./ENGELHARDT/M. HOTTENROTT, K.

NEUMANN, K./PFÜTZNER, A.: Triathlon: Orthopädische und internistische Aspekte. Band 7, 91-99. Hamburg: Czwalina.

NEUMANN, G./MÜLLER, R. (1994). Schwimmstufentest im Triathlon. In: ENGELHARDT, M./ FRANZ, B./NEUMANN, G./PFÜTZNER, A. (Hrsg.): Triathlon: medizinische und methodische Probleme des Trainings. Band 9, 49-61. Hamburg: Czwalina.

NEUMANN, G./PFÜTZNER, A./BERBALK, A./GROßE, ST. (1995). Leistungs- und Trainingsstruktur im Kurztriathlon. In: ENGELHARDT, M./FRANZ, B./NEUMANN, G./PFÜTZNER, A. (Hrsg.): 9. Internationales Triathlon-Symposium 1994 Kiel. Band 10, 173-188. Hamburg: Czwalina.

NEUMANN,G./SCHÜLER, K.P. (1994). Sportmedizinische Funktionsdiagnostik. 2.Aufl. Leipzig: Barth.

NEUMANN, G./PFÜTZNER, A./HOTTENROTT, K. (1995). Alles unter Kontrolle. 3. Aufl. Aachen Meyer & Meyer.

NEUMANN, G. (1996). Ernährung im Sport. Aachen: Meyer & Meyer.

NEWSHOLME, E.A. (1995). Possible Biochemical Causes of Failure of the Immune and of Fatigue in the Overtraining Syndrome. In: Coching focus. Leeds 28,14-16.

NIEMAN, D.C. (1994). Exercise, Upper Respiratory Tract Infections, and the Immune System. In: Med. Sci. Exerc. 26, 128-139.

NOAKES, T. (1992). The Hyponatriämie of Exercise. In: Int. J. Sports Nutr. 2, 205-228.

NOAKES, T. (1991). Lore of Running. Cape Town: Oxford University Press.

PARRY-BILLINGS, M./BUDGETT, R./KOUTEDAKIS, Y./BLOMSTRAND, E./BROOKS, S./WILLIAMS, C./OLLING, S./BAIGRIE,R./NEWSHOLME, E.A.(1992). Plasma Amino Acid Concentration in the Overtraining Syndrome: Possible Effects on the Immune System. In: Med. Sci. Exerc. 24, 1353-1358.

PAFFENBERGER, R.S./WING, A.L./HYDE, R.T. (1978). Physical Activity of Longshoremen as Related to Death from Coronary Heart Disease and Stroke. In: Am. J. Epidemiol. 108, 161-175.

PEDERSEN, B.K./TVEDE, N./CHRISENSEN, L.D./KARLAND, K./KRAGBAK, S./HLKJR-KRISTENSEN J. (1989). Natural Killer Cell Acticity in Peripheral Blood of Highly Trained and Untrained Persons. In: Int .J. Sports Med. 10, 129.131.

PETERS, A.J./DRESSENDORFER, R.H./RIMAR, J./KEEN, C.L. (1986). Diets of Endurance Runners Competing in a 20 Day Road Race. In: Phys. Sports Med. 14, 63-70.

PIEPER, K.-S./SCHARSCHMIDT, F. (1981). Das biologische Funktionsmodell der konditionellen Fähigkeiten von Hochleistungssportlern. Habil. Schrift, Universität Leipzig.

PFÜTZNER, A. (1990). Zu grundlegenden Problemen der Erhöhung der Leistungswirksamkeit des Vorbereitungssystems im Skilanglauf - Ein Beitrag für eine auf Weltspitzenleistungen gerichtete Entwicklungskonzeption. Dissertation B. Deutsche Hochschule für Körperkultur Leipzig.

PFÜTZNER, A./NEUMANN, G. (1992). Wettkampfsimulationstest im Triathlon. In: BREMER, D./ENGELHARDT, M./NEUMANN, G./WODICK, R. (Hrsg.). Band 6, 137-145. Hamburg: Czwalina.

PFÜTZNER, A./ REIß, M. (1996). Entwicklungstendenzen der Trainings- und Wettkampfsysteme in den Ausdauersportarten mit Folgerungen für den Olympiazyklus 1996-2000. In: Schriftenreihe zur Angewandten Trainingswissenschaft 4, Aachen: Meyer & Meyer

PFÜTZNER, A. (1995). Ausgewählte Aspekte einer Prozeßanalyse als Grundlage für die Erstellung einer Trainingskonzeption 1996-2000 im Triathlon Olympische Distanz. In: ENGELHARDT, M./FRANZ, B./NEUMANN, G./PFÜTZNER, A. (Hrsg.): Triathlon: medizinische und methodische Probleme des Trainings. Band 10,197-220. Hamburg: Czwalina.

PFÜTZNER, A./GROßE, ST./BALDAUF, K./GOHLITZ, D./WITT, M. (1994). Koppeltraining - Hauptbestandteil einer triathlonspezifischen Fähigkeitsentwicklung. In: ENGELHARDT, M./FRANZ, B./ NEUMANN, G./PFÜTZNER, A. (Hrsg.): Triathlon: medizinische und methodische Probleme des Trainings. Band 9, 101-122. Hamburg: Czwalina.

PFÜTZNER; A. (1995). Entwicklungstendenz und Trainingskonzept im Triathlon Olympische Dis-tanz. In: Zeitschrift für Angewandte Trainingswissenschaft 2, 50-66. Aachen: Meyer & Meyer.

POORTMANS, J.R. (1988). Protein Metabolism. In: POORTMANS, J.R. (ed.) Principles of Exercise Biochemistry.164-193. Basel: Karger.

RASCHKA, C./ PLATH, M. (1997). Das Verhalten von Körpergewicht, Fettanteil und Energieaufnahme während eines 20-tägigen Ultralangstreckenlaufs über 1000 km. In: Dtsch. Z. Sportmed. 48, 165-173.

REGUERO, R.J.J./CUBERO, G.I./de la GLESIS. J.L./TERRADOS, N./GONZALEZ, V./CORTINA, R./CORTINA, A. (1995). Prevalence and Upper Limit of Cardiac Hypertrophy in Professional Cyclists. In: Europ. J. Appl. Physiol. 70, 375-378.

REINDELL, H./KÖNIG, H./ROSKAMM, H. (1967). Funktionsdiagnostik des gesunden und kranken Herzens. Stuttgart: Thieme.

REIß, M./ PFEIFFER, U. (1991). Leistungsreserven im Ausdauertraining. Berlin: Sportverlag.

Reiß, M. (1991). Grundprobleme der Steigerung der Wirksamkeit des Hochleistungstrainings in den Ausdauersportarten. In: Leistungssport 21, 33-40.

REIß, M. (1992). Steigerung der Kraftausdauerfähigkeiten durch wirkungsvolles Kraftausdauertraining. Leistungssport, 22, 15-20.

REIß, M./ PFÜTZNER, A. (1993). Tendenzen der Leistungsentwicklung in den Ausdauersportarten. In: Leistungssport 23, 9-14.

REIß, M., LÖFFLER, P., SCHMIDT, P./ SCHÖN, R. (1993): Schlüsselprobleme des langfristigen Leistungsaufbaus. In: Leistungssport 23 12-16.

REIß, M./GOHLITZ, D. (1994). Schlüsselprobleme der Leistungsdiagnostik im Hochleistungstraining der Ausdauersportarten (dargestellt am Beispiel der leichtathletischen Lauf- und Gehdisziplinen). In: Schriftenreihe zur Angewandten Trainingswissenschaft 1, 30-48. Aachen: Meyer & Meyer.

REIß, M./GOHLITZ, D./ERNST, O. (1994). Untersuchungen zur wirksamen Gestaltung des kraftbetonten Grundlagenausdauertrainings. Ergebnisbericht. Institut für Angewandte Trainingswissenschaft, Leipzig.

REIß, M./ERNST, O./GOHLITZ, D. (1996). Leistungsniveau und Entwicklungstendenzen in den leichtathletischen Laufdisziplinen aus der Perspektive der Olympischen Spiele 1996. In: Zeitschrift für Angewandte Trainingswissenschaft 3, 46-75.

ROST, R./GERHARDUS, H./SCHMIDT, K. (1985). Auswirkungen eines Hochleistungstrainings im Schwimmsport mit Beginn im Kindesalter auf das Herz-Kreislauf-System. In: Med. Welt 36, 65-71.

ROST, R. (1990). Herz und Sport. Erlangen: Perimed Verlag.

SARIS W.H.M.: Nutrition and Top Sport (1989). In: Int. J. Sport Med. 10, Suppl. S1-S76.

SCHMIDTBLEICHER, D. (1987). Motorische Beanspruchungsform Kraft: Struktur und Einfluß-größen, Adaption, Trainingsmethoden, Diagnose und Trainingssteuerung. In: Dtsch. Z. Sportmedizin, Köln 38, 356-372.

SCHNABEL, G./THIEß, G./HARRE, D. (1995). Trainingswissenschaft, Leistung, Training, Wettkampf. Berlin: Sportverlag.

SHERMAN W.M./COSTILL D.L./FINK W.J./HAGERMAN F.C./ARMSTRONG L.W./MURRAY T.F. (1983). Effect of a 42,2 km Footrace and Subsequent Rest or Exercise on Muscle Glycogen and Enzymes. In: J. Appl. Physiol. 55, 1219-1224.

SLEAMAKER, R. (1991). Systematisches Leistungstraining. Aachen: Meyer & Meyer.

STEGMANN, H./KINDERMANN; W./SCHNABEL, A. (1981). Lactate Kinetics and Individual Anaerobic Threshold. In: J. Sports Med. 2, 160-165.

SPRIET, L. N./GLEDHILL, A.B./FROESE, D.L./WILKES (1986). Effect of Graded Erythrocythemia on Cardiovascular and Metabolic Response to Exercise. In: J. Appl. Physiol. 61, 1942-1948.

STEINACKER, J.M./ANGELE, M./LIU, Y./LORMES, W./REIßNECKER, S./MENOLD, E./WHIPP B.J. (1994). Atmungsmechanik beim Rudern. In: KINDERMANN,W./ SCHWARZ, L. (Hrsg.): Bewegung und Sport - eine Herausforderung für die Medizin. Wehr: Ciba Geigy Verlag.

STEINACKER, J.M./HALDER, A., LIU, Y./THOMAS, A. (1996). Hypoxic Ventilatory Response during Rest and Exercise after a Himalayan Expedition. In: Eur. J. Appl. Physiol. 73, 202-209.

SVEDENHAG, J. et al. (1996). Zit : SALTIN, B. (1997) The Physiology of Competitive c.c.Skiing across a Four Decade Perspective; with on Training Induced Adaptations and Role of Training at Medium Altitude. S. 435-469. In: MÜLLER, E./SCHWAMEDER, H./KORNEXL E./RASCHER C. (eds.). Science and Skiing, London: E & FN SPON.

THOMSON, J./STONE, J. A./GINSBURG, A.D./HAMILTON, P. (1982). O_2-Transport during Exercise Following Blood Reinfusion. In: J. Appl. Physiol. 53, 1213-1219.

VERCHOSHANSKIJ, J. (1992). Ein neues Trainingssystem für zyklische Sportarten. Trainerbibliothek des DSB 29, Köln.

WEIß, M. (1994). Anamnestische, klinische und laborchemische Daten von 1300 Sporttauglichkeitsuntersuchungen im Hinblick auf Infekte und deren Prophylaxe bei Leistungssportlern. In: LIESEN, H./WEIß, M./ BAUM, M. Regulations- und Repairmechanismen. S.399-402. Köln: Deutscher Ärzteverlag.

WILMORE J.H./ COSTILL D.L. (1994). Physiology of Sport and Exercise. Champaign: Human Kinetics.

WORM, N. (1992). Ratgeber Ernährung. 2.Aufl. München: TR-Verlagsunion.

ZINTL, F.(1990). Ausdauertraining. Grundlagen, Methoden, Trainingssteuerung. 2. Aufl., München: BLV-Verlagsgesellschaft

18 Index